Obstetrical Events and Developmental Sequelae

Editor

Nergesh Tejani, M.D.

Director
Division of Maternal-Fetal Medicine
Department of Obstetrics and Gynecology
Westchester County Medical Center
New York Medical College
Valhalla, New York

CRC Press, Inc.
Boca Raton, Florida

Library of Congress Cataloging-in-Publication Data

Obstetrical events and developmental sequelae/editor, Nergesh
  Tejani.
      p.   cm.
    Includes bibliographies and index.
    ISBN 0-8493-5762-4
    1. Fetus—Diseases—complications and sequelae.   2. Pregnancy,
  Complications of.   I. Tejani, Nergesh, 1933-   .
    [DNLM: 1. Blood Transfusion, Intrauterine.   2. Breech
  Presentation.   3. Child Development.   4. Extraction, Obstetrical.
  5. Fetus—drug effects.   6. Infant, Low Birth Weight.   7. Pregnancy
  Complications.   WS 105 014]
    RG627.027 1989
    618.3—dc20
    DNLM/DLC
    for Library of Congress   89-9859
                                                                              CIP

This book represents information obtained from authentic and highly regarded sources. Reprinted material is quoted with permission, and sources are indicated. A wide variety of references are listed. Every reasonable effort has been made to give reliable data and information, but the author and the publisher cannot assume responsibility for the validity of all materials or for the consequences of their use.

Direct all inquiries to CRC Press, Inc., 2000 Corporate Blvd., N.W., Boca Raton, Florida 33431.

© 1990 by CRC Press, Inc.

International Standard Book Number 0-8493-5762-4

Library of Congress Card Number 89-9859
Printed in the United States

To Col. K. M. Bharucha, A.M.C.

ACKNOWLEDGMENT

To Stella Torres for her many hours of help in the organization of this book

PREFACE

Growth and developmental findings in infancy and early childhood are dependent on a complex variety of factors in which the environment plays a major role. Voluminous literature has accumulated on long-term development related to pediatric problems, with special reference to neonatal intensive care unit graduates; however, information on development related to obstetrical factors is presently sparse. The few reports that do exist are scattered and not easily available to the obstetrician. The purpose of this volume is to accumulate and consolidate such information. The long-term significance of selected obstetric situations will be presented by authors who have personally investigated these problems.

This is by no means an all-inclusive text on this topic; several areas of concern are left uncovered. However, I feel that the obstetrician and all those in allied fields will find useful information on the long-term significance of tocolytic agents, steroids, subgroups of growth retardation, fetal hypoxia, acidosis, malpresentation, intrauterine transfusion, and premature rupture of membranes. This represents a beginning which hopefully may be extended in the future.

Nergesh Tejani, M.D.
January 1989

THE EDITOR

Nergesh Tejani, M.D., is Director, Division of Maternal-Fetal Medicine, Westchester County Medical Center, Valhalla, New York and Professor of Obstetrics and Gynecology at New York Medical College.

Dr. Tejani received her premedical and medical degrees from Bombay University, Bombay, India and has practiced and taught obstetrics in India, Uganda, the U.K., and the U.S. Her long association with the Nassau County Medical Center in East Meadow, Long Island, New York furthered an interest in the effect of obstetrical conditions and practices on the growth and development of the children resulting from these pregnancies. Much of her effort in this area was carried out with graduate students in the Ph.D. program at Hofstra University, Hempstead, New York.

This book represents a culmination of this all important but often neglected area in obstetrical literature.

CONTRIBUTORS

S. Arulkumaran, M.D., M.R.C.O.G.
Senior Lecturer and Consultant
Department of Obstetrics and Gynecology
National University Hospital
National University of Singapore
Singapore

Richard Depp, M.D.
Professor and Chair
Department of Obstetrics and Gynecology
Jefferson Medical College
Philadelphia, Pennsylvania

Anne DeZoete, Ph.D.
Developmental Psychologist
Pediatric Department
National Women's Hospital
Auckland, New Zealand

John Elkins, Ph.D.
Professor
Schonell Educational Research Centre
University of Queensland
St. Lucia, Queensland,
Australia

Eric Garfinkel, Ph.D.
Professor
Department of Psychology
Hofstra University
Hempstead, New York

Victor Halitsky, M.D.
Acting Chairman
Department of Obstetrics and Gynecology
Nassau County Medical Center
East Meadow, New York

Ross N. Howie, F.R.A.C.P.
Associate Professor
Department of Pediatrics
University of Auckland
National Women's Hospital
Auckland, New Zealand

I. Ingemarsson, M.D., Ph.D.
Associate Professor
Department of Obstetrics and Gynecology
University Hospital
University of Lund
Lund, Sweden

Niels H. Lauersen, M.D., Ph.D.
Department of Obstetrics and Gynecology
Lenox Hill Hospital
New York, New York

Allen Y. L. Liang, F.R.A.C.P.
Pediatrician
Auckland Hospital
Auckland, New Zealand

James A. Low, M.D.
Professor
Department of Obstetrics and Gynecology
Queen's University
Kingston, Ontario
Canada

Barton MacArthur, M.A., Ph.D.
Senior Lecturer
Department of Education
University of Auckland
Auckland, New Zealand

Walter J. Morales, M.D., Ph.D.
Director of Maternal and Fetal Medicine
Department of Obstetrics and Gynecology
The Arnold Palmer Children's Hospital
 and Perinatal Center
Orlando, Florida

Patricia O'Donoghue, Ph.D.
Acting Academic Dean
Department of Academic Affairs
Carlow College
Pittsburgh, Pennsylvania

Michael J. Painter, M.D.
Chief
Division of Child Neurology
Children's Hospital of Pittsburgh
Pittsburgh, Pennsylvania

Richard P. Perkins, M.D.
Professor
Department of Obstetrics and Gynecology
Creighton University School of Medicine
Omaha, Nebraska

Dianne Polowczyk, Ph.D.
Associate Psychologist
Outpatient Division
Kings Park Psychiatric Center
Kings Park, New York

Florence E. Sisenwein, Ph.D.
Adjunct Clinical Professor
Department of Psychology
St. John's University
Flushing, New York

Nergesh Tejani, M.D.
Director
Division of Maternal-Fetal Medicine
Department of Obstetrics and Gynecology
Westchester County Medical Center
New York Medical College
Valhalla, New York

Uma L. Verma, M.D.
Attending Physician
Division of Maternal-Fetal Medicine
Department of Obstetrics and Gynecology
Westchester County Medical Center
New York Medical College
Valhalla, New York

M. Westgren, M.D., Ph.D.
Associate Professor
Department of Obstetrics and Gynecology
Karolinska Institute
Danderyds Hospital
Danderyd, Sweden

Eve K. Winer, Ph.D.
Psychologist
Great Neck Public Schools
Great Neck, New York

TABLE OF CONTENTS

INTRODUCTION

Nergesh Tejani

Little[1] and Freud,[2] in the 19th century, wrote on their observations linking cerebral palsy and mental retardation to the events of birth. The temporal relationship of static neurological and psychometric impairment in infancy and childhood to the process of birth has entrenched the belief that these are cause and effect. Obstetricians are continuously placed on the defensive where the ill-defined term "birth asphyxia" is used to explain much of this pathology. Since asphyxia is a specific term applied to hypoxia, hypercarbia, and acidosis, it becomes evident that what is being expressed is either a low Apgar score or a retrospective judgment after developmental sequelae are discovered.

In the face of this type of misconception and misrepresentation, it is surprising that investigation in the area of the long-term effects of obstetrical situations on the developing child is sparse. The classic attempt in this country, the United Cerebral Palsy study, is now several decades removed from present-day methods and cannot be regarded as representative of obstetrical practice in the 1980s. Several other criticisms may be applied to it. As one example, while it is necessary to use representative centers to obtain a cross-sectional sample, this precludes method uniformity, and information is often massed together from disparate cohorts; appropriate selection of control populations is a constant problem and a source of fallacy. A careful analysis of the problems in this study as applied to forceps deliveries is presented by Verma in Chapter 11.

While much information on long-term sequelae is accumulating from varied neonatal aspects, little has been done in the intrapartum area and even less in the antepartum area. Additionally, much of the information is scattered and difficult to assimilate. This volume is a step toward correcting this void. It is far from being all-inclusive and endeavors to present long-term sequelae and considerations in certain selected obstetrically oriented perinatal events.

Pharmacological agents for the treatment of preterm labor have been in use now for two decades. Ethanol, although presently not used, was in wide usage for this purpose in the 1970s. The adverse fetal effects of chronic alcohol abuse in pregnancy are now well established. It followed from this that it was of greatest concern to examine the long-term effect of this tocolytic agent in a controlled situation. Sisenwein and Tejani deal with this topic in Chapter 4. Some extrapolation to binge patterns of drinking in pregnancy may be valid, since information in this area is sparse. Ritodrine HCl, a beta-agonist, is the only tocolytic agent approved by the U.S. Food and Drug Administration. Its widespread use obligates some knowledge of the long-term outcome on the children who have been exposed to this agent *in utero*. In Chapter 3, Polowczyk and Lauersen present their own experience and review the limited literature in this area.

Corticosteroids were shown to enhance fetal lung maturity by Liggins and Howie in 1972.[3] The frequency of usage of corticosteroids for this purpose varies, most centers administering them at least selectively. Concern about the effects of corticosteroids on developing tissue, particularly on cerebellar function and growth, has been expressed. MacArthur and other members of the New Zealand group who first investigated this agent present their own findings and a review of the literature on this issue in Chapter 5.

Intrauterine growth retardation is now a widely recognized problem in obstetrics. An awareness of the condition, sonographic confirmation and evaluation of the situation, and application of fetal functional tests to preempt intrauterine demise are now widely accepted management strategies. Further study of this situation has revealed its heterogeneity. At least two prototypes of intrauterine growth patterns are recognized. An asymmetrical type, where the brain is preferentially perfused, results in the least compromise of the brain and head and is typically seen with maternal vascular disorders. A symmetrical type, where all organs suffer retarded growth from an early stage of development, has also been recognized. The etiology of this condition is almost certainly multifactorial. Chronic fetal intrauterine infection, gross chromosomal abnormalities, and other genetic defects are known to result in this condition; however, most cases are "idiopathic" and are of unknown origin, possibly related to nutritional or trace metal deficiency. The study of long-term sequelae obviously would be of limited value unless the subsets within growth-retarded infants were examined separately. Surprisingly few investigators have designed studies in this manner. In Chapter 6, Winer and Tejani present their work and review the literature on sequelae of subsets of small-for-gestational-age children.

Kernicterus, the result of the detrimental effect of unconjugated bilirubin on the basal ganglia of the neonate, is widely recognized. In cases of severe fetal isoimmunization where intrauterine fetal intraperitoneal transfusions have been used, long-term follow-up of sequelae is difficult to interpret because of overlapping variables of hyperbilirubinemia and effects inherent to immaturity which often coexist. Halitsky presents an exhaustive analysis of the available literature on this topic in Chapter 7. His analysis is especially directed toward the elimination of the confounding variables of hyperbilirubinemia and immaturity.

Conservative management of cases of preterm premature rupture of membranes, with the hope of allowing time to gain maturity, is widely practiced. With expectant management, signs of intrauterine infection are looked for and regarded as indications to terminate pregnancy. Immediate success in gaining maturity in a proportion of these cases is the experience of most obstetricians; however, the long-term sequelae of prolonged membrane rupture, with and without intrauterine infection, are unknown. Morales presents his work, probably unique in this area, in Chapter 8 and gives his conclusions on a 1-year follow-up of cases who experienced *in utero* prolonged rupture of membranes.

The problems of delivery of a fetus presenting as breech have been the subject of obstetrical debate, with an escalated number of cases now being delivered by cesarean section in the belief that this improves neonatal mortality and morbidity. In Chapter 10 Ingemarsson et al. discuss this topic, with the especially provocative message that the fetus presenting as breech is a symptom of inherent and preexisting problems, the route of delivery being of lesser importance.

Continuous fetal heart rate monitoring is now widely practiced and regarded as a standard of intrapartum care. The immediate benefits of fetal heart rate monitoring specifically in patients not at risk are unclear. Certainly the sensitivity of abnormal fetal heart rate patterns to identify a distressed fetus is very low. As may be expected, the long-term sequelae of intrapartum fetal heart rate patterns have been largely unexplored. Painter et al. present their findings and review the literature on this topic in Chapter 9.

True birth asphyxia is represented by hypoxia, hypercarbia, and acidosis in fetal scalp and umbilical arterial blood. Low presents a scholarly examination of the implications of fetal hypoxia in Chapter 2. The long-term sequelae of established fetal hypoxia/acidosis are shown by him to be unpredictable. Little wonder, then, that the term "birth asphyxia" is used loosely and imprecisely; it has only imprecise long-term significance.

The long-term sequelae of forceps deliveries are reviewed and presented by Verma in Chapter 11. Multiple confounding variables are scrutinized and presented.

Although neonatal periventricular/intraventricular hemorrhage is manifested in the neonatal period, the obstetrical antecedents to this condition have been examined and are summarized in Chapter 12 by Garfinkel and Verma. The long-term sequelae of periventricular/intraventricular hemorrhage, including the authors' own experiences, are described. This chapter includes an examination of the sequelae of cases of isolated ventricular dilatation in the absence of hemorrhage. The sequelae following periventricular leucomalacia have recently been recognized and are reviewed by the authors. Although this information is limited, it is impressive and persuasive that this lesion predicts long-term deficits better than almost any other manifestation in the newborn. With both established and newer imaging techniques, it appears that accurate long-term prognostication in the preterm neonate may soon become a reality.

The opening chapter by Perkins is a tour de force of a variety of perinatal situations where long-term sequelae may be known or, if not investigated, may be a potential problem waiting to be resolved — an invitation from Dr. Perkins to interested investigators.

In the interpretation of long-term sequelae, several difficulties should be recognized. With mobile populations, attrition of original study groups may occur to the extent of invalidity. Additionally, self-selection due to a high level of compliance in caring and intact homes as opposed to troubled situations is problematic. The enormous number of variables during the antepartum, intrapartum, and neonatal periods and in the subsequent environment makes interpretation difficult and perfectly matched controls virtually impossible. The factor of socioeconomic status may not be ignored; however, its assessment presents problems. This assessment usually takes the form of questionnaires which vary in detail. The shorter, less detailed ones lack finer points, but are usually filled out accurately. Questionnaires that are more detailed are often tiresome and exacting to complete, and their supposed accuracy is offset by the quality of information supplied.

In view of the multiplicity of variables involved in examination of long-term sequelae, the choice of control populations presents unusual difficulties and sources for misinterpretation. In examining the effects of forceps deliveries from the United Cerebral Palsy study data, Verma points out conflicting conclusions made by different investigators studying the same data base due to selection and to differences in the control groups. In considering the long-term significance of obstetrical factors, controlling for birth weight, birth weight percentile, gestational age, age at examination, and socioeconomic status may be considered minimum requisites.

The relative merits of continuous and categorical outcomes deserve some thought. A few points of difference in mean values on the various psychometric scales are of much less practical significance than the comparison of numbers of "affected" children to the "unaffected". This might appear self-evident; however, it is possible to apply undue importance to differences in mean scores because of the facility with which these can be manipulated statistically. Application of this to individual cases is of far less significance than a comparison of categorical outcomes.

This book represents a small beginning. Obstetricians have come to the painful realization that their responsibility does not end upon delivery of a live infant. Investigation into this area is essential to the well-being of both patient and physician. The good news is that the limited information to date shows predominantly negative findings.

REFERENCES

1. **Little, W. J.,** On the influence of abnormal parturition, difficult labors, premature birth, and asphyxia neonatorum on the mental and physical condition of the child, especially in relation to deformities, *Trans. Obstet. Soc. London*, 2, 293, 1862.
2. **Freud, S.,** Infantile cerbrallahmung, in *Nothnagel's Specielle Pathologie und Therapie*, Vol. 12, Vienna, 1897, 9.
3. **Liggins, G. C. and Howie, R. N.,** A controlled trial of antepartum glucocorticoid treatment for prevention of the respiratory distress syndrome in premature infants, *Pediatrics*, 50, 515, 1972.

Chapter 1

SELECTED PERINATAL EVENTS AND FOLLOW-UP STUDIES

Richard P. Perkins

TABLE OF CONTENTS

I. INTRODUCTION

The purpose of this chapter is to deal with certain perinatal events commonly encountered in obstetrics and neonatology and how they may impact upon outcome, not only on immediate survival and neonatal well-being, but also on long-term childhood growth and development. Clearly, not all events occurring during pregnancy and the neonatal period can be adequately surveyed, but those which may have a major impact on these areas deserve some exploration in a forum such as this. We will attempt to synthesize what is currently known and, where consensus can be found as to causation and treatment, seek to shed some light on these areas. Regrettably, the most severe problems encountered in many cases remain controversial as to why they arise and how to prevent or treat them. Were this not so, these problems undoubtedly would have been solved long ago.

Other chapters in this book deal with major areas of concern, including breech presentation, intrauterine growth retardation, the long-term implication of tocolytic agents and prenatal corticosteroid therapy, and general implications of fetal hypoxia. These subjects will not be explored in depth in this chapter, except in passing as they relate to the continuity of consideration regarding long-term outcome. These are important perinatal management issues, however, and to leave them totally unaddressed in this chapter would not be entirely appropriate.

II. PRENATAL EVENTS

The value of *prenatal care* and its association with good perinatal outcome can scarcely be denied. Viewpoints differ, however, as to the components which determine the value of prenatal care. The worst perinatal outcomes appear disproportionately represented among populations of patients receiving minimal or no prenatal surveillance and intervention. Lee et al.[1] noted in a recent review that in the 25 years from 1950 to 1975, neonatal mortality in this country progressively declined despite no major change in birth weight distributions. This overall improvement was therefore attributed to the benefits of increasingly sophisticated and available perinatal care. Although the U.S. remains in a disadvantageous position in relation to perinatal mortality rates reported from many other developed countries, this fact can be addressed by two major observations. First, this country reports perinatal mortality in very liberal terms in comparison to other countries, choosing to include babies with birth weights as low as 500 g and extending the statistical period for neonatal mortality through the 28th day of life. Second, this country maintains a higher rate of preterm birth than other countries with more favorable statistics. Within this latter frame of reference, results from this country on survival by narrow birth weight and gestational age categories exceed those of most other parts of the globe. Nonetheless, preterm birth, with all of its ramifications for perinatal mortality and morbidity, remains our preeminent unsolved problem.

Factors predisposing to adverse pregnancy outcome can often be anticipated, but not always ameliorated, even prior to conception. Poor control of *maternal diabetes mellitus* is a prime example of a remediable problem. Although data are conflicting regarding the impact of *prior pregnancy outcome* on subsequent successful childbearing, most studies suggest that, with reference to prior pregnancy loss, associations can be made with subsequent adversity. This holds even when such prior loss occurred voluntarily, especially if such loss was induced following the first trimester of pregnancy.[2] The degree to which the reproductive apparatus is mechanically traumatized may have considerable impact, even in the first-trimester abortion. The factor of *involuntary infertility* also has been repeatedly found in studies seeking associations between prenatal influences and cerebral palsy. Recurrence risks for preterm and growth-retarded infants remain two to three times those of the normal population after adjustments for intervening factors.

The impact of *birth order* and the interval between pregnancies has until recently been a neglected area of inquiry. On a population basis it can be shown that if one disregards for the moment the greater morbidity and mortality intrinsic to the first pregnancies, enhanced adverse outcomes can be demonstrated among fourth, fifth, and sixth pregnancies and beyond.[3,4] Dowding[3] noted that birth order statistics are largely reflective of socioeconomic status, advanced multiparity being a feature of socioeconomic disadvantage, reflecting itself in suboptimal birth weight among first and fifth pregnancies and beyond. The factor of advanced maternal age and the acquisition of age-related medical complications must also be recognized. Bakketeig and Hoffman[4] also noted an increased overall risk of adverse outcome to fourth pregnancies and beyond on a population basis, but in given families perinatal mortality progressively decreased with increasing parity. The importance of the spacing of gestations was noted, adverse outcomes largely occurring in those pregnancies in close proximity to prior gestations. Siegel and Morris[5] acknowledged the adverse effect of close spacing of pregnancies and the enhancement of risk if the pregnancy was recognized to be at high risk socioeconomically. These considerations reflected themselves in an increased risk of both maternal and perinatal mortality, preterm birth, and a subsequent correlation with poor child care, child abuse, increased rates of infections among mothers and babies, diminished relative height and growth among the children, diminished childhood intelligence, and other related matters.

Some attention in the past has been focused on the magnitude of *maternal weight gain* and its impact on perinatal well-being. Tavris and Read[6] recently reported correlations between maternal weight gain and ultimate outcome for the pregnancy. It was noted that if pregnancies continued beyond 35 weeks and maternal weight gain fell within the range of 5 to 29 lb, no associations with ultimate adverse effect could be demonstrated with the child. Increased risks of fetal, infant, and childhood death as well as an increased frequency of cognitive defects could be demonstrated at age 5 among children born of pregnancies in which weight gain was <5 or >29 lb. Similar results were found during analysis of weight gain data derived from the National Collaborative Perinatal Project (NCPP),[7] with the additional observation that optimal outcomes in initially obese women occurred with lesser degrees of weight gain. Although maternal height, prepregnancy weight, and weight gain have been correlated with ultimate fetal size, recent data also suggest that a genetic component may also be expressed by correlations with the birth weight of the mother.[8] These and other generalizations are made with the understanding that maternal conditions independently influencing weight gain, such as hypertension, twins, and diabetes, are excluded.

Maternal smoking has long been suspected of having adverse affects on fetal growth and welfare.[9] Babies born of mothers who smoke heavily are smaller than their estimated growth potential would anticipate. Associations have also been made between maternal smoking and placental abruption, preterm birth, and other types of pregnancy wastage. These effects have largely been attributed to the vascular effects of smoking on the maternal-fetal-placental relationship. Kelly et al.,[10] in a study on tobacco and nontobacco cigarette smoking, observed maternal and fetal cardiovascular responses in comparison to those of nonsmokers. Smoking tobacco-containing cigarettes resulted in an increase in maternal heart rate, mean arterial pressure, and fetal heart rate, with a decrease in both fetal heart rate variability and fetal movement. This was not seen in nontobacco cigarette smokers, and the author concluded that this effect was related to the nicotine content, which constituted the main difference between the two types of cigarettes. Undoubtedly other chemical differences existed as well.

Although Jouppila et al.[11] noted that smoking one cigarette failed to have any impact on fetal aortic or umbilical vein flow, there is little doubt that chronic smoking can have such effects. In addition, impacts on fetal breathing, movement, and reactivity on antepartum testing have been observed. In terms of long-term effects, Rantakallio[12] followed the status of children of smoking mothers through the age of 14. Observed among these children were an increased incidence of respiratory disease, short stature, and decreased school perform-ance. This difference remained after adjusting for mother's height, age, and socioeconomic status, baby's sex, and the other children in the family. Smoking mothers themselves differed from others in socioeconomic status, but within their socioeconomic class these mothers had diminished quality of health as well as increased rates of unemployment and abandonment of their families. There was no outcome difference for the child if the *father* was the smoking parent, suggesting that passive smoking is as relevant to the observed phenomena as active smoking. Investigators in this country have demonstrated intermediate levels of fetal-neonatal thiocyanate among babies born to mothers where passive smoking constituted the only exposure,[13] whereas others have not observed these same results.[14] Although the maximal birth weight reduction attributable to smoking has been stated to be approximately 300 g, it is clear that maternal smoking is an undesirable facet of the health of the maternal-fetal unit.

Although another chapter in this book addresses the issue of alcohol exposure and the developing fetus, *adverse effects from other agents,* even those potentially required for the maintenance of maternal welfare, have been demonstrated. Although the list of incriminated drugs is substantial and includes not only prescribed therapeutic agents, but other pharma-cological entities illicitly used for recreational purposes, including narcotics, among the most potent high-risk agents are the oral coumarin family of anticoagulants.[15] Chronic exposure to these agents throughout pregnancy has been associated with newborn abnormalities, including abnormal facies, hypoplastic digits, stippled epiphyses, and mental retardation. Exposure limited to the mid-trimester of pregnancy has been associated with an increased frequency of optic atrophy, faulty brain growth and development, and mental retardation. Continuation into the third trimester of pregnancy may result in chronic fetal anticoagulation and spontaneous or trauma-induced hemorrhage.

Other phenotypic and functional abnormalities have been attributed to the family of drugs generally prescribed for anticonvulsant therapy, the most prominent of which are phenytoin or diphenylhydantoin, valproic acid, and trimethadione. Although a retrospective review informally conducted at our institution on 30 mothers chronically ingesting Dilantin® throughout pregnancy failed to reveal an increased frequency of gross morphological ab-normality, such associations clearly have been observed in larger studies.[16] Unfortunately, since defects have been reported at a lower frequency among women exclusively on bar-biturate therapy, the question is frequently raised as to the effect of the basic disease under treatment on these abnormalities vs. the agents used to treat it. There can be little doubt, however, that diphenylhydantoin can result in lowered maternal folic acid levels, potentially interfering with normal fetoplacental development.[17] This drug has also been incriminated in a disturbance in vitamin K availability, potentially resulting in relative disturbances in fetal blood coagulation.[18] Phenobarbital has also been implicated in such developments, although the mechanisms may be different and involve a more rapid turnover of vitamin-K-dependent coagulation factors through enhanced hepatic enzyme activity. The end result is the same, however, in the potential for fetal and neonatal hemorrhage.

The latest addition to anticonvulsant therapeutic programs, valproic acid, has been associated with an increased frequency of neural tube and other defects.[19] Trimethadione has a well-defined phenotypic syndrome and should be avoided during gestation.[20]

A. PRETERM BIRTH

These and many other recognized maternal complications may result in the risk of *preterm birth.* Since the preterm neonate is at high risk for long-term neurological and psychological compromise, these complications, when involving the welfare of mother and baby, must be considered and the decision to prevent preterm birth predicated on the feasibility of its prevention vs. the benefits to mother and baby of allowing the process to continue. If fetal welfare is best served by remaining *in utero* and the treatment designed and predicted to successfully arrest the labor process does not unduly threaten the welfare of the mother or child, this course of action should be undertaken. If, on the other hand, a serious fetal or maternal condition would be alleviated by allowing delivery to occur unimpeded or after only a short delay, then this course of action should be followed.

Presuming that in most cases the benefits of stopping preterm labor outweigh the risks, one must then consider the short- and long-term effects of whatever agent is used to attempt to achieve this end. Nearly all agents for the inhibition of preterm labor studied to this date have been associated with some obvious benefits and some apparent or theoretical risks. In the early era of preterm labor suppression, intravenous (i.v.) ethanol was considered the only available effective agent. Our own studies have suggested that the use of ethanol in inhibiting labor with a growth-retarded fetus may enhance morbidity and mortality. This problem is discussed in this book, the conclusion being that an increase in central nervous system pathology on long-term follow-up of the newborn is noted if delivery occurs within 15 h of stopping administration of the agent.

In a follow-up study of brief exposure to isoxsuprine for labor suppression, Brazy et al.[21] found no major differences in neonatal and childhood behavior between treated and control infants. In a previous study, however, Brazy and Pupkin[22] reported an association between isoxsuprine therapy and increased rates of neonatal hypocalcemia, hypoglycemia, ileus, hypotension, and death if drug exposure was continued to within 48 h of birth. The rate of ultimate neonatal death diminished with increasing duration of therapy, however, presumably attributable in part to the gains realized in the gestational ages of the babies treated. Perinatal death rate increases paralleled the increase in maternal side effects during therapy.

Beta-mimetic therapy has been associated with demonstrable effects on pulmonary surfactant production and release, both *in vitro* and (presumably) in clinical use. It has been postulated that prolonged use of beta-mimetic therapy may result in exhaustion of pulmonary surfactant production, potentially enhancing the risk of pulmonary immaturity following birth.[23] Dudenhausen et al.[24] demonstrated that long-term fenoterol therapy was statistically associated with a decrease in amniotic fluid lecithin content in comparison to control patients. Clearly, any therapy which predisposes to enhanced risks of hyaline membrane disease also involves augmented risks of related complications.

Beta-mimetic drugs have other potential adverse effects on fetal homeostasis as well. Hansen et al.[25] reported on control and study populations of newborns following ritodrine therapy. Treated babies had diminished inulin clearances and increased plasma renin activity and urinary vasopression excretion on the first day following birth, but these changes were resolved by the sixth day of life. Gestational age in the studied population correlated inversely with plasma ritodrine concentration, renin activity, and vasopressin. Despite these observations, there were no differences in urine or serum electrolyte concentration, osmolality, urinary sodium excretion, and volume of urine production. The salt- and water-retaining potentials of these drugs in high dosage and with prolonged use, however, are clearly demonstrable in the mother through a declining hematocrit and the occasional development of pulmonary edema. Our own studies, as well as other reports, have indicated the dramatic effect that these drugs can have on blood glucose, potassium, CO_2, lactate, and pH.[26] These effects seem interrelated, and they quite likely can be enhanced by the concomitant administration of glucose-containing i.v. fluids. Adverse effects appear to be limited by the administration of a balanced electrolyte solution without carbohydrate. These risks can be further augmented by the parallel utilization of corticosteroids to enhance fetal pulmonary maturity.[27] The measure of benefit of this therapy is questionable, however, especially considering that many (if not all) beta-mimetic agents (as well as other nonbeta-mimetic agents, such as aminophylline, ethanol, and magnesium sulfate) have been claimed to enhance pulmonary maturity in the treated pregnancy. The possibility exists that preterm labor itself either enhances the rate of pulmonary maturity or indicates a preexisting but undiagnosed condition which results in pulmonary maturation. Further studies in this area are sorely needed. The potential benefits of corticosteroids to those responsive to their effects seem clear. The potential long-term detriments are still being explored, but do not appear severe with the usual regimens and brief use (see Chapter 5).

Other issues relating to *untimely birth* should be mentioned. In every neonatal intensive care unit in this country, there commonly reside a small number of babies who because of inexpert assessment of prenatal factors prior to elective delivery suffer from avoidable iatrogenic prematurity. With the current availability of technology for determining with reasonable certainty the gestational age, appropriateness of growth, and pulmonary maturity of the fetus, these occurrences should be effectively abolished in appropriate care systems. Abnormally delayed pulmonary maturity in some families is an established risk factor, probably encouraging the adoption of the philosophy that elective intervention should always be preceded by objective evidence of fetal lung maturity. Still, many cases of potentially avoidable iatrogenic prematurity represent examples of inattention to basic obstetric care principles. Iatrogenic preterm delivery should occur only when the welfare of the baby or mother can clearly be demonstrated to be served by early intervention.

B. PERINATAL INFECTION

Congenital infections threaten both fetal life and multisystem integrity. Prelabor infections of greatest concern are cytomegalovirus (CMV), rubella, and toxoplasmosis. All are capable of causing extensive neurological destruction as well as long-term deficit. Rubella carries major risks, but is seen less often now that immunization programs are widespread.

CMV is prevalent in nature, and the notable majority of adults in most societies demonstrate acquired immunity.[28] Although most serious fetal infections result from primary maternal infection, some instances of fetal involvement from recurrent infection have been reported.

Toxoplasmosis varies in prevalence geographically. Only primary maternal infections appear to threaten the fetus. Although the domestic house cat has been named as a putative vector (if allowed to hunt and roam free), proof of this is scant and circumstantial in this country.

Herpesvirus (simplex) in the overwhelming majority of cases appears to threaten the fetus only at delivery or after rupture of membranes. Residual neurological deficit occurs in up to 50% of survivors of neonatal sepsis.[29] This figure can be expected to diminish as more effective antiviral agents appear, and acyclovir may prove to be effective in the future. The protective effects of prior maternal immunity remain to be fully defined.

Prognosis for neurological well-being depends on the agent infecting the fetus, the time of onset *in utero*, treatment (if any is available and effective), and perhaps some factors of fetal-neonatal passive immunity. With rubella, the earlier in gestation the infection is acquired, the more severe and widespread the affliction.[30] If infected in the first month of gestation, over half of the surviving fetuses will manifest ocular, cardiac, and central nervous system (CNS) deficits, and over 80% will have significant hearing loss. These numbers diminish somewhat in the second month, particularly the ocular involvement, which drops to <10% by the third month, but the frequencies of reported cardiac and general neurological involvement are still at 20 to 25% in the third month and two thirds are deaf. If affected as late as the fourth month, half are deaf and one fourth show some CNS deficit, usually microcephaly as well as functional and cognitive difficulties. The "congenital rubella syndrome" has been well described.[31]

CMV infection still occurs in 3 to 6% of women during pregnancy, and up to 2% of newborns excrete the virus. The development of the infection is slow, and many acquiring the virus at delivery may be asymptomatic. Microcephaly may be present at birth, associated with intracranial (typically periventricular) calcifications and chorioretinitis, or may develop later.[32] Hepatosplenomegaly and other signs of generalized viral infection may be seen, as with rubella and others. Over 90% of those with intracranial findings either die or are left with mental retardation, motor defects, deafness, and seizures. Late-acquired CMV may also contribute to the pool of unattributed hearing loss in childhood.[33]

Toxoplasmosis can result in intracranial calcification (more commonly diffuse), hydrocephalus, and, rarely, porencephaly or hydranencephaly. Microcephaly is also common among survivors of serious involvement. Although deafness is not common among survivors, mental retardation, seizures, spastic motor deficits, and ocular involvement are prevalent.[32]

Congenital herpes is rare, as the infection rarely crosses the placenta, but when acquired at delivery (or *in utero* after rupture of membranes) the disease has a fairly rapid onset (7 to 10 days) and is global in distribution. Over half of untreated, at-risk babies exposed will die, and at least half of the survivors will be damaged, showing intra- and extracranial pathology.[29] Acyclovir seems to be very promising as an agent likely to ameliorate these dismal outcome prognoses.

Many other viral agents have been associated with neonatal evidence of injury. The role of these agents in stillbirth and idiopathic symmetric growth retardation, as well as in the instigation of maternal multisystemic "toxemia" syndromes, awaits further study. Varicella, Coxsackie B, and the encephalitis virus family remain rarely identified noxious agents. Hepatitis B virus appears to be nearly completely avoidable as a neonatal infectious agent by proper identification and newborn administration of specific immune globulin.[34]

C. ANTEPARTUM TESTING

Prenatal assessment in the form of nonstress testing is widely practiced and used as evidence of fetal well-being. The long-term significance of abnormal tests is unknown and would be of great interest. Controversy still exists in this country regarding the relative merits of contraction-provoked vs. passive observation of signs of fetal welfare or jeopardy.[35-37] Although proponents of each philosophy report extremely low rates of fetal-neonatal morbidity and mortality through the use of stress or nonstress testing, the issue of which is the better method of achieving an optimal outcome in high-risk circumstances has not been resolved. While stress-testing-mediated programs report good results, it cannot be retrospectively determined with accuracy how many babies delivered as a result of nonreassuring stress testing would have continued satisfactorily *in utero* had intervention not occurred.

Alternatively, if nonstress testing is utilized as the *only* method of antenatal surveillance, a high frequency of falsely nonreassuring tests resulting in intervention will clearly be recognized. If rational approaches utilizing the relatively simplistic nonstress testing protocol are backed up (when nonreassuring) with contraction stress testing for further proof of apparent lack of fetal welfare, the lowest rate of unjustified intervention may be realized. In the series by Solum and Sjoberg[36] over 10,000 nonstress tests on 1455 patients were reported, with only 5 fetal deaths resulting, all preceded by abnormal tests. In the large comparative series of stress vs. nonstress testing reported by Freeman et al.,[37] somewhat better results were achieved if contraction stress testing was utilized as the decision-making screening procedure. In contrast, other series utilizing nonstress testing backed up by contraction stress testing have shown similar results. Although protocols depending on contraction stress testing can clearly be simplified in many cases by the use of breast stimulation instead of exogenous oxytocin-induced contractions,[38] future studies comparing these two methods are needed, especially in terms of long-term morbidity, in order for a clearer view of the appropriate regimen for uteroplacental insufficiency to be determined. It must also be realized that the standard of excellence of antenatal testing need not be the absence of labor intolerance, but rather the quality of ultimate outcome and the gains in extending pregnancy to the best achieved gestational age.

III. LABOR AND DELIVERY EVENTS

Adverse intrapartum events, whether occurring at appropriate or inappropriate gestational ages, have some potential for creating fetal injury resulting in long-term neurological and functional handicap.[39,40] The degree to which the intrapartum period is truly responsible for subsequent handicap, however, is undoubtedly substantially less than current opinion would indicate. The potential adverse consequences of preterm birth are acknowledged. What remains to be clarified, however, are the nature and severity of circumstances which result in preterm birth, either by elective intervention or by spontaneous preterm labor. Although the avoidance of preterm birth and its related consequences are admirable objectives, we must never lose sight of the fact that the cause of labor remains undefined and, therefore, the message to be heard when it occurs must be meticulously analyzed and understood. Identified high-risk circumstances frequently lead to an indicated pregnancy intervention and delivery at a time other than at full term. Meticulous scientific endeavor must be applied to distinguish between those factors which *result in* preterm delivery and the impact on subsequent handicap of circumstances which *result from* preterm delivery. We must also extend our inquiries further to determine the critically important distinction between those conditions which *predispose to* fetal intolerance of labor and those consequences which *result from* fetal distress.

Despite numerous suggestions that factors occurring *prior* to labor and delivery may be involved in at least half of the subsequent neurological and other functional morbidity and handicap,[39] the intrapartum period remains that portion of the pregnancy exposed to the greatest public scrutiny and at risk for medicolegal litigation. Many of the issues surrounding pertinent aspects of labor and delivery will be covered in other chapters; therefore, this portion of this chapter will be somewhat concise.

A. PERINATAL "ASPHYXIA"

Several recent reports have appeared concerning the causes and ultimate complications associated with fetal intolerance of labor. Low et al.,[41,42] in a series of publications utilizing umbilical arterial buffer base as a reference for intrapartum asphyxia, have studied the consequences of such presumed asphyxia on ultimate neurological well-being. In a substantial study comparing 242 high-risk obstetric pregnancies[42] (126 of which were preterm) with 47 low-risk controls, the incidence of diminished umbilical arterial buffer base (presumably reflecting asphyxia) was studied along with neonatal evidence of encephalopathy and infection. High-risk pregnancies in this series were defined by growth retardation, gestational age <34 weeks, birth weight <1500 g, birth weight >1500 g with intrauterine growth retardation, and metabolic disease exclusive of diabetes. In a brief follow-up,[41] the incidence of provisional deficits among the low-risk patients was 10% and among the high-risk patients was 17% if neither infection nor encephalopathy was present. If evidence of infection was found, 30% of pregnancies were associated with ultimate deficit — 40% if encephalopathy was diagnosed. In similar prior studies, Low had shown a minimal impact of reduced umbilical arterial buffer base alone on ultimate handicap.[42] It is suggested, therefore, by these studies that perinatal-neonatal complications of these sorts have an enhancing effect on the risk of injury.

Westgren et al.[43] studied fetal heart rate and fetal scalp blood pH determinations and their impact on preterm delivery. The pH sampling was conducted at 5 cm and complete cervical dilation, and these findings were correlated with ominous fetal heart rate patterns and the presence of acidosis (defined as a pH <7.25). Ominous patterns and pH correlated well at 5 cm dilation, but not at complete dilation, presumably reflecting the brief interval between the latter determination and delivery. Acidosis discovered by these means correlated with neonatal hypotonia and seizure behavior. No long-term follow-up data were given.

In data from the NCPP, Niswander et al.[44] compared survivors following such highly distressful circumstances in labor as abruptio, placenta previa with hemorrhage, and prolapsed umbilical cord to patients without these complications. On examination at 4 years of age utilizing computer-matched controls, there were no differences in cognitive function and fine motor coordination between the two groups. These findings supported the opinions of Myers[45] and others that acute severe asphyxia is tolerated reasonably well by the otherwise normal baby, possibly in contrast to the impact of long-term partial asphyxia on ultimate neurological excellence.

Painter and co-workers[46] studied the results of 50 high-risk labors in terms of fetal heart rate irregularities and ultimate handicap through a minimum of 12 months after birth. Of the patients studied, 12 had normal fetal heart rate patterns retrospectively judged to have existed throughout the labor, whereas 16 had moderate to severe variable decelerations and 22 had severe variable and/or late decelerations. On brief follow-up, a developmental bias was observed favoring those with normal fetal heart rate patterns compared to those with abnormal patterns; those with the more severe abnormalities appeared to have the higher incidence of ultimate neurological abnormality. In these instances, the Apgar scores were not reflective of ultimate handicaps found.

The lack of relevance of Apgar scores to ultimate neurological well-being has been repeatedly demonstrated recently. Sykes and associates,[47] studying predominantly term deliveries, found no more than 15 to 20% correlation between low Apgar scores at 1 and 5 min and low umbilical arterial pH. In these studies, low scores were infrequently associated with evidence of acidosis, and, conversely, acidosis was equally infrequently associated with Apgar score depression. Others have more recently shown similar findings.[48] This correlation is even less reliable in the preterm baby, as shown by Goldenberg et al.[49] In his study of preterm birth and correlation between Apgar scores and pH at birth, the more premature the baby, the more likely the Apgar scores were to be low despite normal umbilical arterial pH. Also, in this study, the closer to term, the more likely it was that the Apgar score was normal even with a diminished pH. Although the NCPP clearly showed a correspondence between prolonged Apgar depression and ultimate neurological handicap,[50] only among near-term babies did this relationship exist exclusive of complications of prematurity and other related issues. Even in this monumental data base, not all outcomes were investigated for other predisposing factors, nor was the data base completely secure in terms of gestational age determinations, since all of these were made based only on the maternal last menstrual period.

Perinatal acidosis is acknowledged to have an association with the potential induction of neonatal instability and regression in certain characteristics of fetal maturity. The most notable of these is the association between perinatal asphyxia and neonatal hyaline membrane disease. Kenny et al.[51] studied 110 babies of various gestational ages for umbilical artery pH, pCO_2, lactate, and bicarbonate. In the study population, 33 of the 110 had hyaline membrane disease, 16 had transient tachypnea, and 61 were normal. The occurrence of hyaline membrane disease was based largely on diminished gestational age and (presumably related) diminished Apgar score, but bore no relationship to either neonatal pH or to other parameters of acid-base status. These data conflicted somewhat with those of Hobel et al.,[52] who showed a significant relationship between neonatal asphyxia and the induction of respiratory distress.

The mode of delivery must be considered when determining the potential causes of fetal acidosis and neonatal depression. Gilstrap et al.[53] observed no difference in the incidence of acidosis and ultimate outcome among those delivered by low forceps vs. midforceps. No difference also was found between those delivered by elective low forceps and those delivered spontaneously. Among those delivered by midforceps, an increased frequency of vaginal lacerations and a diminished maternal hematocrit were found, but no other differences could be demonstrated. Most other studies, however, have demonstrated an increased frequency of neonatal depression following midforceps delivery, although most cases were not correlated with umbilical arterial pH determinations. Whenever mode of delivery is considered, careful attention must be paid to the circumstances resulting in the choice of that mode of delivery vs. the influence of mode of delivery itself and its attendant anesthesia. As mentioned above, under many circumstances usually involving preterm birth, cesarean section delivery mechanically can pose risks of traumatic injury nearly equivalent to those of vaginal delivery. In light of this consideration, one must not compare abdominal delivery with vaginal delivery on the tacit assumption that cesarean section always results in gentler handling of the fetus. To extend this insight to the extreme of advocating a prophylactic classic cesarean section for all preterm births may represent an overzealous compensation for effects which can be adequately anticipated by better alternative planning.

Despite evidence to the contrary, continual attention appears to be paid to associating fetal "asphyxia" and ultimate neurological handicap. In many cases, "asphyxia" and neonatal depression have been considered synonymous, even though previously cited evidence would obviate this conclusion. In a careful analysis of this potential connection, Dijxhoorn et al.[54] examined over 800 normally grown, vaginally delivered babies at term for associations between umbilical artery pH and neonatal neurological status as assessed by the "optimality scoring system". In this study, the neonatal optimality score was related to the umbilical artery pH as well as to the difference between the umbilical artery pH and the maternal venous pH difference (accounting for passively acquired fetal acidosis). Babies who clearly seemed affected, as well as those considered suspect, were associated with the above-indicated parameters; however, the variance demonstrated by this analysis accounted for only 1 to 4% of all abnormal newborns. The authors were forced to conclude that little or no relationship exists between perinatal acidemia and neonatal neurological status.

Further extending the possible association between duration of abnormality and outcome, Katz and associates[55] studied the relationship between deep and sustained end-stage fetal heart rate decelerations occurring in the second stage of labor and ultimate outcome. Of 55 babies with this finding, 6 demonstrated a 1-min Apgar score of <7 and an acidotic umbilical venous pH. In all babies where the deceleration persisted for >15 min, umbilical venous pH was diminished. The authors did not explain their choice of umbilical *venous* pH as a point of reference, since although this may constitute a rough reflection of fetal arterial status it is actually more an index of placental function and maternal perfusion.

Many authors have demonstrated that the growth-retarded infant possesses a much more limited capacity to compensate for hypoxic stress in labor than does the normally grown baby. In a study of fetal heart rate tracings before cesarean section in 72 infants, Henson et al.[56] studied the correlation between fetal heart rate abnormalities and ultimate evidence of asphyxia. In this series, 23 cesarean sections were performed for abnormal fetal heart pattern characteristics, whereas 49 were performed for other reasons not involving evidence of fetal distress. There was no difference in base excess between the two populations. Almost all babies manifesting distress were found to have had intrauterine growth retardation. The authors concluded that abnormal fetal heart rate tracings do not correlate reliably with fetal acidosis, but may be related to other factors ultimately resulting in intrauterine growth retardation. These and other studies emphasize how important it is to diagnose intrauterine growth retardation, not only from the point of view of conducting careful and appropriate antenatal surveillance, but also for appropriately aggressive responses to evidences of the occurrence of fetal intolerance of labor in these uniquely sensitive infants. Although intrauterine growth retardation may be suspected of exemplifying preexisting injury or, possibly of equal importance, of predisposing to perinatal-neonatal harm, careful analysis of data resulting from pregnancies involving intrauterine growth retardation leaves a distinct impression that aggressive supportive care of the growth-retarded infant during labor and after delivery may determine the potential for neurological normality well beyond factors involved in causing intrauterine growth retardation per se,[57] if careful attention is paid to excluding those infants whose inadequate growth results from chronic, irreparable, intrinsic abnormality. This subject is dealt with extensively in a separate chapter in this book.

Finally, the influence of *obstetric anesthesia* and its contribution to perinatal well-being must also be considered. It has been well demonstrated that, even in the normal baby, vigorous maternal prehydration with dextrose-containing i.v. fluids results in an increased incidence of elevated umbilical cord insulin and glucose levels, an increased frequency of neonatal hypoglycemia, and an enhanced risk of neonatal jaundice.[58] The authors propose that predelivery glucose infusion rates by any means should be limited to ≤6 g/h. Although this management principle has previously been vigorously applied to the management of the carbohydrate-intolerant mother, it seems clear that this represents a risk factor in all deliveries. The impact of various anesthetic techniques has been reviewed extensively by Swanstrom and Bratteby[59-61] in a three-part series. In this study, high glucose levels were strongly associated with signs of asphyxia (diminished Apgar score, base deficit, and elevated lactate levels), irrespective of mode of anesthesia. In those observed under epidural anesthesia, glucose was found to be elevated in 20% and was also associated with fetal distress. Low levels of glucose were noted in 27%. In those also managed by regional anesthesia, levels of glycerol and free fatty acids were not normalized until 2 h after delivery, whereas values reached a steady state within 1 h in those managed by local anesthesia. In those subject to asphyxia, however, a steady state was reached in the first 10 min of life. In the 30- to 120-min interval, ketone bodies increased in controls, decreased among those with asphyxia, and remained steady among those with regional anesthesia who lacked evidence of asphyxia. In the asphyxiated group, metabolic acidosis diminished and the pH normalized within 10 to 30 min after birth, as was observed among normal patients in other studies. During this interval, pO_2 values were greater than those without asphyxia and pCO_2 values were normal. Among those managed by regional anesthesia, pCO_2 values were greater than controls, metabolic acidosis was less frequent, and pCO_2 values remained steady. Asphyxia and regional anesthesia were found to be associated with lower umbilical cord hematocrit values compared to nonasphyxiated babies and those managed without regional anesthesia. In the final analysis, the authors concluded that maintenance of normal glucose infusions under the various types of anesthesia resulted in better evidence of maintenance of normal fetal glucose homeostasis and a concomitant decrease in the finding of elevated base deficit and lactate levels.

With the use of regional anesthesia in obstetrics, associated disturbances in uterine perfusion, as well as the provision of large amounts of glucose in the supportive intravenous fluid administrations, must always be kept in mind. Although the long-term implications of these findings remain to be further explored, the fundamental principles involved in the maintenance of normal fetal homeostasis must always be respected during labor, and interventions designed to provide appropriate fetal support must constantly be examined for unexpected adverse effects. Clearly, no optimal form of anesthesia-analgesia can be said to be intrinsically better for preservation of fetal-neonatal welfare than any other until all aspects of the care of the mother and baby during labor are taken into account. The obvious association with mode of delivery, including traumatic influences, must be considered, as well as the potential impact of general anesthesia on transient neonatal depression without long-term adverse effects if the baby is well supported during this time.

B. OBSTETRIC TRAUMA

Some comment must be offered as to the risks of traumatic birth and its role in the production of neonatal and childhood handicap. Some reference already has been made to the contributions of breech, forceps, and preterm birth. Here we will primarily focus on term (or postterm) vertex vaginal delivery, especially related to mechanical problems such as shoulder dystocia and the still contentious area of midforceps delivery.

1. Birth "Trauma"

In postulating the causal relationship between dystotic events and adverse outcome, one must consider the relative contributions of physical-mechanical factors, fetal susceptibility to harm (fragility), timing and duration of the noxious event, and unknown contributors.

Although it is unquestionably possible to harm the normal fetus and newborn through physical stress, this occurs with surprising infrequency and the resultant injury usually resolves, albeit slowly, if it involves peripheral nerves. Shoulder dystocia is a reflection of a positional and size disproportion between mother and child, being more commonly seen, therefore, in large and bulky babies than among those born preterm. Incidences of 1 to 3% have commonly been quoted for babies up to 4000 or 4500 g, rising to 10% or more in those over 4500 g.[62] Infants of diabetic mothers seem more prone, gram for gram, to this complication.[63] A protracted active phase of labor and protracted descent can often be clues to imminent mechanical delivery problems, and the perceived need for midpelvic forceps delivery is an added predictor.[64] The risks in delivery are primarily for cervicothoracic nerve damage, resulting in Erb's palsy (or Klumpke's palsy in <5% of all instances of peripheral nerve injury). The former, although distressing, will resolve in almost all instances within 12 to 18 months;[65] the latter has a poor resolution rate. They both result from relatively excessive force compared to the fetal ability to resist injury, in the interest of disimpacting the shoulder and subsequently assisting delivery of (usually) the anterior shoulder and arm. In some instances, though, because the alternative is death, the resultant injury is unavoidable. If retained too long in a partially delivered state, any fetus will expire due to lack of ability to respire, as concomitant cord compression is common.

Survivors of near-miss acute neonatal lifelessness show over a 75% frequency of neurological integrity, regardless of the cause of the compromise, so the effort is usually justified if resuscitation is proposed. The residual rate of handicap may reflect the proportion of survivors previously compromised or unpredictably fragile. Further work on this matter is desperately needed, as the same logic can be applied to the predisposition to fetal intolerance of labor, as previously discussed (see Table 1).

Midforceps delivery, once the hallmark of the obstetrician's technical expertise, has lately come under attack as an independent source of fetal morbidity. The argument rages, and it is likely, as with most polarized views, that the truth lies in an intermediate position.[71,72]

Although we shall not attempt to define the appropriate view to be taken on this unresolved matter, there can be little doubt that the artful (and surely the less than artful) use of midpelvic instrumental delivery can result in maternal and fetal traumatic harm. Vaginal and contiguous tissues can be torn from one another, and fetal cranial trauma (both comprehensive and excoriative) is an ever-present risk. The degree to which intracranial pathology may result from such events, whether by classic forceps or vacuum apparatus,[73] is controversial, save those instances associated with skull fracture. In the absence of a pathognomonic lesion, it can only be said that for any given baby there are limits to be observed, both in forceps applied and diameters to be negotiated. Neonatal depression is common, and its consequences are tied to depth and duration of that depression, as well as to the fragility of the fetus, which in turn involves features of prematurity, size, forces applied, and quality of neonatal care, both immediate and distant. The unquestioned ability of meconium aspiration, frequently a concomitant risk factor among large (older) fetuses, to enhance stabilization and oxygenation difficulties in the newborn can also attribute to an adverse outcome.[74] When faced with overwhelming evidence of such risks, serious consideration of alternative modes of delivery is advisable, if circumstances permit. Planning for maternal and neonatal needs in advance of crisis is the sign of the conscientious provider.

TABLE 1
Survival and Normality after Perinatal Death or Severe Depression

Study	Steiner[a]	Dweck[b]	Thomson[c]	Scott[d]	DeSouza[e]	Total[f]	
Total	39	51	86	48	#	223	
Survived	22	20	43	23	(53)	108	(48.4%)
Follow-up	22	13	31	23	53	142 of 161 (88.2%)	
Normal	18	10	29	17	49	121 of 142 (85.2%)	
Abnormal	4	3	2	6	4	21 of 142 (14.8%)	
% abnormal	18.1	23.0	6.5	26.1	8.3		
Total M & M[g]	53.8	66.7+	52.3+	64.5	#	135 of 276 (48.9%)	

[a] All cardiac arrests in perinatal period. Four of four damaged had not reestablished respirations after 30 min. Data from Reference 66.

[b] All had Apgars @ 1 min of ≤3; two had Apgars @ 5 min of >6 and were excluded; several very premature; all three with residual abnormalities were SGA. Data from Reference 67.

[c] All had Apgars @ 1 min of 0 (4; 2 survived) or Apgars @ 5 min of <4 (82; 41 survived); not all could be located for follow-up. Data from Reference 68.

[d] Nonsurvivors: apparent stillbirth (15) or failed to establish respiration by 20 min; 33 had Apgars @ 1 min of 1 to 2; 9 of 15 stillborns would have also fit into second group; of 6 with cerebral palsy, 4 had chronic stress (and 2 of 4 SGA), and 4 of 6 had athetoid cerebral palsy; 20 of 23 were abnormal for up to 6 weeks. Data from Reference 69.

[e] Only survivors studied (#); 42% established respirations by 5 min; all had severe neurological abnormalities neonatally; of four abnormal, $^3/_4$ were of doubtful importance. Data from Reference 70.

[f] Mixture of study data; where fractions appear, study "#" included; total = 276 with "#", 223 without.

[g] M & M = morbidity and mortality.

The foregoing has been a brief review of many of the more important term peripartum concerns regarding ultimate neurological injury. Since several other chapters in this book are concerned more specifically with these events, no further commentary will be offered at this time. What remains is to deal with neonatal complications as events unique to this time period, with or without predisposition by predelivery events. By necessity, because of rampant controversy many such perinatal influences will be discussed under the specific entities to be explored.

IV. NEONATAL EVENTS

This section will concern itself with major neonatal complications, especially those of the preterm child. As stated above, much controversy exists surrounding the predispositions to as well as the ultimate consequences of these unfortunate occurrences. Finally, a brief discussion of cerebral palsy and mental retardation will conclude this chapter of the book.

A. INTRACRANIAL HEMORRHAGE
One of the most devastating neonatal events from the point of view of survival as well as that of neurological injury is the development of intracranial hemorrhage. A vast amount of recent literature has been dedicated to debating the appropriate mode of diagnosis of this event, not only in terms of timing of studies, but also the diagnostic modalities to be considered optimal for this purpose. Early studies concerned themselves with the clinical diagnosis of intracranial hemorrhage based on obvious signs of deterioration in the newborn, including falling hematocrit, signs of increasing intracranial pressure, and cardiorespiratory instability. Many, but not all, of these studies involved the ultimate confirmation of diagnosis at autopsy. This diagnostic period was followed by an era of utilization of neonatal computerized axial tomography (CT), and this in turn was followed by the current widespread utilization of neonatal cranial ultrasonography.

The diagnosis of intracranial hemorrhage varies widely in frequency depending upon the modality utilized for its determination.[75] It is clear that, except in the most devastating hemorrhages, clinical recognition of this event occurs with relatively low frequency. Although the current popular grading system, based on the work of Papile et al.,[76] was conceived utilizing CT criteria, this has been greatly extended into the field of ultrasonographically derived diagnoses, perhaps to the detriment of the comparability of studies of this entity. It is acknowledged that CT scanning, although potentially of great utility because of its clarity, will not detect the presence of blood within a fluid medium until the concentration reaches a hematocrit of approximately 15%. Far greater acuity can be achieved with ultrasound, which is capable of diagnosing bleeding with perhaps as low a concentration as a hematocrit of 1 to 2%.[75] The importance of making the diagnosis of scanty hemorrhagic events remains somewhat controversial, however. This is particularly true in light of the data from Papile et al.[77] suggesting that hemorrhages of less than Grade III are infrequently associated with ultimately significant neurological disability. Bejar and associates[78] were able to determine the presence of intracranial hemorrhage in 90% of babies of <34 weeks gestation. This finding, however, has not been correlated with a similarly disturbing frequency of neurological abnormality.

It is generally agreed that the vast majority of intracranial hemorrhages occurring prior to 36 weeks gestation emanate from the subependymal germinal matrix, which lies over the head of the caudate nucleus in the lateral walls of the lateral ventricles.[78] A very small number of hemorrhages occurring in the preterm baby arise from the choroid plexus or in the subarachnoid space and other areas. In contrast, hemorrhages in the term baby largely appear to originate from these latter locations.[79] The implications of these different sites of origin are significant in their relationship to neurological harm.

Although much speculation has been offered about the origins of deficits associated with subependymal hemorrhage (SEH), most of the attention has been devoted to local pathology resulting from extension of the bleeding into adjacent neurological tissue and tissue tracts. Since one limb of the internal capsule passes close to this site of bleeding, it has been thought that its association with spastic diplegia (the predominant motor neurological injury of prematurity) results from injury to this tract. Extending concerns for the more global implication of this event, Volpe et al.,[80] in a study of patients with intracranial bleeding established by positron emission tomography (PET), showed that flow was markedly diminished not only at the site of bleeding, but was two to four times more limited throughout the entire affected cerebral hemisphere. In one baby restudied at 3 months of age, the degree of blood flow attenuation remained severely compromised. These observations, if borne out in similar studies in larger populations, can only enhance concern for the implications of such events and must more vigorously spur on the efforts toward its ultimate prevention.

Other than its association with preterm birth, no definitive single cause for this event has been unequivocally proven to date. In an early study by Simmons et al.[81] an association was noted between the occurrence of intraventricular hemorrhage and the administration of therapeutic sodium bicarbonate. Subsequent speculations surrounding this association have centered on differentiating between the administration of bicarbonate itself vs. the indications and circumstances under which it is given, the rate of infusion, and its osmolality. In a study by Papile et al.,[82] intraventricular hemorrhage was not found to be related to either sodium concentration or to the amount of bicarbonate given, but only to the rate of infusion of the hyperosmolar solution. In a subsequent study by Clark et al.[83] centering on low birth weight infants (weighing <1250 g) with hemorrhage confirmed by CT or autopsy, a significant association was noted between intraventricular hemorrhage and bicarbonate administration, as well as with any fluid administration, arterial blood gas monitoring and stabilization, and with the absence of steroid administration. In this study, no association could be made between intraventricular hemorrhage and predisposing obstetric or asphyxial factors, and no correlation was found between neonatal events and intraventricular hemorrhage.

From another perspective, Meidell et al[84] studied 40 babies of <35 weeks gestation with serial ultrasound examinations. Of those studied, 15 of 17 with bleeds were observed to have had hemorrhages within the first 2 h after birth. There was no correlation in this small study with mode of delivery, bicarbonate or fluid administration, or the first blood pressure determined. An association was made with reduced 1- and 5-min Apgar scores. The lesions progressed in most cases over the first 3 days of life and were associated with increased ventilatory requirements.

The association between intracranial hemorrhage and respiratory distress has been a relatively constant one. It has not been established, however, if requiring ventilatory assistance is a reflection of a common set of circumstances or is in some way etiologically related to intracranial hemorrhage. In the study by Garcia-Prats et al.[85] among babies weighing <1500 g who were <32 weeks gestation, intraventricular hemorrhage and hyaline membrane disease were found to be associated; 56% of patients had intraventricular hemorrhage if hyaline membrane disease was present, 31% if it was absent. There was no difference in incidence, however, among those weighing <1000 g. In a report from Beverley et al.,[86] who studied 150 babies of <34 weeks gestation using ultrasound for diagnosis, the incidence of intracranial hemorrhage was 26% overall and 51% among babies weighing <1500 g. Half of these babies had signs of hemorrhage within the first 8 h of life. Respiratory distress and other complications were increased in frequency among afflicted infants. Birth by outlet forceps or cesarean section was associated with a decreased incidence, but there was no evidence of acidosis at birth among those with hemorrhage. The overall mortality in this series was 27%.

A possible causative association between the need for ventilatory support and the occurrence of intracranial hemorrhage was suggested by Hill et al.[87] In this study, respiratory distress and intrathoracic air leaks were found to be associated with increased flow velocities in the anterior cerebral artery during diastole, which resolved with resolution of the intrathoracic problem. Systemic arterial pressure alterations were noted to occur simultaneously. Associations with blood pressure fluctuations were also noted by McDonald et al.[88] Among 50 babies of <33 weeks gestation studied by ultrasound, 30% experienced intraventricular hemorrhage; the overall incidence of intracranial bleeding of all sorts was 40%. In this series, Grade III hemorrhages were associated with a 5-min Apgar score of ≤5, vaginal delivery, the presence of labor, and intrapartum maternal vaginal hemorrhage. Associations were also made with neonatal blood pressure fluctuations and with rapid colloid administration.

Associations between hemorrhage and diminished Apgar score are difficult to sort out with regard to the possible cause-and-effect relationship involved. Since hemorrhage is more frequent among very low birth weight babies, the association may be circumstantial. Other studies, however, have tended to dispute the premise of a coincidental association, attributing increased risk to low Apgar scores among babies compared to uninvolved controls of similar birth weight and gestational age. Factors such as mode of delivery and condition at birth have also been implicated. In the study by Strauss et al.[89] involving 119 babies weighing <1500 g, 24% were found by ultrasound to have hemorrhage, including 4.4% with Grade III or IV hemorrhage. Ominous fetal monitoring tracings were found in 50% of those with ultimate hemorrhage and in only 8% of those without subsequent bleeding. Reassuring fetal monitoring patterns were also significantly more frequent among the uninvolved. Apgar scores were significantly more frequently diminished among those with serious hemorrhage, even though umbilical arterial pH values of <7.20 did not occur more frequently among the afflicted. The factors of fetal position, mode of delivery, and presence of labor have all been examined by several authors. The results are conflicting.

Horbar et al.[90] studied 77 babies of <1200 g, with a 42% incidence of intracranial hemorrhage discovered by ultrasound or at autopsy. Univariate analysis revealed associations with gestational age, duration of labor, and vaginal delivery. Multivariate analysis, however, revealed no obstetric factors to be associated with hemorrhage. Logistic analysis, accounting for 70% of the associated factors, revealed a correlation with vertex presentation, pregnancies of <30 weeks gestation, and labor lasting >6 h. In the absence of vertex presentation, only duration of labor was associated with the occurrence of intracranial hemorrhage. Tejani et al.[91] studied 126 babies weighing <2000 g at birth, all within the first 24 h of life. At this point the incidence of intracranial hemorrhage was 21%. The presence of labor was significantly associated with an increased risk of hemorrhage, and cesarean section was not demonstrated to be protective. Umbilical arterial pH values and fetal monitoring abnormalities were not related to outcome.

Lebed et al.[92] reported the results of 357 ultrasound scans of 176 newborns studied from 1 to 3 days after birth. In many cases, results were confirmed by CT, spinal tap, or autopsy. The overall incidence of some degree of hemorrhage was 72%, while it was 90% among breech-presenting babies of <33 weeks gestation and 45% among those of >36 weeks. In further studies of the interaction between presentation and the presence of labor, 100% of breeches had hemorrhage if labor occurred. Mode of delivery appeared to have no influence on the incidence of hemorrhage irrespective of presentation, and, specifically, no benefit to cesarean section could be demonstrated if labor occurred. In this as well as other studies, babies of advanced gestational age were more likely to have experienced subarachnoid hemorrhage, whereas preterm babies more commonly experienced intraventricular bleeding. These results were similar to those of Bejar et al.[78]

Kenny et al.[93] focused on the association between hemorrhage and acid-base studies at birth. Umbilical arterial blood values were examined among babies of 26 to 29 weeks in this series. Intraventricular hemorrhage was associated with decreased Apgar scores and increased pCO_2, but not with pH, bicarbonate, or lactate values.

Rayburn et al.[94] investigated the association between obstetric factors and the incidence of hemorrhage. In this study, 103 babies of <1500 g were studied by ultrasound. No association could be found with maternal hypertension, antepartum hemorrhage, breech presentation, mode of delivery, preterm rupture of membranes, or birth outside the Level III center; only immaturity and neonatal complications were associated with hemorrhage. Similar results were recorded by Papile and co-workers[76] among 46 consecutive babies weighing <1500 g and studied by CT. The overall incidence of hemorrhage was 43%, without association with birth weight, gestational age, Apgar scores, the need for resuscitation, or respiratory assistance. Other data from Burstein et al.[95,96] established risk factors for an increased incidence of hemorrhage — male fetus, twin, initial Apgar score <4, birth weight <1500 g if born elsewhere or <1200 g if born at the Level III center, and the need for assisted ventilation. Any two criteria served as an indication for CT study with a reasonable expectation of finding an abnormality.

Risk factors involving the adequacy of fetal growth have also been examined. Procianoy et al.[97] studied growth-retarded and normally grown babies of <32 weeks matched for gestational age. Among small-for-gestational-age babies, a marked reduction in both hyaline membrane disease and intraventricular hemorrhage was noted. In somewhat contradictory findings, Bada et al.[98] studied 155 babies of <1500 g with daily ultrasonography; 55% of the babies demonstrated hemorrhage within the first 24 h and an additional 24% after this time. No maternal variables were related to the incidence of hemorrhage, and there were no differences found based on Apgar score, duration of labor, or presentation. Hemorrhage was significantly related to immediate condition in the neonatal period, as well as to birth weight and gestational age. The relative risk of hemorrhage was 1.3 among those with intrauterine growth retardation. Dykes et al.[99] also noted an increased risk of hemorrhage with intrauterine growth retardation, as well as with respiratory complications involving air leak, diminished pO_2, increased pCO_2, increased ventilatory requirements involving peak pressures of >25 and an inspiratory/expiratory (I/E) ratio of greater than 1:1, bicarbonate and volume administration, hypotension, severe hyaline membrane disease, and intrauterine growth retardation. No associations could be established with Apgar score, birth weight, gestational age, male gender, increased osmolality or sodium concentration, hypothermia, increased continuous positive airway pressure (CPAP) or positive end-expiratory pressure (PEEP) requirements, birth outside the Level III center, birth trauma, or coagulation disturbances.

Increased interest has developed recently in the association between subtle coagulation abnormalities in the newborn and the advent of intracranial hemorrhage. Beverley et al.[100] administered prophylactic fresh frozen plasma to a group of newborns of <32 weeks gestation weighing under 1500 g. In comparison to controls, the rate of intraventricular hemorrhage was 14% among those treated at birth and again at 24 h of age, whereas the incidence was 41% among those not treated. Coagulation parameters in the two groups did not differ at birth. In contrast, McDonald et al.[101] demonstrated subtle evidence of hypocoagulability in the first 4 h of life among those with hemorrhage; differences demonstrated in the at-risk patients were diminished fibrinogen, platelets, antithrombin-III, and Factor VIII. Other findings included increased concentrations of fibrin monomer and an increased clotting time. Risk was increased among babies with amnionitis, but was diminished in maternal toxemia cases. No associations could be found with prior aspirin ingestion by the mother.

The influence of corticosteroid administration has been investigated by various authors, with differing results. As mentioned earlier, steroid administration was associated with a lowered incidence of hemorrhage in the study population of Clark et al.[83] Whether or not this influence is an independent one or is mediated through a diminished frequency of respiratory distress is unknown. In studies by Worthington et al.,[102] no effect from mode of delivery could be demonstrated, and birth weight was the most important factor in determining survival. Other significant associations were found with a more nearly optimal 5-min Apgar score, the absence of respiratory distress and intraventricular hemorrhage, and the presence of prior steroid administration and intrauterine growth retardation. Respiratory distress was significantly less frequent among intrauterine-growth-retarded babies, those with good 5-min Apgar scores, and females. Intraventricular hemorrhage was associated with lesser gestational age, the presence of severe respiratory distress, and steroid administration (an unusual association in this series). Pursuing this element further, it was noted that steroids were associated with an increased survival while also being associated with an increased incidence of intraventricular hemorrhage and did not bear a relationship to diminished respiratory distress.

In contrast, Hoskins et al.,[103] studying 106 babies of <1000 g over a 2-year interval, demonstrated a 68% survival rate. Survival was associated with greater birth weight and gestational age, the presence of intrauterine growth retardation, the administration of steroids, and the absence of hyaline membrane disease, seizures, and intracranial hemorrhage. Only a 13% incidence of significant handicap was noted in this population.

Great speculation has been offered about the etiology of intracranial hemorrhage. Several facts have been established. It is known that the vasculature serving the germinal matrix is fragile and poorly supported. This renders it susceptible to injury by significant fluctuations in the blood flow velocity at times of increased flow, while at the same time the general blood supply to the area is in a "watershed" area of the brain, rendering it susceptible to ischemia at times of reduced flow. Autoregulation of cerebral blood flow is relatively poor in immature infants, and this is further impaired by asphyxia. These factors, combined with subtle but potentially significant alterations in blood coagulation in preterm infants, may predispose to ischemia and/or hemorrhage.[104]

Factors intrinsic to preterm infants requiring ventilatory assistance include periodic endotracheal tube suctioning. Perlman and Volpe[105] have noted an increase in anterior cerebral arterial flow velocity during suctioning procedures, associated with systemic hypertension and increased intracranial pressure. These authors questioned the safety and necessity of routine suctioning procedures. As mentioned earlier, increased pressures are also associated with intrathoracic air leak problems, which are rarely encountered unless ventilatory assistance has been rendered.

Attempts to reduce these fluctuations and their impacts on hemorrhage have involved sedation with phenobarbital (reducing neonatal responsiveness as well as cerebral oxygen consumption). Neonatal phenobarbital administration has been reported by Donn et al.[106] to reduce intracranial hemorrhage in their study population from 47% among controls to 13% among treated babies. In contrast, however, Bedard et al.[107] were unable to demonstrate any benefit to newborns from phenobarbital administration. Perlman et al.[108] also reported a potential benefit from neonatal paralysis induced by curare; prevention of severe intracranial hemorrhage and a significant reduction of most lesser degrees and other types of hemorrhage were shown.

Finally, intracranial hemorrhage, although generally thought of as occurring within the first few days of life, has been found by Mitchell and O'Tuama[109] in older children of 2 weeks to 3 months of age. Significant associations were noted with hypoxemia, acidosis, cerebral ischemia, and increased sodium concentrations.

Excellent reviews of associations and speculations as to causation have been published by Wigglesworth and Pape[110,111] and by Allan and Volpe.[104]

Long-term follow-up of children with intracranial hemorrhage has revealed various observations. Baerts and Meradji,[112] in serial ultrasonic examinations among premature infants, were unable to demonstrate any perceptible changes in intracranial findings after 2 months of age. In a study designed to differentiate between changes resulting from periventricular hemorrhage and ischemic lesions, Sinha et al.[113] observed that ischemic lesions develop later (around 7 days after birth), as contrasted with hemorrhage (usually occurring within 2 days). In this population, significant associations were found between persistent ventricular enlargement and ultimate mortality. Patients with these lesions were found to have been predisposed by antepartum maternal hemorrhage, birth "asphyxia", apneic spells, and sepsis. These findings, although significant, were generally not associated with periventricular hemorrhage alone.

Nelson and Broman,[114] utilizing data from the NCPP, noted that of all perinatal events, intracranial hemorrhage and seizures were the best indicators of mental and motor handicap among children examined at age 7. The incidence of handicap was not increased among growth-retarded babies, but was significantly greater among preterm infants than in term babies. This was true despite the fact that almost 70% of all babies with ultimate neurological handicap were near term at birth. Increased associations were also found with peripheral and cranial nerve abnormalities and "brain abnormalities" noted in the neonatal period. In a follow-up of babies weighing <1500 g at birth, Papile et al.[76] noted that the incidence of handicap was only 9% among those with Grade I lesions and 11% among those with Grade II, but it increased to 36% among those with Grade III and 76% with Grade IV lesions. The presence or absence of hydrocephalus did not influence the incidence of abnormality. Our own studies[115] confirm the high correlation between normal CT studies and normal outcome.

Finally, in a study of babies of <33 weeks gestation with a 1-year follow up, Graziani et al.[116] attempted to differentiate between changes related to intracranial hemorrhage and those possibly resulting from other causes. Three groups were studied. In group I, 29 babies without intracranial hemorrhage or other problems were studied. In group II were 22 babies with intracranial hemorrhage lacking ventricular dilatation. Group III was made up of ten babies with intraventricular hemorrhage and ventricular enlargement. In group III, a decrease in occipitofrontal growth and an increased ventricular ratio and ventricular index were noted. These data were interpreted as indicating that atrophy rather than hydrocephalus exists in these babies and is associated with a decreased Bayley motor score and a 40% incidence of cerebral palsy.

B. RESPIRATORY DISTRESS SYNDROMES

A more common complication of preterm birth, significant respiratory distress appears to constitute a more manageable complication with less severe neurological implications as a pure condition than intracranial hemorrhage. Although respiratory distress has been linked to intracranial hemorrhage as outlined above, we will discuss this circumstance as though it was a separate entity unrelated to other problems except those relating to pulmonary injury.

It has long been noted that male infants predominate in neonatal mortality over females of the same gestational age.[117] Khoury et al.[118] demonstrated that the male dominance was primarily due to respiratory disorders, which were primarily concentrated among babies of 1500 to 2500 g. Below that birth weight category, the incidences appeared to be approximately the same.

Besides birth weight and gestational age, other factors predisposing preterm babies to respiratory distress include potential fetal distress during labor. Douvas et al.[119] surveyed the results of babies weighing <1800 g during monitored labor. Asphyxia was defined as depression at birth or a low pH determined in the nursery. In those studied, hyaline membrane disease was higher in frequency among those with abnormal intrapartum fetal monitoring tracings, as previously suggested by Hobel et al.[52] and Martin et al.[120] In contrast, Kenny et al.,[121] studying preterm twin births, noted that Apgar scores among second-born twins were regularly lower than those of first-born twins without relationship to pH changes unless the interval between births was >8 min. In this circumstance, pH and Apgar score were both diminished in the second baby. In the overall study, hyaline membrane disease was statistically associated with diminished Apgar scores, but not with diminished pH determinations. Studies previously quoted in this chapter have also divorced the association between Apgar score and acidosis.

Perelman and Farrell[122] cited the diminishing mortality from hyaline membrane disease over the course of time, while they noted that it remains the leading cause of death in preterm birth. This diminished mortality was attributed to improved management of "asphyxia". Over the last 20 years, the major impacts on the management of neonatal respiratory distress have occurred with the institution of CPAP and the introduction of antenatal corticosteroids in appropriately selected babies. Since significant hyaline membrane disease is thought to be attributable to a lack of normal alveolar surfactant production, release, or recycling, several approaches have been offered. Since mature surfactant in small amounts can be demonstrated in infants as early as 24 weeks gestation, several complex factors may be involved in its absence among affected infants. Friedman and Rosenberg[123] noted that in sick newborns a deficiency of essential fatty acids was associated with abnormal surfactant production. Correction of essential fatty acid deficiencies resulted in improved surfactant production and overall clinical status.

Perinatal conditions also related to respiratory distress were investigated by Linderkamp et al.,[124] associating red cell mass as determined by radioiodinated human serum albumin studies at various gestational ages between 26 and 36 weeks. Lower Apgar scores and red cell masses were noted in patients afflicted with respiratory distress than among comparable babies without respiratory distress. The incidence of respiratory distress was significantly increased among babies with low 1-min Apgar scores and red cell masses of <35 ml/kg. At the same gestational ages, respiratory distress was increased with reduced red cell mass, even among those with similar Apgar scores. A concomitant influence was also demonstrated in that among those with similar red cell masses, respiratory distress was increased with diminished Apgar score. Since red cell mass may be a factor of chronic hypoxia as well as volume constriction in response to asphyxia, all of these factors may be interrelated.

Over the history of the management of preterm labor and birth, many therapies have been associated with apparent diminutions in risk of respiratory distress. Early studies involving ethanol therapy[125] demonstrated a reduction in respiratory distress, but not without complications, as demonstrated in the work of Sisenwein et al.[126] Other studies have shown beneficial effects from aminophylline administration,[127] fetal thyroid hormone therapy,[128] and prolactin[129] in promoting surfactant release in pulmonary alveolar cells in tissue culture. Even human surfactant therapy administered to the newborn has been shown by Hallman et al.[130] to reduce the impact of respiratory distress as well as its severity. In general, however, such measures instituted only during the neonatal period have been of dubious benefit once respiratory distress is established. Whether or not aggressive intervention through early prophylactic intubation is effective in reducing the severity or the duration of respiratory distress among babies at risk was discussed by Drew.[131] This study appeared to show an advantage to early prophylactic intubation; however, others have disputed the value of this approach, claiming no obvious benefit and an increased risk of tube-related complications.

A serious complication associated with hyaline membrane disease is the ultimate development of *bronchopulmonary dysplasia (BPD)*. This condition, although chronically disabling, generally has a tendency to ameliorate over a period of time in early childhood; its presence is associated with prolonged requirements for increased oxygen administration. In a study by Lindroth et al.,[132] 135 infants were examined following mechanical ventilation. Over the 6-year period of study, BPD was found to increase with hyaline membrane disease, but over the study interval there was a decrease in apnea and bradycardia spells, and neurological and developmental sequelae diminished from 22 to 13%, reaching 11% among babies under 1500 g.

Long-term follow-up implications about the presence of neonatal respiratory distress have been reported by a large number of investigators. Reynolds and Taghizadeh[133] reported that a group of children treated from 1967 to 1972 showed no benefit from the neonatal administration of corticosteroids. It was noted during the study, however, that increasing I/E ratios were associated with a better outcome. Based on these results, Reynolds proposed that the successful management of hyaline membrane disease was probably related more to mechanical factors than to oxygen requirements.

In a study of respiratory distress patients managed after the institution of CPAP therapy, Kamper and Moller[134] reported 51 survivors. Of these, one had serious tetraplegia and mental retardation and six others had speech retardation. These seven children also had significantly reduced gestational ages and birth weights, lower Apgar scores, and increased pCO_2 before the institution of ventilatory therapy. On long-term follow-up, three of the seven affected infants resolved their deficits. By comparison, Bennett et al.[135] noted that hyaline membrane disease influenced mental and motor development at 4 months of age, but not at 12 and 24 months. Reduced gestational age was related to reduced mental performance characteristics at 24 months. There was no relationship in this population between hyaline membrane disease and CNS handicaps, these being entirely related to birth weight and gestational age. Finally, in a prior excellent review of the consequences of respiratory distress to long-term outcome, Thompson and Reynolds[136,137] noted that most previous studies had shown some increased motor, but not mental, sequelae to respiratory distress. The existence of high-risk factors increased the risk of mental and motor handicap, especially among males and those with hyperbilirubinemia.

The interaction between premature rupture of membranes and respiratory distress has been the subject of numerous investigations, with some varying results. Although the prevailing opinion holds that preterm rupture of membranes may ameliorate respiratory distress or improve survival among very low birth weight infants, studies vary as to the relative impacts of these two events on outcome. The influence of corticosteroid administration on these results has also been considered, the vast majority of studies suggesting that corticosteroids have no observable beneficial effects following preterm rupture of membranes.[138] Despite this rather consistent observation, steroid administration continues to occur regularly in this clinical circumstance. Since infection is a recognized risk factor following or related to preterm rupture of membranes, one must seriously question the addition of steroid therapy to this risk circumstance.

Herschel et al.[139] studied 136 babies between 24 and 28 weeks gestation, comparing outcome with and without premature rupture of membranes. In the study population, steroids were administered by protocol to all pregnancies expected to terminate between 27 and 34 weeks gestation. Although no babies were ventilated at 24 weeks and only some at 26, three variables emerged as important in determining survival. Gestational age had a threefold impact on survival, steroids given at least 24 h prior to birth a twofold impact, and a lack of a requirement for resuscitation at birth was also influential. These three factors together predicted 80% of the outcomes. No unique benefit to ruptured membranes could be demonstrated.

Lee et al.,[140] studying the incidence of respiratory distress following premature rupture of membranes and with maternal hypertension, noted a reduction in respiratory distress only among pregnancies of >32 weeks gestation or birth weights of >1500 g. If membranes had been ruptured at least 24 h in this study, no additional improvement was noted thereafter.

In our reported series of premature rupture of membranes,[141] we were able to demonstrate increased survival following premature rupture of membranes before 30 weeks gestation or with birth weights of <1200 g, without any significant reduction in the incidence of respiratory complications. Following these birth weight and gestational age points, no differences were noted. These results were at sharp variance with those of Berkowitz et al.[142] who demonstrated a reduction in respiratory distress without improvement in survival prior to 32 weeks gestation and improved survival without change in respiratory distress after 32 weeks. Although studies concerning these issues are commonplace, there is little disagreement that premature rupture of membranes in the presence of an otherwise normal baby is generally associated with improvement in ultimate neonatal welfare, in the absence of complications such as cord prolapse or infection. The citations demonstrating these conclusions are too numerous for inclusion in this review.

The presence of infection before or following rupture of membranes remains a serious potential complication, limiting the optimism otherwise appropriate to this event. A primary offending agent from which the fetus appears to be at greatest risk is the Group B streptococcus. Controversy rages as to the timing of exposure of the fetus to this organism in relation to rupture of membranes. Many believe, as does this author, that the organism finds its way to the fetus substantially in advance of spontaneous rupture of membranes, which may be a manifestation of a later stage in the infectious process. Since in the laboratory circumstance the organism has been found to cross intact membranes readily,[143] it may be an exception to the general supposition that the membranes pose a protective barrier to the presence of serious bacterial penetration of the amniotic cavity from below.

Faix and Donn[144] reported four infants surviving Group B streptococcal septic shock and who manifested evidence of periventricular leukomalacia. This finding was not demonstrated in infants surviving other septic conditions, and the incidence was only 11% among other babies with shock secondary to noninfectious complications. It was concluded that the risk of this neurological complication was exceptionally high with this infectious agent.

Evidence of the dissemination capabilities of the organism was offered by Edwards et al.,[145] who noted that the second twin in studied pregnancies was at risk if the first twin was infected with the organism. This was true even in the absence of ruptured membranes with the second twin. Experimental evidence derived from studies exposing fetal lambs to toxins derived from Group B streptococcus has demonstrated persistence of pulmonary hypotension and shock among the exposed animals, resulting in serious circulatory compromise.[146] This condition could be prevented by pretreatment of the lambs with prostaglandin synthetase inhibiting agents, and it could be ameliorated by concomitant or subsequent administration of these agents. These observations, if borne out in human studies, may represent a significant lifesaving therapy in this devastating disease, which carries a mortality risk of 50 to 80% in its early-onset form.

The potential adverse influences of amniotic fluid infections and their frequencies have been extensively reviewed by Naeye.[147] Utilizing data from the NCPP, infection was found to be associated with diminished Apgar scores and neonatal death, the 5-min score correlating with mortality. He noted (based on histological and autopsy studies) nearly a 50% incidence of amniotic fluid infection among preterm births and a 25% incidence among term pregnancies. These incidences far exceed those of any other studies reported to date.

Although most studies on newborns following premature rupture of the membranes have suggested a high frequency of infectious agents in the environment, the general impression has been that these events are infrequently associated with neonatal morbidity (in the absence of *Listeria* or Group B streptococcus), even when the environment appears to be heavily colonized. An exception to the general state of optimism was offered by Hardt et al.[148] in a study of 127 babies weighing <2000 g. Long-term outcome was compared among those with combinations of chorioamnionitis, preterm labor, preterm rupture without infection, and abruptio placentae. Analysis of variance revealed that, in comparing cases of uncomplicated premature rupture with those involving chorioamnionitis, a significant reduction in mental Bayley scores could be shown in those with infection. As additional evidence for this possible risk factor, Naeye has suggested in another study[149] a synergistic relationship between amniotic infection and hyperbilirubinemia in the risk of visual, hearing, mental, and motor impairment on subsequent follow-up.

Although most amniotic fluid infections have been assumed to result from bacterial cases, Martin et al.[150] reported that careful cervical culturing revealed the presence of chlamydia in 67% of 268 women studied before 19 weeks gestation. Among those with chlamydial colonization, stillbirth or neonatal death occurred in 33%, as opposed to 3.4% among controls. In addition, the mean gestational age at birth among colonized women was significantly lower than among those free of infection. It may well be that infection with this organism requires further study and greater attention in the future.

Finally, Hill et al.,[151] in studying the consequences of neonatal infection, concluded that a lack of certain humoral and cellular aspects of acute inflammatory response may contribute to the high morbidity and mortality observed in certain babies. If this can be shown in subsequent studies, fetal factors not considered in the past may emerge as more important than previously realized in determining susceptibility to infectious complications.

C. OTHER NEONATAL COMPLICATIONS

Other complications for which the premature newborn is at risk include *necrotizing enterocolitis (NEC)*. Although this complication has been studied extensively and its etiology speculated upon liberally, with the exception of occasional outbreaks associated with infectious agents no single causation has been determined. The impact on ultimate welfare can be significant, however. Stevenson et al.,[152] in reporting 40 survivors of NEC, were able to demonstrate only 19 normal babies; 21 had various functional abnormalities, including 6 with neurological handicap. However, this 15% incidence is not unusually high for the gestational age group usually considered to be at risk for this complication.

Controversy rages as to the significance of *hyperviscosity* in the newborn of any gestational age, central hematocrits of $\geq 63\%$ usually being associated with this finding. Black et al.,[153] reporting a small series of babies with demonstrated hyperviscosity, noted a 38%

neurological motor abnormality rate on follow-up as well as an increased frequency with hypoglycemia, which was itself significantly increased in frequency with this condition. If both abnormalities were present, 55% of babies appeared neurologically abnormal on follow-up. The timing of intervention in this condition may not influence the incidence of abnormalities associated with it. Also, the etiology of hyperviscosity, which may itself result in handicap or an increased susceptibility to injury from such events as hypoglycemia, has not been thoroughly investigated. Early intervention with reduction of hematocrit and viscosity seems indicated, even if no long-term benefit may occur.[154]

Other adverse neonatal developments, including hypocalcemia, hypotension, electrolyte imbalances of other sorts, and hypothermia, may in themselves be associated with ultimate harm or may be part of a constellation of events which in concert cause injury to the baby. *Hyperbilirubinemia*, a frequent minor problem of preterm birth currently manageable by exchange transfusion and/or phototherapy, has largely disappeared in association with ultimate neurological injury under these modern treatment approaches. Passing attention must be paid to the previously mentioned suggestion by Naeye[149] of a potential synergistic relationship between bilirubin toxicity and infection resulting in neurological injury at serum bilirubin levels below those independently associated with harm. Further work on this potential association seems indicated. With these modern approaches and the aggressive handling of conditions resulting in severe neonatal bilirubin elevations, neurological injuries commonly associated with a diagnosis of "kernicterus" have all but been eliminated. With the disappearance of this problem, there has been an associated gradual decline in the incidence of ataxic forms of cerebral palsy. It is hoped that this trend will continue and that we will see the total disappearance of bilirubin-related neurological lesions in the future.

The long-term effects of hyperbilirubinemia in fetal isoimmunization syndromes are discussed elsewhere in this book (see Chapter 7).

V. OVERALL OUTCOMES OF LOW BIRTH WEIGHT BIRTH

In recent years, a steady improvement in survival rates of low birth weight (<2500 g) and very low birth weight (<1500 g) infants has been observed. In the very lowest birth weight categories, much of this improvement can be attributed to a combination of good obstetric and neonatal care and the application of appropriate optimism in the handling of pregnancies destined to result in preterm birth. Paul and associates[155] have shown that babies in their population weighing <1500 g contribute two thirds of all neonatal deaths, even though they represent only 1.5% of all births. The chief factor in determining outcome appears to have been an accurate estimation of ultimate birth weight, those thought to weigh ≥1000 g showing better survival than those of equal weight who are managed as though they were of lesser birth weight and viability potential. The potential impact of attitude on outcome was also demonstrated by Goldenberg et al.[156] in a survey of physicians in the southeastern U.S. In this survey, physicians were asked to state the expected survival of babies of various gestational ages and to designate the point at which 50% of babies would survive. A large proportion of those surveyed were less optimistic than current perinatal survival figures would justify. The authors' suggestion was that these underestimations of survival potential might influence patterns of management as well as referral to regional medical centers, thereby resulting in compromised survival of the babies involved.

Shennan and Milligan[157] surveyed the results of 124 babies born over a 2-year period weighing 1000 to 2000 g. In this study reported in 1980, only a 9% neonatal mortality was observed and only 3 of 73 babies showed evidence of neurological damage on follow-up. Mean Bayley scores for the population were normal and comparable to those of older babies. Similar results were reported by these authors in a later study,[158] stressing that aggressive supportive obstetric care results in improved survival and neurological welfare.

Buckswold et al.[159] reported on two different eras of perinatal care of babies weighing 500 to 800 g. The first period was $2^1/_2$ years of a pessimistic approach to these babies and the second a $4^1/_2$-year period of optimistic and aggressive management. In the second time period a 44% survival was noted, among which 43% were normal on follow-up, 22% were mildly impaired, and 35% were significantly handicapped. Of these last 19 babies, 1 was profoundly and 4 were severely compromised. The authors stressed that these figures supported an aggressive approach.

Dillon and Egan,[160] reporting on babies 24 to 27 weeks in gestation, indicated that aggressive management and the use of prenatal steroids along with alcohol or terbutaline therapy to delay delivery significantly improved survival over prior comparison periods. Gilstrap et al.[161] noted that handicap was inversely proportional to birth weight. In his series, 29% of 24- to 29-week fetuses had significant morbidity as opposed to 6% of those born at 30 to 32 weeks. These figures have been echoed by several other authors, although the incidence of ultimate neurological disability has not uniformly been found to be inversely related to birth weight.

Intervening neonatal complications may have a significant impact on this potential. Astbury et al.[162] reported on 213 babies weighing <1500 g. Of these, 34% showed attention deficits on long-term follow-up. Those with deficits had demonstrated significantly increased frequencies of NEC, BPD, apnea, and duration of fat feedings and a decrease in weight percentile at discharge. These babies also had significantly decreased mental Bayley scores, diminished head circumferences, increased tonic disorders, diminished visuomotor and fine and gross motor coordination, and generally greater incidences of physical and neurological disabilities. These authors have proposed that behavior is a reasonably good index of the presence of perinatal problems and general neurological difficulties.

Considerable attention has been paid to the immediate newborn state and its association with ultimate handicap as influenced by birth weight and gestational age. Brown et al.[163] noted that the early newborn status of tone was an important predictor of ultimate death and damage. In this series, babies with neonatal hypotonia which persisted beyond 7 days had the highest incidence of death and handicap, with minimal normality among survivors. Among those with hypotonia progressing to extensor hypertonus the incidence of abnormality was still considerable, but some babies ultimately resolved these deficits. Those with initial hypertonus had a lower frequency of ultimate abnormality, and normal tone indicated few abnormalities.

In a slightly different view, Shennan et al.[164] reported results of babies at 26 to 30 weeks gestation over a 1-year follow-up. Poor condition at birth was associated with death, but did not relate to ultimate handicap. Death was correlated with short neonatal stays, steroid administration <36 h before birth, abnormal fetal heart rate patterns before delivery, diminished 1- and 5-min Apgar scores, diminished umbilical venous pH, and increased umbilical venous base deficit. Among those who survived, however, there was no difference in condition at birth between normal and handicapped individuals, but those with ultimate handicap had increased oxygen requirements, higher rates of ventilatory assistance, and greater incidence of intraventricular hemorrhage. In analyzing the populations during the prenatal stage of care, few if any prenatal differences and obstetric factors could be defined. Among breech-presenting babies, an increase in handicap was noted irrespective of mode of delivery. The possibility of undiagnosable prenatal determinants of ultimate handicap was also raised by Touwen et al.[165] In reviewing the spectrum of care of 1507 babies, 80 were defined as abnormal and were subsequently followed. Of these, 61 of 80 were normal at 4 years, 10 mildly abnormal, 8 were severely abnormal, and 1 died. The immediate neonatal state, in retrospect, did not predict outcome, including Apgar score, birth weight, gestational age, and the presence of acidosis. In fact, no obstetric factors were defined in association with ultimate abnormality. The authors stated the opinion that neonatal events may significantly affect the extent of and recovery from abnormality.

Peacock and Hirata[166] were also unable to demonstrate recognizable obstetric factors influencing outcome for the newborn. In studying 164 babies weighing 750 to 1000 g from 1972 to 1975, a 62% survival was noted, diminished survival being associated with low birth weight, reduced Apgar scores, severe respiratory distress, intracranial hemorrhage, seizures, and sepsis. Of the 82 babies followed, 7 had cerebral palsy, 7 had less serious neurological abnormalities, and 82% were normal over 4 years. Neonatal events associated with ultimate handicap were respiratory distress and seizures.

In a similar population, Driscoll et al.[167] reported data collected prior to 1982 on 54 babies weighing <1000 g. Of these, 26 survived, and 24 of the 26 weighed >750 g. Of the survivors, neurological deficit was demonstrated in 17%, intellectual deficit in 13%, and "birth asphyxia" (neonatal depression) correlated with a bad outcome. In this study, perinatal mortality among intrauterine growth-retarded babies was the same as those infants of equal birth weight who had grown normally.

Other prenatal predispositions to abnormal outcome uncontrollable by obstetric care were suggested by Shapiro et al.[168] In a large study of 390,425 live births, correlations with neonatal deaths included advanced maternal age and prior fetal loss. Incidentally noted was an increased survival of babies weighing <2000 g born by cesarean section. This latter finding is in sharp contrast to earlier reports suggesting the potential for enhanced respiratory distress, morbidity, and mortality from cesarean birth. Levkoff et al.[169] indicated that risk factors for birth of babies weighing <1500 g were not the same as for babies weighing 1500 to 2500 g. Among the populations studied, risk factors for very low birth weight birth were prior abortion, prior fetal death, and the presence of maternal hypertension. For the low birth weight infants of >1500 g, reduced maternal weight, height, and nonwhite race were the major associated factors.

Neonatal and childhood head growth can be related to neurological handicap. In the early neonatal period, excessive growth may indicate hemorrhage and/or hydrocephalus. This complication frequently requires surgical intervention. On long-term follow-up, however, handicap is more commonly associated with inadequate head growth. Gross et al.,[170] in a study of 118 babies weighing <2000 g at birth and followed over 5 years, showed that a head circumference of less than the tenth percentile at birth and abnormal neonatal neurological examination correlated highly with morbidity at 5 years. These associations with microcephaly included neurological deficits and poor subsequent somatic growth as well as poor intellect, intrauterine growth retardation, diminished Apgar scores, and lower socioeconomic status. Georgieff et al.[171] noted that head growth in sick neonates normally lags, rebounds above the normal growth rate on achieving relative wellness, and thereafter reassumes a normal rate of growth. The period of lag depends on the length of caloric deprivation associated with mechanical ventilation and other neonatal complications. If the lag period extends beyond 4 weeks, an association with developmental delay at age 1 year is noted.

There is abundant evidence that very low birth weight babies maintain abnormal growth rates for prolonged periods of time. Pape et al.,[172] reporting on 43 babies of <1000 g who were followed for 2 years, noted that height was generally between the 10th and 25th percentiles for adjusted age and weight between the third and tenth percentiles. Other associated complications were a 35% rate of lower respiratory infections, a 16% incidence of retrolental fibroplasia, a 9% incidence of major motor deficits, and a 21% incidence of severe developmental delay. Vohr and Garcia Coll[173] reported on 42 babies weighing <1500 g followed from 1 to 7 years. At 1 year of age, 22 babies were normal, 12 were suspect, and 8 were abnormal. At 7 years, the categorization was the same in 77% of normals, 58% of suspect babies, and 100% of abnormals, despite the fact that abnormals showed the greatest degree of improvement. The incidence of visuomotor problems was high in all groups. In addition, 50% of suspects and 87% of abnormals had reading problems, all functioning below their age levels; 54% of all babies in the study required special education.

Michelsson et al.[174] has noted that although survival has increased among babies of <1500 g in recent times, definable dysfunctions exist among those without major handicaps. These are chiefly impaired motor function and school performance. He points out that these problems can be recognized and, with appropriate childhood intervention, considerable improvement may be expected.

Finally, in an extensive review of neurological handicap from the NCPP, univariate analysis of predictors of low birth weight birth were numerous, as outlined by Nelson and Ellenberg.[175] A similarly wide variety was demonstrated for very low birth weight birth. On multivariate analysis, however, the only factors which emerged were a last baby with low birth weight and two factors noted only in primigravid pregnancies: nonwhite race and smoking. This reference elegantly reviews predisposing factors from a very large data base.

VI. TERM NEONATAL COMPLICATIONS

Numerous references have been made regarding this area in previous sections of this chapter and in other chapters in this book. Still, since this time is one that is very often carefully scrutinized for signs of events predisposing an infant to ultimate handicap, a few words are in order on this important phase in the continuum of human life.

Careful physical examination of the apparently normal newborn is advisable in all instances. This important time requires more than a cursory glance and an overly optimistic satisfaction with the reassurances from movement and vocalization; the quiet child is not always a testimonial to the appropriateness of his early handling.

Narcotic depression of the normal term newborn is rarely appreciated in the 1-min score. Birth suffices to rouse all but the most abnormally somnolent infant. At length, however, once early stimuli are past, residual narcotic trapped in the slowly metabolizing newborn may exert its effects in producing a return to drowsiness and respiratory inadequacy. Vigilance, not pharmacology, may be the best answer, especially since narcotic antagonists placed in depots poorly accessible by sluggish circulations may be wasted. Also, one must always be wary in the age of illicit drug use of the woman who arrives with her own medication on board and an addicted neonate, for whom full reversal of narcotic effects may be fatal. This caution would include the use of agents intrinsically antagonistic to narcotics, exogenous and endogenous (endorphins), including the newer synthetic narcotic alternatives such as pentazocine, butorphanol, and nalbuphine.

In general, a careful distinction must be made between *depression* (a generic state of general lack of vigor and responsiveness with a wide range of possible causes) and *asphyxia* (a specific depressed state due to inadequacy of prior and present respiratory effort and hypoxia-hypercarbia-acidosis). Naturally, any child depressed at birth, if not properly supported, can become asphyxiated, but to use the term interchangeably with low Apgar scores is scientifically irresponsible and medicolegally pejorative.

The truly "asphyxiated" baby newly born from chronic hypoxic and acidotic circumstances presents a classic picture that is truly rarely seen. The child is limp and pale. Heart rate and respiration are seriously depressed and do not respond readily to ordinary resuscitative effort. If somewhat stabilized, the child spends the first few days of life in a deep and flaccid coma if true brain injury has been sustained. Seizures may supervene. Characteristically, since brain injury usually involves and results from cardiac depression, myocardial and renal function are both impaired. Recovery, in the comparatively rare circumstances in which it occurs, is partial, delayed, and usually associated with severe and permanent loss of most normal neurological function.

This is in sharp contrast to the usual circumstances of birth ultimately associated with global neurological deficit in the usual case of quadriplegic cerebral palsy, and it bears no relationship to that found with lesser forms. These children, though often quite abnormal at birth, stabilize and are responsive more rapidly than the acutely compromised child. Characteristically, no cardiac or excretory abnormality is noted, attesting to the chronic state of the injury and to the reluctance of the already injured child to attempt to appear more generally competent than he truly is.

With these observations in mind, any neonate with functional or behavioral characteristics suggestive of chronic injury deserves a full and complete evaluation during the neonatal period. It is still noted that a significant minority of cerebral palsy-afflicted children leave the hospital undiagnosed. Although tragic from the point of view of early information and intervention, it highlights the fact of the lack of proximate cause.

VII. CEREBRAL PALSY, MENTAL RETARDATION, AND THE FUTURE

Much of the foregoing discussion has concerned itself with reviews of more recent studies concerning survival and complications related to low birth weight and term birth. Most physical sequelae associated with complications of pregnancy, birth, and the neonatal period are resolvable if a congenital anomaly is not involved. Liberal reference has been made to adverse neurological outcome where this was encountered in specific studies, but the spectrum is wide and the perspective of each article concerned is primarily with the studied population.

Neurological handicap, cognitive and motor, represents the most dreaded of adverse outcomes. Not only are these deficits the source of substantial sorrow and inconvenience for the parents of such affected children, but they also represent one of the major medical and financial drains upon family and society. It is therefore not surprising that they form the primary source of contention in malpractice litigation currently directed against the obstetrician. Although the spectrum of feasibility of these contentions has been elegantly addressed in two reviews by Illingworth,[176,177] clearly illustrating the inappropriateness of addressing the obstetrician as the usual cause of the perinatally acquired handicap, these law suits continue to appear regularly.

As pointed out earlier, although low birth weight babies represent a minority of all births, they have the majority of all morbidity and long-term handicaps observed in the population that are not associated with congenital anomalies or childhood accidents. Avoidance of preterm birth where possible and appropriate constitutes the main objective in attempting to reduce these handicaps, even though the majority of lesions leading to these handicaps may well be predestined by factors beyond the diagnosis and/or control of the medical care team.

Cerebral palsy, defined as a motor dysfunction of relatively fixed nature usually present since birth (although often missed), is among the most feared of adverse outcomes. In an extensive review from the NCPP, Nelson and Ellenberg[178] subjected the large data base to univariate analysis for three stages of pregnancy: prenatal, labor and delivery, and neonatal factors. Among *prenatal* factors, the highest univariate associations were found with mental retardation in the mother and maternal epilepsy. Other associations were with white race, a prior history of hyperthyroidism, prolonged and/or unusual menstrual cycles, history of low birth weight birth in the past, history of neonatal death, a prior baby with a deficit, heavy proteinuria in the second half of pregnancy, incompetent cervix, third-trimester bleeding, polyhydramnios, decreased weight gain, and estrogen or thyroid hormone therapy.

Factors associated with *labor and delivery* were third-trimester bleeding among low birth weight babies, ruptured membranes >24 h with birth weight <2500 g, amniotic infection, abnormal presentation, lowest fetal heart rate <60, very low Apgar score (highest association), male gender, gestational age, birth weight, delayed onset of spontaneous respiration, asymmetric intrauterine growth retardation, and one or more anomalies not involving the central nervous system. *Neonatal* factors included respiratory depression, altered homeostasis, seizures, special care requirements among babies weighing >2500 g, respiratory distress (especially among those weighing >2500 g), aspiration, anemia with hematocrit <40%, hyperbilirubinemia, infection, and antibiotic therapy. Multivariate analysis was not offered for these data.

We reported on a series of 78 babies weighing <2000 g at birth who were carefully followed and closely examined for mental and motor handicap.[179] Of the large number of factors examined, motor abnormalities correlated by multiple regression analysis with the presence of meconium and short labor with rapid delivery. Mental abnormalities were associated with low birth weight and the absence of hypocalcemia. Overall scoring, combining mental and motor handicaps and a general impression of welfare, showed the presence of meconium and the absence of fetal distress as being associated with poor overall outcome. We concluded that the presence of meconium staining, unusual among preterm babies, was a particularly bad sign. All babies with known infections and anomalies were excluded.

Other studies have examined a wide variety of possible associations. Nelson and Ellenberg,[180] again from the NCPP, examined obstetric factors and their association with cerebral palsy and seizures. Despite the large data base, no factors were associated with cerebral palsy rates of >2% if the baby weighed at least 2500 g. Highest associations with ultimate cerebral palsy were among those with a 5-min Apgar score of ≤3. If the 5-min score was ≥7, the risk was not increased. No associations could be found between obstetric factors and seizures.

Rantakallio[181] examined 12,000 babies by quartile of birth weight, followed to age 14. Mortality was highest among those more than two standard deviations from the mean and in the 10th to 25th percentile. Mental retardation was increased among those in the lowest 25th percentile. Major neurologic dysfunction without abnormal school performance problems did not distribute abnormally. Height at age 14 was proportional to the birth weight quartile in boys, preterm born children being shorter than term-born children, suggesting persistent growth and developmental factors at work.

Taking another approach, Mayer and Wingate[182] made contact with 605 victims of cerebral palsy who were registered through assistance programs, or with their parents; a total of 158 responses were examined. In comparison to the unaffected normal population, associations between cerebral palsy and other factors were a maternal history of increased reproductive losses, prematurity, term vaginal breech delivery, vaginal bleeding, low birth weight, and precipitous delivery. Of interest, only 7.6% of affected children were the firstborn of their families. There was no difference in the incidence of hypertension, anemia, hyperemesis, preterm rupture of membranes, isoimmunization, and type of anesthesia used for delivery. Spontaneous delivery occurred in 60.5%, and the length of labor was unrelated to complications. The incidence was increased in the presence of anomalies and possibly among twins. The overall incidence in the study population of babies weighing <2500 g was 32.5%.

Stanley[183] noted that the male sex predominates in abnormal neurological outcome in most studies. It was noted in her study, however, that neurological outcome among males by birth weight and gestational age had recently improved substantially in Australia, as had the overall rate of cerebral palsy.

Westgren et al.[184] examined the mode of delivery as a factor among babies weighing <2000 g, 59 born vaginally and 59 by cesarean section. Vaginal delivery was associated with an increased frequency of acidosis and hypothermia, without a difference in incidence of respiratory disorders or ventilatory requirements. Follow-up indicated no difference in incidence of cerebral palsy between the two groups. Vaginal delivery was, however, significantly associated with an increased frequency of psychomotor retardation.

A. TYPES OF CEREBRAL PALSY

Spastic diplegia is most commonly associated with preterm birth and subependymal germinal matrix hemorrhage. Fluctuations in its frequency within populations over the last few decades have reflected the survival rates of very low birth weight babies, therefore demonstrating recent increases in the frequency of this form of cerebral palsy. Bennett et al.[185] examined differences in perinatal and neonatal factors among those affected and unaffected by spastic diplegia. No differences could be found. By gestational age, spastic diplegia patients had smaller heads, weighed less, and had increased frequencies of brief neurological depression, intracranial hemorrhage, and seizures. It was concluded that prenatal factors were largely responsible for this adverse outcome. On a sobering note, of the 18 babies studied, 15 had been discharged from the nursery as neurologically normal.

The literature on other forms of cerebral palsy, including the more devastating *spastic quadriplegia (tetraplegia),* frequently associated with mental retardation, is substantial and confusing. To attempt to review and synthesize this literature is beyond the scope of this chapter. Evidence to suggest that this most serious complication reflects global prenatal damage occurring before labor is increasing.

Over the last 20 to 30 years, the overall incidence of cerebral palsy has diminished somewhat, but not to the extent that one might expect with the advances in perinatal technology. In fact, as previously noted, the incidence of spastic diplegia may be increasing as greater numbers and proportions of babies of low birth weight and very low birth weight survive the perinatal period. The incidences of the rarer types of cerebral palsy have remained relatively stable or have diminished only slightly, with the exception of *ataxic disorders,* which have in the past been largely associated with genetic predispositions[186] or, more commonly, with bilirubin-associated brain injury secondary to isoimmunization. With improved means of caring for the isoimmunized mother, including amniocentesis, fetal transfusion, early delivery, and aggressive neonatal management, the incidence of this long-term neurological problem has decreased sharply. In point of fact, most follow-up studies of babies with erythroblastosis born in the modern era show no increase in neurological dysfunction.[187]

Spastic hemiplegia remains a mystery, but may well be attributable to a circulatory accident occurring *in utero,* probably before birth. Churchill[188] was able to show a striking association between hemiplegia and fetal head position during labor and delivery.

Suggestions that prenatal conditioning to perinatal injury must exist have come from various observations. Babies born of obstetric events leading to preterm birth are regularly found among the lower 50th percentile of birth weight for their gestational age. There is a persistent though as yet unproven sentiment that fetal intolerance of labor reflects factors not unique to the labor process, but predisposed to by sensitivity or fragility existing before labor. Evidence for this hypothesis came first from the NCPP,[59,189] which showed that severe neonatal depression and failure to initiate spontaneous respirations did not result in significant neurological injury unless prolonged beyond 10 min of age. Babies with prolonged, severe depression of these sorts ultimately suffered a 50% neonatal mortality; yet, among survivors, 75% were neurologically intact at 7 years of age, and the resolution rates of lesser neonatal neurological abnormalities were very high.[189]

Several articles have appeared concerning the ultimate outcome for babies born dead but successfully resuscitated, maintaining very low Apgar scores beyond 5 min, or suffering neonatal dying spells with successful resuscitation.[73-77] These studies and their outcomes are summarized in Table 1 (see Section III.B.1). In brief, analysis of these studies indicates that although the mortality rate collectively exemplified in these studies is close to 50%, over 85% of survivors were neurologically normal. This suggests a high threshold for damage, which certainly cannot be explained by brief intolerance of hypoxia and circulatory disturbances during the labor process. It also suggests the presence of a small segment of the population with unusual susceptibility, perhaps exemplifying Myers' example of prolonged partial asphyxia. Whether these causes are within the reach of obstetrical care is highly speculative.

B. MENTAL RETARDATION

Mental retardation can be most simply described as occurring in two forms. In one form, resulting in severe mental handicap, most causations (when definable) are attributed to anomaly, infection, postnatal trauma, karyotype irregularity, or congenital metabolic disease. The causes for these, although rare, are numerous.

Far more common are mild to moderate degrees of mental retardation, the causes of which appear more obscure. Mounting evidence exists, however, for these being associated with low socioeconomic status and unstimulating home environments, frequently associated as well with parental mental subnormality. Examples of the latter thesis were offered by Escalona,[190] who studied two populations of patients born in the same medical center. In dividing the follow-up of these patients into the highest and lowest socioeconomic groups, intelligence testing results were similar up through approximately 18 months of age. Thereafter, results in the lower socioeconomic subset diminished, while those in the upper subset remained stable. It is apparent that the concept of mental retardation is not an easily defined one, either through testing or in determination of etiology. There are suggestions, though, that mild retardation may be remediable with early and aggressive intervention.

C. THE FUTURE

Tasks for the future regarding neurological handicap center around defining and avoiding causation. The vast majority of effort at present, however, is being made in treatment, which is a worthy objective, but does not reduce the frequency of such problems or their economic impact on parents and society.

Defining the nature and timing of injury will be difficult. Certain clues can be looked for, however, and these have largely been neglected in the past. For example, the enamelization of deciduous teeth progresses at a predictable pace during fetal life. The presence of enamel hypoplasia of specific teeth may be associated with the timing of a major fetal insult undetected during gestation which may correlate with neurological susceptibility at a similar time.[191] Bone and cartilage abnormalities can be detected similarly, and these should be sought.[192] Clues such as these and others to be defined later may be of enormous assistance, not only in increasing our knowledge as to the avoidance of injury, but also in protecting the obstetrician against unwarranted accusations of negligent care.

The primary breakthroughs, however, in avoidance of most ultimate handicaps must be in two areas: the definition of the nature and timing of noxious events resulting in injury, and in the safe and successful prevention of preterm birth. We suggest that the current assignment of available resources to treatment and rehabilitation, although needed for these purposes, does nothing for prevention. Until we as a society are willing to consider preventive medicine to be as meritorious as restorative efforts, the solutions will not be found, and the simplistic view of perinatal morbidity which constitutes the basis for the current malpractice pogrom will persevere, to the detriment of the quality and economy of medical care throughout this land.

35

REFERENCES

1. **Lee, K.-S., Paneth, N., Gartner, L. M., Pearlman, M. A., and Gruss, L.,** Neonatal mortality: analysis of the recent improvement in the United States, *Am. J. Public Health,* 70, 15, 1980.
2. **Bracken, M. B.,** Induced abortion as a risk factor for perinatal complications: a review, *Yale J. Biol. Med.,* 51, 539, 1978.
3. **Dowding, V. M.,** New assessment of the effects of birth order and socioeconomic status on birth weight, *Br. Med. J.,* 282, 683, 1981.
4. **Bakketeig, L. S. and Hoffman, H. J.,** Perinatal mortality by birth order within cohorts based on sibship size, *Br. Med. J.,* 2, 693, 1979.
5. **Seigel, E. and Morris, N. M.,** Family planning: its health rationale, *Am. J. Obstet. Gynecol.,* 118, 995, 1974.
6. **Tavris, D. R. and Read, J. A.,** Effect of maternal weight gain on fetal, infant, and childhood death and on cognitive development, *Obstet. Gynecol.,* 60, 689, 1982.
7. **Niswander, K. and Jackson, E. C.,** Physical characteristics of the gravida and their association with birth weight and perinatal death, *Am. J. Obstet. Gynecol.,* 119, 306, 1974.
8. **Klebanoff, M. A., Mills, J. L., and Berendes, H. W.,** Mother's birth weight as a predictor of macrosomia, *Am. J. Obstet. Gynecol.,* 153, 253, 1985.
9. **Naeye, R. L. and Peters, E. C.,** Mental development of children whose mothers smoked during pregnancy, *Obstet. Gynecol.,* 64, 601, 1984.
10. **Kelly, J., Mathews, K. A., and O'Conor, M.,** Smoking in pregnancy: effects on mother and fetus, *Br. J. Obstet. Gynaecol.,* 91, 111, 1984.
11. **Jouppila, P., Kirkinin, P., and Eik-Nes, S.,** Acute effect of maternal smoking on the human fetal blood flow, *Br. J. Obstet. Gynaecol.,* 90, 7, 1983.
12. **Rantakallio, P.,** A follow-up study up to the age of 14 of children whose mothers smoked during pregnancy, *Acta Paediatr. Scand.,* 72, 747, 1983.
13. **Bottoms, S. F., Kuhnert, B. R., Kuhnert, P. M., and Reese, A. L.,** Maternal passive smoking and fetal serum thiocyanate levels, *Am. J. Obstet. Gynecol.,* 144, 787, 1982.
14. **Hauth, J. C., Hauth, J., Drawbaugh, R. B., and Gilstrap, L. C., III,** Passive smoking and thiocyanate concentrations in pregnant women and newborns, *Obstet. Gynecol.,* 63, 519, 1984.
15. **Stevenson, R. E., Burton, O. M., Ferlauto, G. J., and Taylor, H. A.,** Hazards of oral anticoagulants during pregnancy, *JAMA,* 243, 1549, 1980.
16. **Hanson, J. W. and Smith, D. W.,** The fetal hydantoin syndrome, *J. Pediatr.,* 87, 285, 1975.
17. **Kochenour, N. K., Emery, M. G., and Sawchuk, R. J.,** Phenytoin metabolism during pregnancy, *Obstet. Gynecol.,* 56, 577, 1980.
18. **Solomon, G. E., Hilgartner, M. W., and Kutt, H.,** Coagulation deficits caused by diphenylhydantoin, *Neurology,* 22, 1165, 1972.
19. **DiLiberti, J. H., Farndon, P. A., Dennis, N. R., and Curry, C. J. R.,** The fetal valproate syndrome, *Am. J. Hum. Genet.,* 19, 473, 1984.
20. **Fabro, S. and Brown, N. A.,** Teratogenic potential of anticonvulsants, *N. Engl. J. Med.,* 300, 1280, 1979.
21. **Brazy, J. E., Eckerman, C. O., and Gross, S. J.,** Follow-up of infants of <1500 grams birth weight with antenatal isoxsuprine exposure, *J. Pediatr.,* 102, 611, 1983.
22. **Brazy, J. E. and Pupkin, M. J.,** Effects of maternal isoxsuprine administration on preterm infants, *J. Pediatr.,* 94, 444, 1979.
23. **Ekelund, L., Burgoyne, R., and Enhorning, G.,** Pulmonary surfactant release in fetal rabbits: immediate and delayed response to terbutaline, *Am. J. Obstet. Gynecol.,* 147, 437, 1983.
24. **Dudenhausen, J. W., Kynast, G., Lange-Lindberg, A.-M., and Saling, E.,** Influence of long-term beta-mimetic therapy on lecithin content of amniotic fluid, *Gynecol. Obstet. Invest.,* 9, 205, 1978.
25. **Hansen, N. B., Oh, W., Larochelle, F., and Stonestreet, B. S.,** Effects of maternal ritodrine administration on neonatal renal function, *J. Pediatr.,* 103, 774, 1983.
26. **Perkins, R. P., Varela-Gittings, F. H., Dunn, T. S., Argubright, K. F., and Skipper, B. J.,** The influence of IV solution content on ritodrine-induced metabolic changes, *Obstet. Gynecol.,* 70, 892, 1987.
27. **Kirkpatrick, C., Quenon, M., and Desir, D.,** Blood anions and electrolytes during ritodrine infusion in preterm labor, *Am. J. Obstet. Gynecol.,* 138, 523, 1980.
28. **Alford, C. A., Reynolds, D. W., and Stagno, S.,** Current concepts of chronic perinatal infections, in *Modern Perinatal Medicine,* Gluck, L., Ed., Year Book Medical Publishers, Chicago, 1974, 285.
29. **Volpe, J. J.,** *Neurology of the Newborn,* W.B. Saunders, Philadelphia, 1987, 575.
30. **Cooper, L. Z., Ziring, P. R., Ockerase, A. B., et al.,** Rubella, *Am. J. Dis. Child.,* 18, 118, 1969.
31. **Smith, D. W.,** *Recognizable Patterns of Human Malformation,* 3rd ed., W.B. Saunders, Philadelphia, 1982, 424.

32. **Feldman, H. A.,** Cytomegalovirus, in *Obstetric and Perinatal Infections,* Finland, C. D., Ed., Lea & Febiger, Philadelphia, 1973, 19.
33. **Davis, L. E., Johnsson, L.-G., and Kornfeld, M.,** Cytomegalovirus labyrinthitis in an infant: morphological, virological, and immunofluorescent studies, *J. Neuropathol. Exp. Neurol.,* 40, 9, 1981.
34. **Reesink, H. W., Reerine-Brongers, E. E., Lafeber-Schut, B. J. T., Kalshoven-Benschop, J., and Brummelhuis, H. G.,** Prevention of chronic HBsAg carrier state in infants of HBsAg-positive mothers by hepatitis B immunoglobulin, *Lancet,* 2, 1129, 1979.
35. **Staisch, K. J., Westlake, J. R., and Bashore, R. A.,** Blinded oxytocin challenge test and perinatal outcome, *Am. J. Obstet. Gynecol.,* 138, 399, 1980.
36. **Solum, T. and Sjoberg, N.-O.,** Antenatal cardiotocography and intrauterine death, *Acta Obstet. Gynecol. Scand.,* 59, 481, 1980.
37. **Freeman, R. K., Anderson, G., and Dorchester, W.,** A prospective multi-institutional study of antepartum fetal heart rate monitoring. II. Contraction stress test versus nonstress test for primary surveillance, *Am. J. Obstet. Gynecol.,* 143, 778, 1982.
38. **Capeless, E. I. and Mann, L. I.,** Use of breast stimulation for antepartum stress testing, *Obstet. Gynecol.,* 64, 641, 1984.
39. **Holm, V. A.,** The causes of cerebral palsy: a contemporary perspective, *JAMA,* 247, 1473, 1982.
40. **Wigglesworth, J. S.,** The central nervous system, in *Perinatal Pathology,* W.B. Saunders, Philadelphia, 1984, 243.
41. **Low, J. A., Galbraith, R. S., Muir, D., Killen, H. L., Pater, E. A., and Karchmar, E. J.,** Intrapartum fetal hypoxia: a study of long-term morbidity, *Am. J. Obstet. Gynecol.,* 145, 129, 1983.
42. **Low, J. A., Galbraith, R. S., Muir, D., Killen, H. L., Karchmar, J., and Campbell, D.,** Intrapartum fetal asphyxia: a preliminary report in regard to long-term morbidity, *Am. J. Obstet. Gynecol.,* 130, 525, 1978.
43. **Westgren, M., Hormquist, P., Ingemarsson, I., and Svenningsen, N.,** Intrapartum fetal acidosis in preterm infants: fetal monitoring and long-term morbidity, *Obstet. Gynecol.,* 63, 355, 1984.
44. **Niswander, K. R., Gordon, M., and Drage, J. S.,** The effect of intrauterine hypoxia on the child surviving to 4 years, *Am. J. Obstet. Gynecol.,* 121, 892, 1975.
45. **Myers, R. E.,** Two patterns of perinatal brain damage and their conditions of occurrence, *Am. J. Obstet. Gynecol.,* 112, 246, 1972.
46. **Painter, M. J., Depp, R., and O'Donoghue, P. D.,** Fetal heart rate patterns and development in the first year of life, *Am. J. Obstet. Gynecol.,* 132, 271, 1978.
47. **Sykes, G. S., Molloy, P. M., Johnson, P., Gu, W., Ashworth, F., Stirrat, G. M., and Turnbull, A. C.,** Do Apgar scores indicate asphyxia?, *Lancet,* 1, 494, 1982.
48. **Silverman, F., Suidan, J., Wasserman, J., Antoine, C., and Young, B. K.,** The Apgar score: is it enough?, *Obstet. Gynecol.,* 66, 331, 1985.
49. **Goldenberg, R. L., Huddleston, J. F., and Nelson, K. G.,** Apgar scores and umbilical arterial pH in preterm newborn infants, *Am. J. Obstet. Gynecol.,* 149, 651, 1984.
50. **Nelson, K. B. and Ellenberg, J. H.,** Apgar scores as predictors of chronic neurologic disability, *Pediatrics,* 68, 36, 1981.
51. **Kenny, J. D., Adams, J. M., Corbet, A. J. S., and Rudolph, A. J.,** The role of acidosis at birth in the development of hyaline membrane disease, *Pediatrics,* 58, 184, 1976.
52. **Hobel, C. J., Hyvarinen, M. A., and Oh, W.,** Abnormal fetal heart rate patterns and fetal acid-base balance in low birth weight infants in relation to respiratory distress syndrome, *Obstet. Gynecol.,* 39, 83, 1972.
53. **Gilstrap, L. C., Hauth, J. C., Schiano, S., and Connor, K. D.,** Neonatal acidosis and method of delivery, *Obstet. Gynecol.,* 63, 681, 1984.
54. **Dijxhoorn, M. J., Visser, G. H. A., Huisjes, H. J., Fidler, V., and Touwen, B. C. L.,** The relation between umbilical pH values and neonatal neurological morbidity in full term appropriate-for-dates infants, *Early Human Dev.,* 11, 33, 1985.
55. **Katz, M., Shani, N., Meizner, I., et al.,** Is end-stage deceleration of the fetal heart ominous?, *Br. J. Obstet. Gynaecol.,* 89, 186, 1982.
56. **Henson, G. L., Dawes, G. S., and Redman, C. W. G.,** Antenatal fetal heart-rate variability in relation to fetal acid-base status at caesarean section, *Br. J. Obstet. Gynaecol.,* 90, 516, 1983.
57. **Commey, J. O. O. and Fitzhardinge, P. M.,** Handicap in the preterm small-for-gestational age infant, *J. Pediatr.,* 94, 779, 1979.
58. **Kenepp, N. B., Kumar, S., Shelley, W. C., Stanley, C. A., Gabbe, S. G., and Gutsche, B. B.,** Fetal and neonatal hazards of maternal hydration with 5% dextrose before caesarian section, *Lancet,* 1, 1150, 1982.
59. **Swanstrom, S. and Bratteby, L.-E.,** Metabolic effects of obstetric regional analgesia and of asphyxia in the newborn infant during the first two hours after birth. I. Arterial blood glucose concentrations, *Acta Paediatr. Scand.,* 70, 791, 1981.

60. **Swanstrom, S. and Bratteby, L.-E.,** Metabolic effects of obstetric regional analgesia and of asphyxia in the newborn infant during the first two hours after birth. II. Arterial plasma concentrations of glycerol, free fatty acids and beta-hydroxybutyric acid, *Acta Paediatr. Scand.,* 70, 801, 1981.

61. **Swanstrom, S. and Bratteby, L.-E.,** Metabolic effects of obstetrical regional analgesia and of asphyxia in the newborn infant during the first two hours after birth. III. Adjustment of arterial blood gases and acid-base balance, *Acta Paediatr. Scand.,* 80, 811, 1981.

62. **Lee, C. Y.,** Shoulder dystocia, *Clin. Obstet. Gynecol.,* 30, 77, 1987.

63. **Acker, D. B., Sachs, B. P., and Friedman, E. A.,** Risk factors for shoulder dystocia, *Obstet. Gynecol.,* 66, 762, 1985.

64. **Benedetti, T. J. and Gabbe, S. G.,** Shoulder dystocia: a complication of fetal macrosomia and prolonged second stage of labor with mid-pelvic delivery, *Obstet. Gynecol.,* 52, 526, 1978.

65. **McFarland, L. V., Raskin, M., Daling, J. R., and Benedetti, T. J.,** Erb/Duchenne's palsy: a consequence of fetal macrosomia and method of delivery, *Obstet. Gynecol.,* 68, 784, 1986.

66. **Steiner, H. and Neligan, G.,** Perinatal cardiac arrest: quality of the survivors, *Arch. Dis. Child.,* 50, 696, 1975.

67. **Dweck, H. S., Huggins, W., Dorman, L. P., Saxon, S. A., Benton, J. W., Jr., and Cassady, G.,** Developmental sequelae in infants having suffered severe perinatal asphyxia, *Am. J. Obstet. Gynecol.,* 119, 811, 1974.

68. **Thomson, A. J., Searle, M., and Russell, G.,** Quality of survival after severe birth asphyxia, *Arch. Dis. Child.,* 52, 620, 1977.

69. **Scott, H.,** Outcome of very severe birth asphyxia, *Arch. Dis. Child.,* 51, 712, 1976.

70. **DeSouza, S. W. and Richards, B.,** Neurological sequelae in newborn babies after perinatal asphyxia, *Arch. Dis. Child.,* 53, 564, 1978.

71. **Friedman, E. A.,** Midforceps delivery: no?, *Clin. Obstet. Gynecol.,* 30, 93, 1987.

72. **Hayashi, R. H.,** Midforceps delivery: yes?, *Clin. Obstet. Gynecol.,* 30, 90, 1987.

73. **Plauche, W. C.,** Fetal cranial injuries related to delivery with the Malstrom vacuum extractor, *Obstet. Gynecol.,* 53, 750, 1979.

74. **Carson, B. S., Losey, R. W., Bowes, W. A., Jr., and Simmons, M. A.,** Combined obstetric and pediatric approach to prevent meconium aspiration, *Am. J. Obstet. Gynecol.,* 126, 712, 1976.

75. **Bejar, R., Coen, R. W., and Gluck, L.,** Hypoxic-ischemic and hemorrhagic brain injury in the newborn, *Perinatol./Neonatol.,* July/August, 69, 1982.

76. **Papile, L. A., Burstein, J., Burstein, R., and Koffler, H.,** Incidence and evolution of subependymal and intraventricular hemorrhage: a study of infants with birth weights less than 1500 grams, *J. Pediatr.,* 92, 529, 1978.

77. **Papile, L. A., Munsick-Bruno, G., and Schaefer, A.,** Relationship of cerebral intraventricular hemorrhage and early childhood handicaps, *J. Pediatr.,* 103, 273, 1983.

78. **Bejar, R., Curbelo, V., Coen, R. W., Leopold, G., James, H., and Gluck, L.,** Diagnosis and follow-up of intraventricular and intracerebral hemorrhages by ultrasound studies of infant's brain through the fontanelles and sutures, *Pediatrics,* 66, 661, 1980.

79. **Norman, M. G.,** Perinatal brain damage, *Perspect. Pediatr. Pathol.,* 4, 41, 1978.

80. **Volpe, J. J., Herscovitch, P., Perlman, J. M., and Raichle, M. E.,** Positron emission tomography in the newborn: extensive impairment of regional cerebral blood flow with intraventricular hemorrhage and hemorrhagic intracerebral involvement, *Pediatrics,* 72, 589, 1983.

81. **Simmons, M. A., Adcock, E. W., Bard, H., and Battaglia, F. C.,** Hypernatremia and intracranial hemorrhage in neonates, *N. Engl. J. Med.,* 291, 6, 1974.

82. **Papile, L. A., Burstein, J., Burstein, R., and Koffler, H.,** Relationship of intravenous sodium bicarbonate infusions and cerebral intraventricular hemorrhage, *J. Pediatr.,* 93, 834, 1978.

83. **Clark, C. E., Clyman, R. I., Roth, R. S., Sniderman, S. H., Lane, B., and Ballard, R. A.,** Risk factor analysis of intraventricular hemorrhage in low-birth-weight infants, *J. Pediatr.,* 99, 625, 1981.

84. **Meidell, R., Marinelli, P., and Pettett, G.,** Perinatal factors associated with early-onset intracranial hemorrhage in premature infants, *Am. J. Dis. Child.,* 139, 160, 1985.

85. **Garcia-Prats, J. A., Procianoy, R. S., Adams, J. M., and Rudolph, A. J.,** The hyaline membrane disease-intraventricular hemorrhage relationship in the very low birth weight infant: perinatal aspects, *Acta Paediatr. Scand.,* 71, 79, 1982.

86. **Beverley, D. W., Chance, G. W., and Coates, C. F.,** Intraventricular hemorrhage — timing of occurrence and relationship to perinatal events, *Br. J. Obstet. Gynaecol.,* 91, 1007, 1984.

87. **Hill, A., Perlman, J. M., and Volpe, J. J.,** Relationship of pneumothorax to occurrence of intraventricular hemorrhage in the premature newborn, *Pediatrics,* 69, 144, 1982.

88. **McDonald, M. M., Koops, B. L., Johnson, M. L., Guggenheim, M. A., Rumack, C. M., Mitchell, S. A., and Hathaway, W. E.,** Timing and antecedents of intracranial hemorrhage in the newborn, *Pediatrics,* 74, 32, 1984.

89. **Strauss, A., Kirz, D., Modanlou, H. D., and Freeman, R. K.,** Perinatal events and intraventricular/ subependymal hemorrhage in the very low-birth weight infant, *Am. J. Obstet. Gynecol.,* 151, 1022, 1985.

90. **Horbar, J. D., Pasnick, M., McAuliffe, T. L., and Lucey, J. F.,** Obstetric events and risk of periventricular hemorrhage in premature infants, *Am. J. Dis. Child.,* 137, 678, 1983.

91. **Tejani, N., Rebold, B., Tuck, S., Ditroia, D., Sutro, W., and Verma, U.,** Obstetric factors in the causation of early periventricular-intraventricular hemorrhage, *Obstet. Gynecol.,* 64, 510, 1984.

92. **Lebed, M. R., Schifrin, B. S., Waffran, F., Hohler, C. W., and Afriat, C. I.,** Real-time B scanning in the diagnosis of neonatal intracranial hemorrhage, *Am. J. Obstet. Gynecol.,* 142, 851, 1982.

93. **Kenny, J. D., Garcia-Prats, J. A., Hilliard, J. L., Corbet, A. J. S., and Rudolph, A. J.,** Hypercarbia at birth: a possible role in the pathogenesis of intraventricular hemorrhage, *Pediatrics,* 62, 465, 1978.

94. **Rayburn, W. F., Donn, S. M., Kolin, M. G., and Schork, M. A.,** Obstetric care and intraventricular hemorrhage in the low birth weight infant, *Obstet. Gynecol.,* 61, 408, 1983.

95. **Burstein, J., Papile, L.-A., and Burstein, R.,** Subependymal germinal matrix and intraventricular hemorrhage in premature infants: diagnosis by CT, *Am. J. Roentgenol.,* 128, 971, 1977.

96. **Burstein, J., Papile, L.-A., and Burstein, R.,** Intraventricular hemorrhage in premature newborns: prospective study using computed tomography, *Am. J. Roentgenol.,* 132, 631, 1979.

97. **Procianoy, R. S., Garcia-Prats, J. A., Adams, J. M., Silvers, A., and Rudolph, A. J.,** Hyaline membrane disease and intraventricular haemorrhage in small for gestational age infants, *Arch. Dis. Child.,* 55, 502, 1980.

98. **Bada, H. S., Korones, S. B., Anderson, G. D., Magill, H. L., and Wong, S. P.,** Obstetric factors and relative risk of neonatal germinal layer/intraventricular hemorrhage, *Am. J. Obstet. Gynecol.,* 148, 798, 1984.

99. **Dykes, F. D., Lazzara, A., Ahmann, P., Blumenstein, B., Schwartz, J., and Brann, A. W.,** Intraventricular hemorrhage: a prospective evaluation of etiopathogenesis, *Pediatrics,* 66, 42, 1980.

100. **Beverley, D. W., Pitts-Tucker, T. J., Congdon, P. J., Arthur, R. J., and Tate, G.,** Prevention of intraventricular haemorrhage by fresh frozen plasma, *Arch. Dis. Child.,* 60, 710, 1985.

101. **McDonald, M. M., Johnson, M. L., Rumack, C. M., Koops, B. L., Guggenheim, M. A., Babb, C., and Hathaway, W. E.,** Role of coagulopathy in newborn intracranial hemorrhage, *Pediatrics,* 74, 26, 1984.

102. **Worthington, D., Davis, L. E., Grausz, J. P., and Sobocinski, K.,** Factors influencing survival and morbidity with very low birth weight delivery, *Obstet. Gynecol.,* 62, 550, 1983.

103. **Hoskins, E. M., Elliot, E., Shennan, A. T., Skidmore, M. B., and Keith, E.,** Outcome of very low-birth weight infants born at a perinatal center, *Am. J. Obstet. Gynecol.,* 145, 135, 1983.

104. **Allan, W. C. and Volpe, J. J.,** Periventricular-intraventricular hemorrhage, *Pediatr. Clin. North Am.,* 36, 47, 1986.

105. **Perlman, J. M. and Volpe, J. J.,** Suctioning in the preterm infant: effects on cerebral blood flow velocity, intracranial pressure, and arterial blood pressure, *Pediatrics,* 72, 329, 1983.

106. **Donn, S. M., Roloff, D. W., and Goldstein, G. W.,** Prevention of intraventricular haemorrhage in preterm infants by phenobarbitone: a controlled study, *Lancet,* 2, 215, 1981.

107. **Bedard, M. P., Shankaran, S., Slovis, T. L., Pantoja, A., Dayal, B., and Poland, R. L.,** Effect of prophylactic phenobarbital on intraventricular hemorrhage in high-risk infants, *Pediatrics,* 73, 435, 1984.

108. **Perlman, J. M., Goodman, S., Kreusser, K. L., and Volpe, J. J.,** Reduction in intraventricular hemorrhage by elimination of fluctuating cerebral blood-flow velocity in preterm infants with respiratory distress syndrome, *N. Engl. J. Med.,* 312, 1353, 1985.

109. **Mitchell, W. and O'Tuama, L.,** Cerebral intraventricular hemorrhages in infants: a widening age spectrum, *Pediatrics,* 65, 35, 1980.

110. **Wigglesworth, J. S. and Pape, K. E.,** Pathophysiology of intracranial haemorrhage in the newborn, *J. Perinat. Med.,* 8, 119, 1980.

111. **Wigglesworth, J. S.,** A new look of intraventricular hemorrhage, *Contemp. OB/GYN,* March, 98, 1985.

112. **Baerts, W. and Meradji, M.,** Cranial ultrasound in preterm infants: long term follow-up, *Arch. Dis. Child.,* 60, 702, 1985.

113. **Sinha, S. K., Davies, J. M., Sims, D. G., and Chiswick, M. L.,** Relation between periventricular haemorrhage and ischaemic brain lesions diagnosed by ultrasound in very pre-term infants, *Lancet,* 2, 1154, 1985.

114. **Nelson, K. B. and Broman, S. H.,** Perinatal risk factors in children with serious motor and mental handicaps, *Ann. Neurol.,* 2, 371, 1977.

115. **Perkins, R. P.,** Perinatal observations in a high-risk population managed without intrapartum fetal pH studies, *Am. J. Obstet. Gynecol.,* 149, 327, 1984.

116. **Graziani, L. J., Pasto, M., Stanley, C., Steben, J., Desai, H., Desai, S., Foy, P. M., Branca, P., and Goldberg, B. B.,** Cranial ultrasound and clinical studies in preterm infants, *J. Pediatr.,* 106, 269, 1985.

117. **Manniello, R. L. and Farrell, P. M.,** Analysis of United States neonatal mortality statistics from 1968 to 1974, with specific reference to changing trends in major causalities, *Am. J. Obstet. Gynecol.,* 129, 667, 1977.

118. **Khoury, M. J., Marks, J. S., McCarthy, B. J., and Zaro, S. M.,** Factors affecting the sex differential in neonatal mortality: the role of respiratory distress syndrome, *Am. J. Obstet. Gynecol.,* 151, 777, 1985.

119. **Douvas, S. G., Meeks, G. R., Graves, G., Walsh, D. A., and Morrison, J. C.,** Intrapartum fetal heart rate monitoring as a predictor of fetal distress and immediate neonatal condition in low-birth weight (≤1800 grams) infants, *Am. J. Obstet. Gynecol.,* 148, 300, 1984.

120. **Martin, C. B., Siassi, B., and Hon, E. H.,** Fetal heart rate patterns and neonatal death in low birth weight infants, *Obstet. Gynecol.,* 44, 503, 1974.

121. **Kenny, J. D., Corbet, A. J., Adams, J. M., and Rudolph, A. J.,** Hyaline membrane disease and acidosis at birth in twins, *Obstet. Gynecol.,* 50, 710, 1977.

122. **Perelman, R. H. and Farrell, P. M.,** Analysis of causes of neonatal death in the United States with specific emphasis on fatal hyaline membrane disease, *Pediatrics,* 70, 570, 1982.

123. **Friedman, Z. and Rosenberg, A.,** Abnormal lung surfactant related to essential fatty acid deficiency in a neonate, *Pediatrics,* 63, 855, 1979.

124. **Linderkamp, O., Versmold, H. T., Fendel, H., Riegel, K. P., and Betke, K.,** Association of neonatal respiratory distress with birth asphyxia and deficiency of red cell mass in premature infants, *Eur. J. Pediatr.,* 129, 167, 1978.

125. **Barrada, M. I., Virnig, N. L., Edwards, L. E., and Hakanson, E. Y.,** Maternal intravenous ethanol in the prevention of respiratory distress syndrome, *Am. J. Obstet. Gynecol.,* 129, 25, 1977.

126. **Sisenwein, F. E., Tejani, N. A., Boxer, H. S., and DiGiuseppe, R.,** Effects of maternal ethanol infusion during pregnancy on the growth and development of children at four to seven years of age, *Am. J. Obstet. Gynecol.,* 147, 52, 1983.

127. **Hadjigeorgiou, E., Kitsiou, S., Psaroudakis, A., Segos, C., Nicolopoulos, D., and Kaskarelis, D.,** Antepartum aminophylline treatment for prevention of the respiratory distress syndrome in premature infants, *Am. J. Obstet. Gynecol.,* 135, 257, 1979.

128. **Wu, B., Kikkawa, Y., and Orzalesi, M. M.,** The effects of throxine on the maturation of fetal rabbit lungs, *Biol. Neonate,* 22, 161, 1973.

129. **Hauth, J. C., Parker, C. R., McDonald, P. C., Porter, J. C., and Johnston, J. M.,** A role of fetal prolactin in lung maturation, *Obstet. Gynecol.,* 51, 81, 1978.

130. **Hallman, M., Merritt, T. A., Schneider, H., Epstein, B. L., Mannino, F., Edwards, D. K., and Gluck, L.,** Isolation of human surfactant from amniotic fluid and a pilot study of its efficacy in respiratory distress syndrome, *Pediatrics,* 71, 473, 1983.

131. **Drew, J. H.,** Immediate intubation at birth of the very-low-birth-weight infant, *Am. J. Dis. Child.,* 136, 207, 1982.

132. **Lindroth, M., Svenningsen, N. W., Ahlstrom, H., and Jonson, B.,** Evaluation of mechanical ventilation in newborn infants. II. Pulmonary and neuro-developmental sequelae in relation to original diagnosis, *Acta Paediatr. Scand.,* 69, 151, 1980.

133. **Reynolds, E. O. R. and Taghizadeh, A.,** Improved prognosis of infants mechanically ventilated for hyaline membrane disease, *Arch. Dis. Child.,* 49, 505, 1974.

134. **Kamper, J. and Moller, J.,** Long-term prognosis of infants with idiopathic respiratory distress syndrome: follow-up studies in infants surviving after the introduction of continuous positive airway pressure, *Acta Paediatr. Scand.,* 68, 149, 1979.

135. **Bennett, F. C., Robinson, N. M., and Sells, C. J.,** Hyaline membrane disease, birth weight, and gestational age, *Am. J. Dis. Child.,* 136, 888, 1982.

136. **Thompson, T. and Reynolds, J.,** The results of intensive care therapy for neonates with respiratory distress syndrome. I. Neonatal mortality rates for neonates with RDS, *J. Perinat. Med.,* 5, 149, 1977.

137. **Thompson, T. and Reynolds, J.,** The results of intensive care therapy for neonates with respiratory distress syndrome. II. Long-term prognosis for survivors with RDS, *J. Perinat. Med.,* 5, 160, 1977.

138. **Moore, T. R. and Resnik, R.,** Special problems of VLBW infants, *Contemp. OB/GYN,* June, 174, 1984.

139. **Herschel, M., Kennedy, J. L., Kayne, H. L., Henry, M., and Cetrulo, C. L.,** Survival of infants born at 24 to 28 weeks' gestation, *Obstet. Gynecol.,* 60, 154, 1982.

140. **Lee, K.-S., Eidelman, A. I., Tseng, P.-I., Kandall, S. R., and Gartner, L. M.,** Respiratory distress syndrome of the newborn and complications of pregnancy, *Pediatrics,* 58, 675, 1976.

141. **Perkins, R. P.,** The neonatal significance of selected perinatal events among infants of low birthweight. II. The influence of ruptured membranes, *Am. J. Obstet. Gynecol.,* 142, 7, 1982.

142. **Berkowitz, R. L., Bonta, B. W., and Warshaw, J. E.,** The relationship between premature rupture of the membranes and the respiratory distress syndrome, *Am. J. Obstet. Gynecol.,* 124, 712, 1976.

143. **Galask, R. P., Varner, M. W., Petzold, C. R., and Wilbur, S. L.,** Bacterial attachment to the chorioamniotic membranes, *Am. J. Obstet. Gynecol.,* 148, 915, 1984.

144. **Faix, R. G. and Donn, S. M.,** Association of septic shock caused by early-onset Group B streptococcal sepsis and periventricular leukomalacia in the preterm infant, *Pediatrics*, 76, 415, 1985.

145. **Edwards, M. S., Jackson, C. V., and Baker, C. J.,** Increased risk of Group B streptococcal disease in twins, *JAMA*, 245, 2044, 1981.

146. **O'Brien, W. F., Golden, S. M., Bibro, M. C., Charkobardi, P. K., Davis, S. E., and Hemming, V. G.,** Short-term responses in neonatal lambs after infusion of Group B streptococcal extract, *Obstet. Gynecol.*, 65, 802, 1985.

147. **Naeye, R. L.,** Underlying disorders responsible for the neonatal deaths associated with low apgar scores, *Biol. Neonate*, 35, 150, 1979.

148. **Hardt, N. S., Kostenbauder, M., Ogburn, M., Benhke, M., Resnick, M., and Cruz, A.,** Influence of chorioamnionitis on long-term prognosis in low birth weight infants, *Obstet. Gynecol.*, 65, 5, 1985.

149. **Naeye, R. L.,** Amniotic fluid infections, neonatal hyperbilirubinemia, and psychomotor impairment, *Pediatrics*, 62, 497, 1978.

150. **Martin, D. H., Koutsky, L., Eschenbach, D. A., Daling, J. R., Alexander, E. R., Benedetti, J. K., and Holmes, K. K.,** Prematurity and perinatal mortality in pregnancies complicated by maternal *Chlamydia trachomatis* infections, *JAMA*, 247, 1585, 1982.

151. **Hill, H. R., Shigeoka, A. O., Hall, R. T., and Hemming, V. G.,** Neonatal cellular and humoral immunity to Group B streptococci, *Pediatrics*, Suppl. 64, 787, 1979.

152. **Stevenson, D. K., Kerner, J. A., Malachowski, N., and Sunshine, P.,** Late morbidity among survivors of necrotizing enterocolitis, *Pediatrics*, 66, 925, 1980.

153. **Black, V. D., Lubchenco, L. O., Luckey, D. W., Koops, B. L., McGuinness, G. A., Powell, D. P., and Tomlinson, A. L.,** Developmental and neurologic sequelae of neonatal hyperviscosity syndrome, *Pediatrics*, 69, 426, 1982.

154. **Goldberg, K., Wirth, F. H., Hathaway, W. E., Guggenheim, M. A., Murphy, J. R., Braithwaite, W. R., and Lubchenco, L. O.,** Neonatal hyperviscosity. II. Effect of partial plasma exchange transfusion, *Pediatrics*, 69, 419, 1982.

155. **Paul, R. H., Koh, K. S., and Monfared, A. H.,** Obstetric factors influencing outcome in infants weighing from 1,001 to 1,500 grams, *Am. J. Obstet. Gynecol.*, 133, 503, 1979.

156. **Goldenberg, R. L., Nelson, K. G., Dyer, R. L., and Wayne, J.,** The variability of viability: the effect of physicians' perceptions of viability on the survival of very low-birth weight infants, *Am. J. Obstet. Gynecol.*, 143, 678, 1982.

157. **Shennan, A. T. and Milligan, J. E.,** The growth and development of infants weighing 1,000 to 2,000 grams at birth and delivered in a perinatal unit, *Am. J. Obstet. Gynecol.*, 136, 273, 1980.

158. **Milligan, J. E. and Shennan, A. T.,** Perinatal management and outcome in the infant weighing 1,000 to 2,000 grams, *Am. J. Obstet. Gynecol.*, 136, 269, 1980.

159. **Buckswold, S., Zorn, W. A., and Egan, E. A.,** Mortality and follow-up data for neonates weighing 500 to 800 g at birth, *Am. J. Dis. Child.*, 41, 779, 1984.

160. **Dillon, W. P. and Egan, E. A.,** Aggressive obstetric management in late second-trimester deliveries, *Obstet. Gynecol.*, 58, 685, 1981.

161. **Gilstrap, L. C., Hauth, J. C., Bell, R. E., Ackerman, N. B., Yoder, B. A., and DeLemos, R.,** Survival and short-term morbidity of the premature neonate, *Obstet. Gynecol.*, 65, 37, 1985.

162. **Astbury, J., Orgill, A. A., Bajuk, B., and Yu, V. Y. H.,** Neonatal and neurodevelopmental significance of behavior in very low birthweight children, *Early Human Dev.*, 11, 113, 1985.

163. **Brown, J. K., Purvis, R. J., Forfar, J. O., and Cockburn, F.,** Neurological aspects of perinatal asphyxia, *Dev. Med. Child. Neurol.*, 16, 567, 1974.

164. **Shennan, A. T., Milligan, J. E., and Hoskins, E.,** Perinatal factors associated with death as handicap in very preterm infants, *Am. J. Obstet. Gynecol.*, 151, 231, 1985.

165. **Touwen, B. C. L., Lok-Meijer, T. Y., Huisjes, H. J., and Olinga, A. A.,** The recovery rate of neurologically deviant newborns, *Early Human Dev.*, 7, 131, 1982.

166. **Peacock, W. G. and Hirata, T.,** Outcome in low-birth-weight infants (750 to 1,500 grams): a report on 164 cases managed at Children's Hospital, San Francisco, California, *Am. J. Obstet. Gynecol.*, 140, 165, 1981.

167. **Driscoll, J. M., Driscoll, Y. T., Steir, M. E., Stark, R. I., Dangman, B. C., Perez, A., Wung, J.-T., and Kritz, P.,** Mortality and morbidity in infants less than 1,001 grams birth weight, *Pediatrics*, 69, 21, 1982.

168. **Shapiro, S., McCormick, M. C., Starfield, B. H., Krischer, J. P., and Bross, D.,** Relevance of correlates of infant deaths for significant morbidity at 1 year of age, *Am. J. Obstet. Gynecol.*, 136, 363, 1980.

169. **Levkoff, A. H., Westphal, M., Miller, M. C., and Michel, Y.,** Maternal risk factors in infants with very low birth weight, *Obstet. Gynecol.*, 60, 612, 1982.

170. **Gross, S. J., Kosmetatos, N., Grimes, C. T., and Williams, M. L.,** Newborn head size and neurological status, *Am. J. Dis. Child.*, 132, 753, 1978.

171. **Georgieff, M. K., Hoffman, J. S., Pereira, G. R., Bernbaum, J., and Hoffman-Williamson, M.,** Effect of neonatal caloric deprivation on head growth and 1-year developmental status in preterm infants, *J. Pediatr.,* 107, 581, 1985.

172. **Pape, K. E., Buncic, R. J., Ashby, S., and Fitzhardinge, P. M.,** The status at two years of low-birthweight infants born in 1974 with birth weights of less than 1,001 gm, *J. Pediatr.,* 92, 253, 1978.

173. **Vohr, B. R. and Garcia Coll, C. T.,** Neurodevelopmental and school performance of very low-birthweight infants: a seven-year longitudinal study, *Pediatrics,* 76, 345, 1985.

174. **Michelsson, K., Lindahl, E., Parre, M., and Helenius, M.,** Nine-year follow-up of infants weighing 1500g or less at birth, *Acta Paediatr. Scand.,* 73, 835, 1984.

175. **Nelson, K. B. and Ellenberg, J. H.,** Predictors of low and very low birth weight and the relation of these to cerebral palsy, *JAMA,* 254, 1473, 1985.

176. **Illingworth, R. S.,** Why blame the obstetrician? A review, *Br. Med. J.,* 1, 797, 1979.

177. **Illingworth, R. S.,** A paediatrician asks — why is it called birth injury?, *Br. J. Obstet. Gynaecol.,* 92, 122, 1985.

178. **Nelson, K. B. and Ellenberg, J. H.,** Antecedents of cerebral palsy, *Am. J. Dis. Child.,* 139, 1031, 1985.

179. **Perkins, R. P.,** The neonatal significance of selected perinatal events among infants of low birthweight. III. Follow-up studies, *J. Perinat. Med.,* 12, 193, 1984.

180. **Nelson, K. B. and Ellenberg, J. H.,** Obstetric complications as risk factors for cerebral palsy or seizure disorders, *JAMA,* 251, 1843, 1984.

181. **Rantakallio, P.,** A 14-year follow-up of children with normal and abnormal birth weight for their gestational age, *Acta Paediatr. Scand.,* 74, 62, 1985.

182. **Mayer, P. S. and Wingate, M. B.,** Obstetric factors in cerebral palsy, *Obstet. Gynecol.,* 51, 399, 1978.

183. **Stanley, F. J.,** Improved male neonatal outcome in Western Australia, *Early Human Dev.,* 5, 179, 1981.

184. **Westgren, M., Dolfin, T., Halperin, M., Milligan, J., Shennan, A., Svenningsen, N. W., and Ingemarsson, I.,** Mode of delivery in the low birth weight fetus: delivery by cesarean section independent of fetal life versus vaginal delivery in vertex presentation, *Acta Obstet. Gynecol. Scand.,* 64, 51, 1985.

185. **Bennett, F. C., Chandler, L. S., Robinson, M. N., and Sells, C. J.,** Spastic diplegia in premature infants, *Am. J. Dis. Child.,* 135, 732, 1981.

186. **Colan, R. V., Snead, O. C., and Ceballos, R.,** Olivopontocerebellar atrophy in children: a report of seven cases in two families, *Ann. Neurol.,* 10, 355, 1981.

187. **Knobbe, T., Meier, P., Wenar, C., and Cordero, L.,** Psychological development of children who received intrauterine transfusions, *Am. J. Obstet. Gynecol.,* 133, 877, 1979.

188. **Churchill, J. A.,** A study of hemiplegic cerebral palsy, *Dev. Med. Child. Neurol.,* 10, 453, 1968.

189. **Nelson, K. B. and Ellenberg, J. H.,** Children who "outgrew" cerebral palsy, *Pediatrics,* 69, 529, 1982.

190. **Escalona, S. K.,** Babies at double hazard: early development of infants at biologic and social risk, *Pediatrics,* 70, 670, 1982.

191. **Cohen, H. J. and Diner, H.,** The significance of developmental dental enamel defects in neurological diagnosis, *Pediatrics,* 46, 737, 1970.

192. **Emery, J. L.,** Evidence from bone growth that most of the infants dying in the neonatal period had been ill before birth, *Acta Paediatr. Scand. Suppl.,* 172, 55, 1967.

Chapter 2

THE SIGNIFICANCE OF FETAL ASPHYXIA IN REGARD TO MOTOR AND COGNITIVE DEFICITS IN INFANCY AND CHILDHOOD

James A. Low

TABLE OF CONTENTS

I. INTRODUCTION

The complexity of the factors which contribute to motor and cognitive deficits has been well described in a recent review of the prenatal and perinatal causes of mental retardation, cerebral palsy, and seizure disorder.[1] Freeman, in a summary statement, has emphasized how little we know about the factors controlling, modifying, or altering brain development.

Opinions on the relevant factors associated with motor deficits have changed since Little first observed that there were associated perinatal events, including abnormal parturition, difficult labor, premature birth, and asphyxia neonatorum.[2] Subsequently, prenatal factors were advocated as the most significant factors in the pathogenesis of cerebral palsy.[3] However, opinion again changed, and in the 1950s perinatal events were considered to be the predominant etiological factors.[4,5]

It is now generally recognized that severe mental retardation is due to biological factors, usually genetic or metabolic, which occur with equal frequency in all social classes. However, mild mental retardation has been found to be linked with social and environmental deprivation.[6]

This examination of the relationship between intrapartum fetal asphyxia and subsequent motor and cognitive deficits will consider particularly the criteria used in the diagnosis of fetal asphyxia and the motor and cognitive deficits identified.

II. NEUROPATHOLOGY OF FETAL ASPHYXIA IN ANIMALS

The need for an experimental model for the controlled study of asphyxia during birth, which could demonstrate the relationship to subsequent neurological events, was recognized by Windle and his colleagues. A series of experiments in approximately 100 Rhesus monkeys to examine the effects of an acute asphyxial insult were carried out between 1957 and 1963. The results of these landmark experiments were reported in a series of publications over 15 years beginning in 1959.

The principal findings in these studies were identified in the first publication,[7] where the neuropathology in five asphyxiated monkeys and two controls was reported. Following an acute asphyxial insult of 11 to 16 min, the fetus was intubated and resuscitated by means of positive pressure ventilation. Fetal neuropathology studied 2 to 9 days following delivery showed nonhemorrhagic bilateral focal lesions, mainly in relay nuclei of the somesthetic, auditory, and vestibular systems and extrapyramidal cell groups. Certain nuclei were consistently involved, the most striking lesions being necrosis of the inferior colliculi. Severe damage was seen in the gracile and cuneate nuclei, the oculomotor, vestibular, and spinal trigeminal nuclei, the nuclei of the cerebellum, the superior olivary nucleus, the putamen, the globus pallidus, and the ventral lateral group of the thalamic nuclei. Cytolysis of neurons and, to a lesser extent, the neuroglia was evident within 2 days. The intensity of the phagocytic reaction beginning between 24 and 60 h was related to the degree of cell damage. Reactive changes involving astrocytes and microglia were evident in 7 to 10 days. The symmetry and uniform involvement of the nuclei suggested a regional susceptibility.

These findings were confirmed in approximately 50 subsequent studies in which the neuropathology was examined within 3 months of the insult. In a number of these studies, the newborn experienced major respiratory complications following the asphyxial insult. These complications appeared to increase the severity of the lesions and led to further involvement of the cerebral cortex.

Long-term neuropathology following acute fetal asphyxial insults was also described.[8] Data from 12 animals who lived for 10 months to 9 years following their asphyxial insult as well as data from 5 nonasphyxiated controls were presented. The neuropathology included atrophy and scarring at the primary site of the asphyxial lesions. Additionally, there was

TABLE 1
Fetal Blood Gas and Acid-Base Measures of Animals With and Without Evidence of Neuropathology

	Neuropathology	
	None	Present
pH	$\geq$7.0—7.1	$\leq$6.9—7.0
Base deficit (mmol/l)	13—18	<10—13
pCO_2 (mmhg)	<70	80—90
O_2 saturation (%)	>30	<30

evidence of secondary degeneration, with widespread depletion of nerve cell populations in other regions. This secondary change was most clearly seen in that part of the cerebral cortex served by thalamocortical radiations, the reticular formation in the brain stem, and the dorsal columns of the spinal cord. The nerve cells simply disappeared, with no associated scar.

Functional sequelae were examined in 16 monkeys for 3 years or more.[9] The monkeys appeared to adapt to their environment in spite of severe initial brain damage and subsequent transneuronal atrophy. Early neurological signs disappeared or were masked, with improvement of physical and behavioral characteristics, plateauing at 3 to 4 years of age. The monkeys at this stage often appeared overtly normal, but were hypoactive and lacked manual dexterity.

Windle concluded that an acute asphyxial insult of <8 min not requiring active resuscitation of the newborn might not cause evidence of brain damage. Asphyxia of >8 min invariably produced at least transient neurological signs. Asphyxia of >10 min invariably resulted in neuropathology, with a gradation of severity which was directly associated with the duration of the asphyxia.

This work was continued by Myers and colleagues, who noted that the neuropathology of the brain stem which had been observed with acute asphyxia did not correspond to the neuropathology in humans following perinatal injury. The long-term neuropathology in children with deficits attributed to perinatal insults includes ulegyria, diffuse white matter sclerosis, and status marmoratus, with only rare involvement of the lower brain stem.[10] The concept of the significance of long-term partial asphyxia emerged from the observation of several random examples of cortical necrosis with status marmoratus in the acute asphyxial experiments.[11]

Therefore, a series of studies were carried out on the effect of prolonged partial hypoxia induced by either oxytocin stimulation or maternal hypotension in term fetal monkeys for periods of 3 to 5 h. The effects on the brain depended on the degree and duration of the hypoxic insult. No neuropathology was observed in many newborns in whom the hypoxic insult was short and the metabolic acidosis was less severe, i.e., a pH > 7.0 to 7.1. However, neuropathology was observed with more prolonged tissue hypoxia, lasting 30 to 120 min, and the concurrent metabolic acidosis was more severe (pH $\leq$ 6.9 to 7.0) (Table 1).

The neuropathology included both generalized and focal cerebral necrosis. The focal necrosis principally occurred in the paracentral regions and the junctional zone between the parietal and occipital lobes. There was also involvement of basal ganglia, including the caudate nucleus, putamen, and occasionally the globus pallidus. Atrophic cortical necrosis, with varying degrees of damage of white matter, was observed in the animals examined 6 months following the insult. This neuropathology closely mimics the neuropathology of children with cerebral palsy.

The importance of systemic hypotension with decreased cerebral blood flow and the

TABLE 2
Normal Fetal Blood Gas and Acid-Base Measures

	Umbilical vein	Umbilican artery
O_2 tension (mm)	28	15
O_2 saturation (%)	65	25
O_2 capacity (vol%)	22	
O_2 content (vol%)	13	5
CO_2 tension (mm)	40	48
pH	7.34	7.26
Buffer base (mmol/l)	43	41
Base excess (mmol/l)	−3	−5
Lactate (mmol/l)	1.7	
Pyruvate (mmol/l)	0.14	

degree of lactic acidosis in the occurrence of central nervous system injury has been implied in subsequent studies in the fetal monkey and fetal lamb. A relationship in hypoxic fetal monkeys between moderate hypotension, serum and central nervous system lactate levels, and brain damage has been observed.[14] A similar study was carried out in 28 midgestational fetal lambs. Each fetus was subjected to a 2-h hypoxic insult, and the neuropathology was examined 3 days following delivery. No neuropathology was observed in 21 lambs, while 7 lambs exhibited well-demarcated areas of cortical necrosis, with extensive damage of the white matter and basal ganglia. The fetuses with neuropathology had a more severe metabolic acidosis, significantly higher lactate concentrations, and more severe hypotension than those with no neuropathology.[15] Similar observations indicating a relationship between cardio-vascular instability and the neuropathology of hypoxia in the fetal lamb have been reported by Mann and colleagues.[16] These observations support the concept that systemic hypotension with reduced cerebral blood flow is an important factor in the occurrence of the neuropath-ology of hypoxia.

III. DIAGNOSIS OF ASPHYXIA IN THE HUMAN FETUS

A. NORMAL BLOOD GAS AND ACID-BASE MEASURES

A definitive diagnosis of fetal asphyxia requires a blood gas and acid-base assessment. Fetal blood can be obtained during labor by scalp sampling and at delivery by sampling the umbilical vein and artery.

Interpretation of blood gas and acid-base assessment of fetal blood requires an under-standing of normal measures. An extensive literature has provided an indication of the normal values in umbilical vein and artery blood[17] (Table 2). Fetal umbilical venous and arterial oxygen tension is significantly lower than corresponding maternal values. This results in a maternal-fetal gradient which is important for the transfer of oxygen from the mother to the fetus. However, oxygen content in the umbilical vein is within the normal adult range, since fetal blood has a greater oxygen affinity and a higher oxygen capacity. Fetal umbilical venous and arterial carbon dioxide tension is of the same order as in the adult, since there is a fetal-maternal gradient due to maternal hyperventilation with hypocapnia. Fetal blood pH in the umbilical vein and artery is lower than maternal arterial and venous blood pH. However, fetal blood buffer base or base deficit in the umbilical vein and artery closely parallels corresponding measures in maternal blood. The best estimates of resting fetal blood lactate and pyruvate, obtained following elective section, indicate that the normal fetus metabolizes aerobically with no accumulation of fixed acids. This has been confirmed by recent acid-base studies of cord blood obtained percutaneously during pregnancy.[18]

TABLE 3
Measures of a Significant Metabolic Acidosis
Due to Fetal Hypoxia

	Umbilical artery	Capillary
pH	<7.150	<7.200
Buffer base (mmol/l)	<34.0	<36.0

B. MEASURES OF FETAL ASPHYXIA

An acid-base assessment of fetal blood with identification of a fetal metabolic acidosis will confirm that an episode of fetal hypoxia has occurred. It is proposed that an umbilical artery buffer base <34 mmol/l represents a significant metabolic acidosis due to fetal hypoxia. A buffer base of 36 mmol/l represents 2 SD below the mean in a normal population.[19] However, one third of the lactic acid accounting for the metabolic acidosis is derived from an increase in pyruvic acid rather than tissue oxygen debt.[20] Therefore, the adjusted umbilical artery buffer base attributable to tissue hypoxia is on the order of 34 mmol/l. The related umbilical artery pH will vary with the degree of respiratory acidosis at the time of sampling. The average equivalent pH is 7.150. Corresponding capillary blood pH is somewhat higher, with the conventional abnormal pH defined as <7.200. These criteria of a significant metabolic acidosis due to hypoxia are presented in Table 3.

C. CLINICAL INDICATORS OF FETAL ASPHYXIA

Much of the literature which examines the relationship between fetal asphyxia and subsequent motor and cognitive development lacks blood gas and acid-base data. The diagnosis of fetal asphyxia is therefore based upon clinical criteria. However, these clinical proxies are affected by a number of other factors as well as fetal hypoxia. The clinical criteria most frequently used include abnormal fetal heart rate, meconium in the amniotic fluid during labor, and low Apgar scores with delayed onset of respiration at delivery.

Baseline fetal heart rate and fetal heart rate accelerations are not predictive of intrapartum fetal hypoxia with metabolic acidosis.[21] Fetal heart rate decelerations are predictive, but not diagnostic, of fetal asphyxia. In the presence of late decelerations, the probability of fetal hypoxia with a significant metabolic acidosis is <50%. Conversely, approximately 50% of hypoxic fetuses will demonstrate late decelerations in the fetal heart rate record.[22]

The relationship between fetal hypoxia with significant metabolic acidosis, as expressed by umbilical vein and artery blood gas and acid-base measures, and meconium in amniotic fluid and the Apgar scores at 1 and 5 min following delivery has been examined in 1773 obstetric patients (Table 4).

Moderate or severe meconium was observed in 262 patients (15%). Moderate or severe meconium was present in 12 (32%) of the fetuses with significant metabolic acidosis at delivery. On the other hand, there were 250 fetuses with moderate or severe meconium who had blood gas and acid-base measures within the normal range, a false-positive rate of 95%.

An Apgar score of 0 to 3 at 1 min was recorded in 115 newborns (6%) and at 5 min in 11 newborns (1%). A low Apgar score (0 to 3) at 1 min was recorded in 18 (46%) of the newborns with significant metabolic acidosis at delivery. A low Apgar score of 0 to 3 at 5 min was recorded in three (8%) of the newborns with significant metabolic acidosis at delivery. On the other hand, the majority of the newborns with low Apgar scores did not have evidence of fetal hypoxia with metabolic acidosis. An Apgar score of 0 to 3 at 1 min was recorded in 97 newborns with blood gas and acid-base measures in the normal range, a false-positive rate of 84%, and an Apgar score of 0 to 3 at 5 min was recorded in 8 newborns with blood gas and acid-base measures in the normal range, a false-positive rate of 73%.

TABLE 4
The Relationship between Meconium and Apgar
Scores at 1 and 5 Min and Umbilical Artery
Buffer Base

	Umbilical artery buffer base	
	≥34 mmol/l	<34 mmol/l
Meconium (n = 1752)		
None/minimal	1464	26
Moderate/severe	250	12
Apgar score at 1 min (n = 1773)		
7—10	1459	13
4—6	178	8
0—3	97	18
Apgar score at 5 min (n = 1405)		
7—10	1348	31
4—6	12	3
0—3	8	3

The concept of hypoxic ischemic encephalopathy has been introduced in order to improve the prediction of deficits in surviving children.[23] Newborn encephalopathy includes the clinical neurological manifestations of newborn central nervous system disorders. Newborn encephalopathy, particularly seizures and recurrent apnea, is an important predictor of subsequent motor and cognitive handicap.[24,25] A relationship between perinatal hypoxia and newborn encephalopathy has been identified in a number of studies. Clinical studies of birth asphyxia with severe newborn depression have demonstrated that most children who survive with neurodevelopmental sequelae have had clinical signs of encephalopathy during the neonatal period.[26] Studies of children mature at birth with clinical markers of intrapartum hypoxia and subsequent encephalopathy have demonstrated deficits in 25 to 50% of surviving children.[27]

The relationship between fetal hypoxia confirmed by blood gas and acid-base assessment and newborn encephalopathy was examined in 303 high-risk children. There was evidence of fetal asphyxia with significant metabolic acidosis in 12% of the newborns with mild-moderate encephalopathy and in 22% of the newborns with severe newborn encephalopathy[28] (Figure 1).

There is an association between meconium in amniotic fluid, fetal heart rate late decelerations, low Apgar scores at 1 and 5 min, and newborn encephalopathy and intrapartum fetal hypoxia as identified by blood gas and acid-base assessment. However, fetal hypoxia with severe metabolic acidosis may occur in the absence of some or all of these fetal/newborn markers. Finally, the frequency of these fetal/newborn markers in the absence of fetal hypoxia (that is, the incidence of false positives) is in each case very high (Table 5).

IV. EPIDEMIOLOGICAL STUDIES OF MOTOR AND COGNITIVE DEFICITS

A. MOTOR DEFICITS

Most studies of motor handicap have been on cerebral palsy. Kiely et al.[29] have reviewed the trend in recent years in countries with comparable health care facilities. The review included data from Bristol, England,[30] Birmingham, England,[31] Iceland,[32] Sweden,[33] Denmark,[34] the U.S.,[35] Ireland,[36] and Australia.[37] No uniform trend is apparent. These reports on cerebral palsy show a mixed pattern with declining, stable, fluctuating, and rising trends. The encouraging decline reported in Sweden between 1959 to 1970 has not continued.

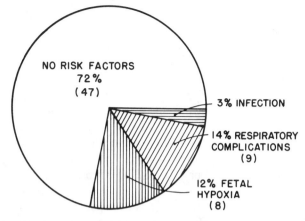

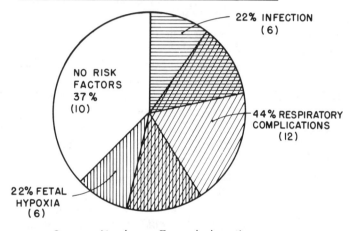

FIGURE 1.   Factors contributing mild-moderate and severe encephalopathy. (From Low, J. A., Galbraith, R. S., Muir, D. W., Killen, H. L., Pater, E. A., and Karchmar, E. J., *Am. J. Obstet. Gynecol.*, 152, 256, 1985. With permission.)

TABLE 5
The Sensitivity and Frequency of False Positives in
Clinical Markers of Fetal Asphyxia

	Fetal asphyxia	
Clinical Markers	**Sensitive (%)**	**False positives (%)**
Late decelerations	50	>50
Moderate/severe meconium	32	95
Apgar score 0—3 at 1 min	46	84
Apgar score 0—3 at 5 min	8	73
Newborn encephalopathy — severe	22	78

The prevalence rate in the 1970s has increased due to an increase in newborns weighing <2500 g, with the incidence of spastic diplegia increasing in parallel with increased survival of low birth weight infants requiring ventilation.[38]

The prevalence rates between countries are not strictly comparable, since the definitions and methods of assessment were not uniform. However, when congenital nervous system anomalies are excluded, prevalence rates for cerebral palsy averaging 2.0 to 2.5 cases per 1000 live births are reported.

The pathologic events responsible for cerebral palsy are assumed to occur in the prenatal and perinatal periods, although a small number have been acquired postnatally. The relevance of these factors has been examined in two major studies, the National Collaborative Perinatal Project (NCPP), a large prospective project in the U.S., and a study from Gothenberg, Sweden which includes a total population in a western region of that country.

The majority of the 202 children with cerebral palsy in the NCPP were of normal birth weight and gestational age. The importance of fetal asphyxia is implied, since the most significant predictors of cerebral palsy were Apgar scores of 0 to 3 at 10 min or later and neonatal seizures.[39]

The Swedish study reported the clinical data of approximately 600 patients with cerebral palsy born between 1954 and 1969.[33] The complications observed in these pregnancies were classified as prenatal, perinatal, postnatal, or untraceable. The perinatal group included obvious complications during delivery and the first 28 days of life in normally grown and low birth weight newborns (≤2500 g); 65% of the children were associated with the perinatal group, which presumably included fetal asphyxia.

The significance of fetal asphyxia has been examined in several separate cerebral palsy syndromes in this Swedish region. The association was examined in 111 selected children with dyskinetic cerebral palsy, of whom 34 were classified as hyperkinetic and 76 dystonic. Fetal asphyxia was defined as moderate (Apgar score ≤7) or severe (Apgar score ≤3 at any time up to 10 min following delivery). Based on these criteria, fetal asphyxia is an important factor in dyskinetic cerebral palsy, occurring in 35% of the hyperkinetic and 54% of the dystonic children.[40] The association was examined in 93 children with spastic diplegia, of whom 49 were term and 44 were preterm at birth. The degree of disability was more severe in term newborns, often being associated with mental retardation and seizure disorders. The criteria of fetal asphyxia included meconium in the amniotic fluid, fetal heart rate ≤100 or ≥160, and delayed onset of respiration (>1 min) requiring active resuscitation. Spastic diplegia in term infants was frequently associated with growth retardation and asphyxia. Birth asphyxia was identified in 31%. It was concluded that prolonged asphyxia was significantly correlated with more severe handicaps.[41]

B. COGNITIVE DEFICITS

Epidemiological studies of mental retardation are based upon IQ scores. Severe mental retardation (IQ <50) and mild mental retardation (IQ 50 to 69) differ in regard to factors contributing to their occurrence and are therefore considered independently.

The expected prevalence rate for severe mental retardation is 3.5 to 4 per 1000 school-age children.[42] Severe mental retardation is assumed to be due to biological complications. The clinical associations were described in 122 children with severe mental retardation born in Sweden between 1959 and 1970.[43] The most common complications associated with severe mental retardation were chromosomal anomalies, congenital malformations, and inborn errors of metabolism, and they were observed in 63% of children. The remaining complications were classified as prenatal (8%), perinatal (8%), infection (6%), and a miscellaneous group (15%). Such observations suggest that fetal asphyxia, as one of a number of perinatal complications, plays a small role in the occurrence of severe mental retardation.

Mild mental retardation is frequently an independent finding correlating with socioenvironmental factors. The anticipated prevalence rate is on the order of 10 to 30 per 1000 school-age children. Mild mental retardation is assumed to represent, in large part, an environmental deprivation.[6]

An exception to this general conclusion was observed in a study of 91 children with mild mental retardation born between 1966 and 1970 in Sweden.[44] The prevalence of mild

TABLE 6
The Relationship between Low Apgar Scores (0—3) and Mortality or Deficits in Survivors in the National Collaborative Perinatal Project[49]

Apgar scores 0—3	Number observed	Mortality (%)	Deficits in survivors (%)
5 min	788	44	5
10 min	362	68	13
15 min	232	81	23
20 min	181	87	38

mental retardation (4 per 1000) was much lower than the usual rate. This was attributed to a high average social standard of the population studied. Mental retardation was commonly associated with other complications in these children, including neurological abnormality (43%), cerebral palsy (9%), clumsiness (23%), and seizure disorder (12%). No clinical complications were observed in 55% of these children. However, prenatal complications were identified in 23%, and perinatal complications, principally fetal asphyxia, occurred in 18%.[45] These findings suggest that fetal asphyxia may play a modest role in the occurrence of mild mental retardation, a relationship which becomes evident in favorable social, environmental, and economic circumstances.

The relationship between perinatal hypoxia and cognitive development in infancy and childhood was examined in the children in the NCPP.[46] The criteria of asphyxia in this analysis included fetal tachycardia in the first stage of labor, low Apgar scores at 1 and 5 min, meconium at delivery, primary apnea, single or multiple apneic spells, resuscitation during and after the first 5 min, and respiratory difficulty in the nursery. Anoxic groups, particularly those with respiratory difficulty as newborns, had lower cognitive scores than normoxic groups in infancy and at the age of 7. Viewed retrospectively, the frequency of signs of hypoxia decreased dramatically as cognitive levels increased in school-age children. These associations were independent of socioeconomic factors.

V. SIGNIFICANCE OF CLINICAL INDICATORS OF FETAL ASPHYXIA

A. APGAR SCORES

Newborn depression, as expressed by low Apgar scores and delayed onset of respiration, has been the most frequently used indicator of fetal asphyxia in studies of subsequent deficits. A relationship between Apgar scores and deficits has been demonstrated in children in the NCPP.[47] Low Apgar scores at 1 min are weakly related to later motor and cognitive development.[48] Therefore, most attention has been directed to low Apgar scores at 5 min or more following delivery. Low Apgar scores at 5 min are independently associated with severe motor and cognitive deficits.[49] The increasing significance of prolonged low Apgar scores was demonstrated in an analysis of 128 children with moderate and severe cerebral palsy[50] (Table 6). This association of prolonged low Apgar scores with deficits is principally in term newborns, reflecting in part the low survival rate of preterm newborns with prolonged low Apgar scores.[51] The association between Apgar scores and deficits is equally true in pregnancies with and without obstetric complications.[52]

Although the association between low Apgar scores and deficits is clear, the majority of children with low Apgar scores are free of handicap. A number of clinical reports have emphasized this point. Steiner and Nelligan[53] reported on the outcome of 22 newborns who experienced perinatal cardiac arrest in whom heart rate was reestablished in 5 min and

TABLE 7
The Relationship between the Severity of
Newborn Encephalopathy and the
Frequency of Handicap[62]

Newborn encephalopathy	Total number observed	Handicap	
		n	%
Mild	66	0	0
Moderate	74	20	27
Severe	7	7	100

spontaneous respiration within 30 min. Major handicaps were observed in four children (20%). Scott[26] reported on the outcome of 23 newborns who had either an Apgar score of 0 or a delay of spontaneous respiration >20 min. Major handicaps were observed in six children (25%). Thomson et al.[54] reported on the outcome of 31 children with Apgar scores of 0 to 3 at 5 min. The interval to sustained respiration ranged from 5 to 60 min. Major handicaps were observed in two children (7%). Mulligan et al.[55] reported on the outcome of 65 children with delayed onset of spontaneous respiration of 2 to >20 min. Major handicaps were observed in 12 children (18%). Ergander and Erikson[56] reported on 81 children with Apgar scores of 0 to 3 at 5 min. Major handicaps were observed in 16 children (20%). The occurrence of handicap was frequently associated with a delay in the onset of respiration of >20 min.

B. NEWBORN ENCEPHALOPATHY

The significance of seizures in the newborn as predictors of subsequent deficit has been well documented.[57,58] Rose and Lombroso,[59] in 137 term newborns with seizures, reported a 20% mortality, and a further 30% survived with serious neurological deficits. Holden et al.,[60] reviewing 181 survivors of neonatal seizures in the NCPP followed to 7 years of age, identified deficits in 30%.

Brown et al.,[61] in a study of 94 asphyxiated newborn infants, emphasized the importance of abnormal tone in the prediction of deficits. The criteria of asphyxia included meconium and/or abnormal fetal heart rate, Apgar scores of <3 at 1 min and/or <5 at 5 min, and resuscitation requiring ventilation. Newborn neurological signs included apnea, apathy, seizures, hypothermia, cerebral cry, persistent vomiting, and abnormal muscle tone. A total of 20 of the asphyxiated newborns with neurological signs died, while 74 survived, of whom 24 had significant handicaps, 15 had minor deficits, and 34 were normal.

Fitzhardinge et al.[62] reported on 62 term infants with postasphyxial encephalopathy. The criteria of asphyxia included meconium and/or abnormal fetal heart rate, Apgar score of <6 at 5 min, or resuscitation requiring ventilation for >2 min. Newborn signs of encephalopathy included seizures, increased intracranial pressure, and abnormal tone. Major handicaps were identified in 29 infants (47%) and minor handicaps in 5 infants (8%).

Robertson and Finer[63] reported on 167 term newborns with evidence of hypoxic-ischemic encephalopathy who were followed 3 to 5 years. The criteria of asphyxia included abnormal fetal heart rate, Apgar score of <5 at 1 min and/or Apgar score of <5 at 5 min, and newborn resuscitation with ventilation for >5 min. Newborn encephalopathy was classified as described by Sarnat, included alterations in consciousness, alterations of muscle tone, and abnormal primitive reflexes. Handicaps were identified in 27 children, with a significant correlation with the severity of the encephalopathy (Table 7). Moderate encephalopathy was more likely to be associated with deficits when accompanied by seizures. All newborns with severe encephalopathy either died or had severe handicaps.

VI. SIGNIFICANCE OF FETAL HYPOXIA WITH METABOLIC ACIDOSIS

Fetal or newborn complications may affect the central nervous system, resulting in motor and cognitive deficits in surviving children. However, it has yet to be determined which complications are most important and how severe they must be to cause deficits. The assessment of individual complications is difficult due to the frequency with which these complications occur concurrently.

A study of an unselected population of 364 preterm and term infants with one or more fetal or newborn complication examined these relationships.[64] Major and/or minor motor and/or cognitive deficits were identified in 24% of the children at 1 year of age. Complications with an independent association with deficits included fetal hypoxia, newborn respiratory complications, and newborn infection. These complications also had an independent association with newborn encephalopathy. These observations support the concept that fetal hypoxia, newborn respiratory complications, and newborn infections may be mechanisms for central nervous system injury and subsequent deficits, while newborn encephalopathy reflects the injury and is an important predictor of such deficits.

An indication of the magnitude of the contribution of these fetal or newborn complications to deficits in this population was obtained by reviewing the 86 children with deficits at 1 year. The importance of complications differed in preterm and term children. The order of frequency in the preterm children was respiratory complications with some infection and occasional fetal hypoxia; these occurred in 29 (58%) of the preterm children. The order of frequency in term children was fetal hypoxia with some infection and occasional respiratory complications; these occurred in 11 (30%) of the term children.

Thus, intrapartum fetal hypoxia with significant metabolic acidosis has a greater association with deficits in term pregnancies than in preterm pregnancies. Fetal hypoxia occurred in two preterm infants with deficits (4%) and in eight of the term infants with deficits (22%).

The relationship between fetal hypoxia (as defined by blood gas and acid-base assessment) and subsequent deficits has been examined in several studies. A prospective follow-up study of 37 children with terminal episodes of fetal hypoxia and a control group of 59 children with no evidence of fetal hypoxia was carried out to 6 years of age.[65] The newborn infants were normally grown and mature at delivery. The infants of the hypoxic group did not display evidence of encephalopathy during the newborn period. There was no significant difference in either the physical growth or the incidence of motor or cognitive deficits in the children of the hypoxic group compared to the children of the control group. This demonstrated that a fetus may experience a terminal episode of fetal hypoxia with significant metabolic acidosis without apparent motor or cognitive deficits in infancy and childhood.

A second study analyzed 60 children with biochemical evidence of intrapartum fetal hypoxia with regard to the question of the degree and duration of fetal hypoxia required to cause central nervous system injury with deficits in surviving children.[66] The objective was to establish what features distinguish the children with deficits from those without deficits at 1 year of age. Eight children (13%) had a major deficit and ten children (16%) had a minor deficit at 1 year. Children with deficits had episodes of hypoxia that were more severe and prolonged and had subsequent to delivery a greater incidence of respiratory complications, apnea, and newborn encephalopathy. These findings suggest that an episode of hypoxia in excess of 1 h may be followed by motor and cognitive deficits.

Again, the relationship between fetal hypoxia and deficits varies in the preterm and term newborns. Of the 18 children with fetal hypoxia and subsequent deficits, 12 (67%) were mature at birth. The significance of the hypoxia to the deficits in these children is emphasized by the absence of other associated risk factors. Of the 18 children with fetal hypoxia and subsequent deficits, 6 (33%) were preterm at birth. Thus, although the frequency of deficits

TABLE 8

The Frequency of Motor and/or Cognitive Deficits in
Infants With and Without Evidence of Fetal Hypoxia and
Significant Metabolic Acidosis at Delivery

Motor and cognitive development	Controls (n = 76)		Hypoxia (n = 36)	
	Total number observed	%	Total number observed	%
Normal	70	93	22	61
Minor deficit	5	6	9	25
Major deficit	1	1	5	14

is increased in preterm and, particularly, very low birth weight infants, fetal hypoxia appears to play only a limited and possibly contributory role in conjunction with newborn respiratory complications occurring following delivery in these children.

The nature of the deficits in mature newborns with fetal hypoxia has been examined in 36 newborns with evidence of fetal hypoxia.[67] Serving as controls were 76 mature newborns without evidence of fetal asphyxia. The incidence of deficits in the hypoxic and control groups is outlined in Table 8. There is an increased incidence of both minor and major deficits in the children with fetal hypoxia.

The minor deficits in the hypoxic group included motor developmental delays with a Bayley Physical Developmental Index in the borderline range (70 to 84). There were no cognitive developmental delays in these children. The five children with major deficits all had motor handicaps. These included two with hemiplegia, one with spastic diplegia, and two with severe hypotonia. Cognitive development was in the normal range for two children. However, one child had a minor deficit and two children had major deficits in cognitive development.

VII. DISCUSSION

The laboratory studies of fetal asphyxia in animals have confirmed the relationship between fetal asphyxia and central nervous system injury. These studies have also provided the best understanding of the definitive characteristics of fetal asphyxia leading to specific neuropathology. Acute total asphyxia for periods in excess of 10 min consistently results in neuropathology in surviving animals. However, these lesions are principally in the brain stem, with limited involvement of the cerebral hemispheres. Prolonged partial hypoxia with developing metabolic acidosis over 30 to 120 min and a pH ≤ 6.9 to 7.0 may result in neuropathology. These lesions characteristically involve the white matter of the cerebral hemispheres and the basal ganglia corresponding to the neuropathology of children with cerebral palsy.

The current confusion in regard to the role of asphyxia in the human fetus was stated by Paneth and Stark in 1983. "Although intrapartum fetal asphyxia is established as an important cause of perinatal loss, there is little consensus as to how much of the burden of neurologic handicap in the community is attributable to intrapartum and neonatal asphyxia as measured clinically."[6] Much of this continuing dilemma is due to two factors. The more important has been the lack of an accurate diagnosis of fetal asphyxia. Most clinical epidemiological studies lack a specific diagnosis for fetal asphyxia. The clinical indicators used have limited sensitivities and high false-positive rates. Thus, they do not provide an accurate indication of the association between fetal asphyxia and subsequent handicaps. Second, many prospective follow-up studies have used differing outcome measures of motor and cognitive development.

Nevertheless, epidemiological studies of cerebral palsy and mental retardation, in spite of their limitations, have provided valuable information. These studies have demonstrated prevalence rates per 1000 live births for cerebral palsy of 2, for severe mental retardation of 4, and for mild mental retardation of 10 to 30. There is compelling evidence that the risk factors differ for different handicaps. Different risk factors may be of particular relevance in separate syndromes of cerebral palsy. Socioeconomic and environmental variables have an impact on the extent of mild mental retardation, but are of limited significance in severe mental retardation. The pathogenesis of major and minor cognitive deficits in children with cerebral palsy may be quite different from that in children without cerebral palsy.

It is evident from these studies that major handicaps are due to mechanisms other than fetal asphyxia. Significant components of cerebral palsy are due to central nervous system anomalies, metabolic disturbances, infection, and postnatal complications. However, perinatal complications which include criteria of fetal asphyxia have been observed in up to 50% of the children with cerebral palsy. From 50 to 60% of children with severe mental retardation have genetically determined abnormalities with perinatal complications, including criteria of fetal asphyxia occurring in <10% of the children with severe mental retardation. Present evidence suggests that the principal factors associated with mild mental retardation are genetic defects and environmental deprivation. Perinatal complications have been observed in approximately 15% of children with mild mental retardation in the Swedish studies.

Current epidemiological studies cannot establish the frequency of major handicaps following an episode of fetal asphyxia. The clinical indicator of fetal asphyxia which has been most carefully examined in regard to its relationship to motor and cognitive deficits is the Apgar score of 0 to 3 at 5 min or more following delivery. The incidence of major handicaps in these children has ranged from 5 to 20%. These observations serve to emphasize that many infants who experience a central nervous system insult will not manifest evidence of a major handicap in infancy or childhood.

A fetal blood gas and acid-base assessment provides an accurate measure of the severity of the hypoxic episode at one point in time. The degree of metabolic acidosis in the fetus may be a reflection of a severe hypoxic episode of short duration or a moderate intermittent hypoxic episode of longer duration. This is due to the slow resolution of fetal fixed acids by the placenta or fetal kidneys.[20] There is no single measure which will indicate the duration of the hypoxic episode in the fetus. Serial blood gas and acid-base measures or the continuous recording of pH could provide the answer. However, at the present time, serial scalp samplings are infrequently available, and a pH electrode appropriate for widespread clinical use has yet to be developed. This question must be resolved if an understanding of fetal asphyxia in the human fetus is to be achieved. Although the clinical indicators are not satisfactory for the diagnosis of fetal asphyxia, they are valuable, complementary signs in conjunction with blood gas and acid-base assessment, providing an indication of the biological impact of asphyxial episodes as defined by the blood gas acid-base assessment. This is particularly true for newborn encephalopathy.

Data are now available in regard to the relationship of fetal asphyxia as identified by blood gas and acid-base assessment and motor and cognitive deficits. These data indicate the importance of the duration as well as the severity of the metabolic acidosis. A terminal episode of fetal asphyxia in mature newborns can occur without evidence of subsequent deficit. However, deficits may result if the hypoxic episode has been present for more than 1 h. Thus, the frequency of deficits attributable to fetal asphyxia depends on the definition of significant fetal asphyxia. The criterion of fetal asphyxia in our center, an umbilical artery buffer base concentration <34 mmol/l, occurs in approximately 2% of newborns. The frequency of major and/or minor deficits at 1 year in these infants is on the order of 20%.

Fetal asphyxia as a cause of deficits is a more frequent factor in term than in preterm children. Motor deficits are most frequent. Major deficits present as one of the syndromes of cerebral palsy. However, minor motor handicaps with motor developmental delay at 1 year of age may occur. Major or minor cognitive deficits may occur. These have been observed in association with cerebral palsy. Whether cognitive deficits occur independent of motor deficits following fetal asphyxia is not yet clear. This has not occurred in our experience. Similarly, Broman,[46] in the review of this association in the NCPP, concluded that few were affected and that many occurred in children with motor disabilities.

Progress has been made in regard to our understanding of the relationship and the magnitude of the contribution of fetal asphyxia to motor and cognitive deficits in surviving children. An accurate diagnosis of the degree and duration of fetal asphyxia, with examination of the association with minor as well as major deficits, is required to further our knowledge of this problem.

REFERENCES

1. **Freeman, J. M., Ed.,** Prenatal and Perinatal Factors Associated with Brain Disorders, NIH Publ. No. 85-1149, U.S. Public Health Service, U.S. Department of Health and Human Services, Washington, D.C., 1985, 111.
2. **Little, W. J.,** On the influence of abnormal parturition, difficult labor, premature birth and asphyxia neonatorum on the mental and physical conditions of the child, especially in relation to deformities, *Trans. London Obstet. Soc.,* 3, 293, 1962.
3. **Collier, J. S.,** The pathogenesis of cerebral diplegia in October 1923, in *Proceedings of the Royal Society of Medicine,* MacAllister, J. Y. S., Ed., Langams Green & Co., London, 1924.
4. **Illingsworth, R. S.,** *The Classification, Incidence and Causation of Cerebral Palsy,* Little, Brown, Boston, 1958.
5. **Crothers, B. and Paine, R. S.,** *The National History of Cerebral Palsy,* Harvard University Press, Cambridge, MA, 1959.
6. **Paneth, N. and Stark, R. I.,** Cerebral palsy and mental retardation in relation to indicators of perinatal asphyxia, an epidemiologic overview, *Am. J. Obstet. Gynecol.,* 147, 960, 1983.
7. **Ranck, J. B. and Windle, W. F.,** Brain damage in the monkey, *Muccaca mulatta* by asphyxia neonatorum, *Exp. Neurol.,* 1, 130, 1959.
8. **Faro, M. G. and Windle, W. F.,** Transneuronal degeneration in brain of monkeys asphyxiated at birth, *Exp. Neurol.,* 24, 38, 1969.
9. **Windle, W. F.,** Brain damage at birth: functional and structural modifications with time, *JAMA,* 206, 1967, 1968.
10. **Malamud, N.,** Sequelae of perinatal trauma, *J. Neuropathol. Exp. Neurol.,* 18, 141, 1959.
11. **Myers, R. E.,** Atrophic cortical necrosis associated with status marmoratus in perinatally damaged monkey, *Neurology,* 19, 1177, 1969.
12. **Myers, R. E., Beard, R., and Adamson, K.,** Brain swelling in the newborn rhesus monkey following prolonged partial asphyxia, *Neurology,* 19, 1012, 1969.
13. **Myers, R. E.,** Fetal Asphyxia and Perinatal Brain Damage Affecting Human Development, PAHO Publ. No. 185, Pan American Health Organization, Washington, D.C., 1969, 205.
14. **Myers, R. E., Wagner, K. R., and DeCourten, G. M.,** Lactic acid accumulation in tissue as a cause of brain injury and death in cardiogenic shock from asphyxia, in *Clinical Perinatal Biochemical Monitoring,* Lauersen, N. and Hochberg, H. M., Eds., Williams & Wilkins, Baltimore, 1981, 11.
15. **Ting, P., Pamaguchi, S., Bache, J. G., Killens, R. H., and Myers, R. E.,** Hypoxic-ischemic cerebral necrosis in mid-gestational sheep fetuses: physiologic correlations, *Exp. Neurol.,* 80, 227, 1983.
16. **Clapp, J. F., Mann, L. I., Peress, N. S., and Szeto, H. H.,** Neuropathology in the chronic fetal lamb preparation: structure-function correlates under different environmental conditions, *Am. J. Obstet. Gynecol.,* 141, 973, 1981.
17. **Low, J. A.,** Maternal and fetal blood gas and acid-base metabolism, in *Scientific Foundations of Obstetrics and Gynaecology,* Barnes, J., Newton, M., and Phillipp, E. E., Eds., Heinemann, London, 1986, 254.
18. **Soothill, P. W., Nicolaides, K. H., Rodeck, C. H., and Gamser, H.,** Blood gases and acid-base status of the human second trimester fetus, *Obstet. Gynecol.,* 68, 173, 1986.
19. **Low, J. A., Pancham, S. R., Worthington, G., and Boston, R. W.,** Acid-base, lactate and pyruvate characteristics of the normal obstetric patient and fetus during the intrapartum period, *Am. J. Obstet. Gynecol.,* 120, 862, 1974.

20. **Low, J. A., Pancham, S. R., Piercy, W. N., Worthington, D., and Karchmar, E. J.,** Maternal and fetal lactate characteristics during labor and delivery, in *Lactate in Acute Conditions,* Bressart, H. and Karger, C., Eds., S. Karger, Basel, 1978, 257.

21. **Low, J. A., Cox, M. J., Karchmar, E. J., McGrath, M. J., Pancham, S. R., and Piercy, W. N.,** The prediction of intrapartum fetal metabolic acidosis by fetal heart rate monitoring, *Am. J. Obstet. Gynecol.,* 139, 299, 1981.

22. **Low, J. A., Pancham, S. R., and Worthington, G.,** Intrapartum fetal heart rate profiles with and without fetal asphyxia, *Am. J. Obstet. Gynecol.,* 127, 729, 1977.

23. **Volpe, J. J.,** *Neurology of the Newborn,* W.B. Saunders, Philadelphia, 1981.

24. **Nelson, K. B. and Ellenberg, J. H.,** Neonatal signs as predictors of cerebral palsy, *Pediatrics,* 64, 225, 1979.

25. **Low, J. A., Galbraith, R. S., Muir, D. W., Killen, H. L., Pater, E. A., and Karchmar, E. J.,** The predictive significance of biological risk factors for deficits in children of a high risk population, *Am. J. Obstet. Gynecol.,* 145, 1059, 1983.

26. **Scott, H.,** Outcome of very severe birth asphyxia, *Arch. Dis. Child.,* 51, 712, 1976.

27. **Hill, A. and Volpe, J. J.,** Seizures, hypoxic-ischemic brain injury and intraventricular hemorrhage in the newborn, *Ann. Neurol.,* 10, 109, 1981.

28. **Low, J. A., Galbraith, R. S., Muir, D. W., Killen, H. L., Pater, E. A., and Karchmar, E. J.,** The relationship between perinatal hypoxia and newborn encephalopathy, *Am. J. Obstet. Gynecol.,* 152, 256, 1985.

29. **Kiely, J., Paneth, N., Stein, Z. A., and Susse, M. S.,** Cerebral palsy and newborn care. I. Secular trends in cerebral palsy, *Dev. Med. Child Neurol.,* 23, 533, 1981.

30. **Woods, G. E.,** A lower incidence of infantile cerebral palsy, *Dev. Med. Child Neurol.,* 5, 449, 1963.

31. **Griffiths, M. I. and Barrett, N. M.,** Cerebral palsy in Birmingham, *Dev. Med. Child Neurol.,* 9, 33, 1967.

32. **Gudmundsson, G.,** Cerebral palsy in Iceland, *Acta Neurol. Scand. Suppl.,* Vol. 34, 1967.

33. **Hagberg, B., Hagberg, G., and Olow, I.,** The changing panorama of cerebral palsy in Sweden 1954—1970. I. Analysis of general changes, *Acta Paediatr. Scand.,* 65, 187, 1975.

34. **Glenting, P.,** Variations in the population of congenital (pre and perinatal) cases of cerebral palsy in Danish countries east of the Little Belt during the years 1950—1969, *Ugeskr. Laeg.,* 138, 2984, 1976.

35. **Nelson, K. B. and Ellenburg, J. H.,** Epidemiology of cerebral palsy, in *Advances in Neurology,* Schomberg, B. L., Ed., Raven Press, New York, 1978, 421.

36. **Cussen, G. H., Barey, J. E., Maloney, A. M., Buckley, N. M., Crowley, M., and Daly, C.,** Cerebral palsy: a regional study, *Ir. Med. J.,* 71, 568, 1978.

37. **Stanley, F. J.,** An epidemiology study of cerebral palsy in Western Australia 1956—1975. I. Changes in total cerebral palsy incidence and associated factors, *Dev. Med. Child Neurol.,* 21, 701, 1979.

38. **Hagberg, B., Hagberg, G., and Olow, I.,** Gains and hazards of intensive neonatal care: an analysis from Swedish cerebral palsy epidemiology, *Dev. Med. Child Neurol.,* 24, 13, 1982.

39. **Nelson, K. B. and Ellenberg, J. H.,** Neonatal signs as predictors of cerebral palsy, *Pediatrics,* 64, 225, 1979.

40. **Kyllerman, M.,** Diskinetic cerebral palsy. II. Pathogenic risk factors and intrauterine growth, *Acta Paediatr. Scand.,* 71, 557, 1982.

41. **Veelken, N., Hagberg, B., Hagberg, G., and Olow, I.,** Diplegia cerebral palsy in Swedish term and preterm children. Differences in reduced optimality, relations to neurology and pathogenetic factors, *Neuropediatrics,* 14, 20, 1983.

42. **Stein, Z. A. and Susser, M. W.,** Mental retardation, in *Public Health and Preventive Medicine,* Last, J. M., Ed., Appleton-Century-Crofts, New York, 1980.

43. **Gustavson, K. H., Hagberg, B., Hagberg, G., and Sars, K.,** Severe mental retardation in a Swedish country. I. Epidemiology, gestational age, birth weight and associated CNS handicaps in children born 1959—70, *Acta Paediatr. Scand.,* 66, 373, 1977.

44. **Hagberg, B., Hagberg, G., Lewerth, A., and Landberg, U.,** Mild mental retardation in Swedish school children. I. Prevalence, *Acta Paediatr. Scand.,* 70, 440, 1981.

45. **Hagberg, B., Hagberg, G., Lewerth, A., and Landberg, U.,** Mild mental retardation in Swedish school children. II. Etiologic and pathogenetic aspects, *Acta Paediatr. Scand.,* 70, 445, 1981.

46. **Broman, S.,** Perinatal anoxia and cognitive development in early childhood, in *Infants Born at Risk,* Field, T., Sostek, A. M., and Goldberg, S., Eds., Spectrum Publications, New York, 1979.

47. **Drage, J. S., Kennedy, C., Berendes, H., Schwarz, B. K., and Weiss, W.,** The Apgar score as an index of infant morbidity. A report from the collaborative study of cerebral palsy, *Dev. Med. Child Neurol.,* 8, 141, 1966.

48. **Broman, S. H., Nicholas, P. L., and Kennedy, W. A.,** *Preschool IQ: Prenatal and Early Developmental Correlates,* Erlbaum, Hillsdale, NJ, 1975.

49. **Nelson, K. B. and Broman, S. H.,** Perinatal risk factors in children with serious motor and mental handicaps, *Ann. Neurol.,* 2, 371, 1977.

50. **Nelson, K. B. and Ellenberg, J. H.,** Neonatal signs as predictors of cerebral palsy, *Pediatrics,* 64, 225, 1979.

51. **Nelson, K. B. and Ellenberg, J. H.,** Apgar scores as predictors of chronic neurologic disability, *Pediatrics,* 63, 36, 1981.

52. **Nelson, K. B. and Ellenberg, J. H.,** Obstetric complications as risk factors for cerebral palsy or seizures disorders, *JAMA,* 251, 1843, 1984.

53. **Steiner, H. and Nelligan, G.,** Perinatal cardiac arrest, *Arch. Dis. Child.,* 50, 696, 1975.

54. **Thomson, A. J., Seale, M., and Russell, G.,** Quality of survival after severe birth asphyxia, *Arch. Dis. Child.,* 52, 620, 1977.

55. **Mulligan, J. C., Painter, M. J., O'Donoghue, P. A., MacDonald, H. M., Allen, A. C., and Taylor, I. M.,** Neonatal asphyxia. II. Neonatal mortality and long-term sequelae, *J. Pediatr.,* 96, 903, 1980.

56. **Ergander, V. and Erikson, H.,** Severe neonatal asphyxia, *Acta Paediatr. Scand.,* 72, 321, 1983.

57. **Amiel-Tison, C.,** Cerebral damage in full-term newborns, aetiological factors, neonatal status and long-term follow-up, *Biol. Neonate,* 14, 234, 1969.

58. **Thorn, I.,** Cerebral symptoms in the newborn, diagnostic and prognostic significance of symptoms of presumed cerebral origin, *Acta Paediatr. Scand. Suppl.,* Vol. 1950, 1969.

59. **Rose, A. L. and Lombroso, C. T.,** Neonatal seizure states, a study of clinical pathological and electroencephalographic features in 137 full-term babies with a long-term follow-up, *Pediatrics,* 45, 404, 1970.

60. **Holden, K. R., Mellits, E. D., and Freeman, J. M.,** Neonatal seizures. I. Correlation of prenatal and perinatal events with outcomes, *Pediatrics,* 70, 165, 1982.

61. **Brown, J. K., Purvis, R. J., Forfar, J. O., and Cockburn, F.,** Neurological aspects of perinatal asphyxia, *Dev. Med. Child Neurol.,* 16, 567, 1974.

62. **Fitzhardinge, P. M., Flodmark, O., Fitz, C. R., and Ashby, S.,** The prognostic value of computed tomography as an adjunct to assessment of the term infant with post asphyxial encephalopathy, *J. Pediatr.,* 99, 777, 1981.

63. **Robertson, C. and Finer, N.,** Term infants with hypoxic-ischemic encephalopathy: outcome at 3—5 years, *Dev. Med. Child Neurol.,* 27, 473, 1985.

64. **Low, J. A., Galbaith, R. S., Muir, D. W., Broekhoven, L. H., Wilkinson, J. W., and Karchmar, E. J.,** The contribution of fetal-newborn complications to motor and cognitive deficits, *Dev. Med. Child Neurol.,* 27, 578, 1985.

65. **Low, J. A., Galbraith, R. S., Muir, D. W., Killen, H. L., Pater, E. A., and Karchmar, E. J.,** Intrapartum fetal hypoxia: a study of long-term morbidity, *Am. J. Obstet. Gynecol.,* 145, 129, 1983.

66. **Low, J. A., Galbraith, R. S., Muir, D. W., Killen, H. L., Pater, E. A., and Karchmar, E. J.,** Factors associated with motor and cognitive deficits in children after intrapartum fetal hypoxia, *Am. J. Obstet. Gynecol.,* 148, 533, 1984.

67. **Low, J. A., Galbraith, R. S., Muir, D. W., Killen, H. L., Pater, E. A., and Karchmar, E. J.,** Motor and cognitive deficits after intrapartum asphyxia in the mature fetus, *Am. J. Obstet. Gynecol.,* 158, 356, 1988.

Chapter 3

LONG-TERM FOLLOW-UP OF INFANTS EXPOSED TO RITODRINE *IN UTERO*

Dianne Polowczyk and Niels H. Lauersen

TABLE OF CONTENTS

I. INTRODUCTION

Ritodrine, a betasympathomimetic drug, is presently the only Food and Drug Administration (FDA)-approved medication for the treatment of premature labor. It is widely used in the U.S. and throughout the world. As the demand for control of premature labor continues, the use of ritodrine is expected to rise. While ritodrine's efficacy as a tocolytic agent has been well established,[1,2] the consequences of human *in utero* exposure have not been well known until recently.

Studies assessing the effect of ritodrine on the fetus are few, and they yield some interesting and conflicting data. Thiery et al.[3] found that babies born after ritodrine exposure were heavier and taller than control infants. No significant differences were found between the experimental and control groups with respect to Apgar scores in that study. Seidel et al.,[4] on the other hand, found no significant difference in birth weight between ritodrine-exposed and control infants. The studies of Karlsson et al.[5] also revealed no significant difference in birth weight or Apgar score between infants delivered of mothers successfully treated with ritodrine and those of normal controls. Huisjes and Touwen[6] compared ritodrine-exposed infants born at term with matched controls and found no difference in umbilical pH, Apgar score, head circumference, and neonatal neurological condition. Some studies have shown an increase in respiratory distress syndrome (RDS) in newborns exposed to ritodrine[7] or an increase in the severity of RDS without the classical signs of hyaline membrane disease.[8] Other researchers, however, have found a decrease in RDS after treatment with ritodrine.[9,10] Rosanelli and co-workers[11] found that 4 out of 18 babies exposed to ritodrine showed postnatal hypoglycemia, a well-known association of the high glucose levels in ritodrine-treated mothers.

The only studies, prior to our own, tracing ritodrine-exposed infants beyond the neonatal stage were those of Karlsson et al.[5] and Freyz et al.[12] Karlsson's study followed ritodrine-exposed infants through 18 months of age in a comparison of three betamimetic agents: isoxsuprine, ritodrine, and terbutaline. The study found no evidence of retarded growth at 18 months of age in any group. Freyz studied children from 12 to 36 months of age. Using the Denver Screening Test and the mothers' reports of developmental milestones, the progress of 42 children was assessed. This study found no significant difference between experimental and control groups on the dependent measures. However, there were actual, though small, differences in attainment of developmental milestones. The ritodrine-exposed group reached milestones at a later date than the control group subjects.

Control for the long-term effect of ritodrine on the development of exposed children arises from the knowledge of the cardiovascular and metabolic side effects of ritodrine to the mothers. Ritodrine-exposed mothers develop more than average hypotension[2,13] and show increased glucose[14-16] and lactate levels.[17] It is known that these situations may compromise fetal brain development.

Although ritodrine is not used clinically in early pregnancy during embryonic organogenesis, this drug is used at a time when vital fetal neurological development is still taking place. Ritodrine is used mainly between the 24th and 34th weeks of gestation, when the brain is undergoing its second growth spurt[18] (Figure 1). This growth spurt begins at mid-pregnancy and continues into the third year of life. During this time, neuroblasts form, glial cells multiply, and myelinization continues, as do the branching of dendrites and formation of synapses. Current theory suggests that any growth-restricting or toxic effects at this time of development will result in permanent structural and behavioral defects.[19,20]

In view of the possible fetal effects of ritodrine and the paucity of data about its long-term effects, the authors studied children who were exposed to ritodrine *in utero* when their mothers participated in a collaborative study during the years 1974 to 1976. The original study compared the effects of ritodrine and ethanol in preventing premature labor and involved

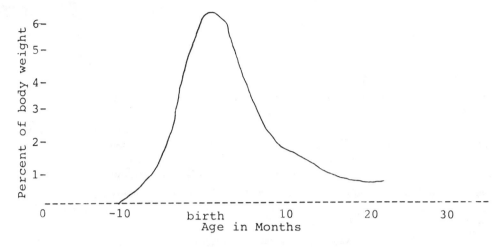

FIGURE 1. Perinatal human brain growth spurt.[19]

TABLE 1
Table of Demographic Characteristics

	Experimental		Control		
	Mean	**SD**	**Mean**	**SD**	*p*
Age	8.34	0.66	8.94	0.62	NS
Gestational age at birth (weeks)	38.10	0.59	37.85	0.62	NS
Birth weight (g)	2690.35	655.32	2793.05	682.46	NS
Race (black/white)	12/8		12/8		NS
Sex (male/female)	10/10		10/10		NS
Socioeconomic status[a]	3.75	0.91	2.85	0.76	0.025

Note: NS = not significant; SD = standard deviation.

[a] Hollingshead two-factor index — a higher score denotes a lower socioeconomic status.

medical centers in the metropolitan New York area (New York Hospital and the Nassau County Medical Center).[2]

II. MATERIALS AND METHODS

Between 1974 and 1976 at the Nassau County Medical Center and New York Hospital, 100 women who were in premature labor participated in a study designed to assess the effects of ethanol and ritodrine as tocolytic agents. As a part of that study, 49 mothers and their fetuses were exposed to ritodrine. A total of 43 of the infants were delivered and lived. For the follow-up study, 20 of these 43 mothers were contacted, and all 20 agreed to participate in the study of long-term effects of *in utero* ritodrine exposure. At the time of the author's study, the children ranged in age from 7 to 9 years, with a mean of 8.64. Each experimental subject was matched with a control from the same population on the basis of sex, race, gestational age (±2 weeks), and birth weight (±500 g). In each group, 14 came from New York Hospital and 6 from the Nassau County Medical Center. Mothers of these children were both clinic and private patients (Table 1).

Each subject was given a battery of psychological tests by a licensed school psychologist to determine functioning in the areas of intelligence, visual motor ability, and academic achievement. Socioemotional adjustment was determined by a personality inventory filled out by the mother. A pediatric examination was given to each child by a licensed pediatrician. It included measures of overall general health, neurologic assessment (cranial nerves, motor/ sensory, and cerebellar functions), and growth factors of height and weight (reported in percentiles from height and weight charts in the *Textbook of Pediatrics*[21]). The group membership (ritodrine-exposed or control) was not known to the examiners.

Intellectual functioning was measured by the Wechsler Intelligence Scale for Children — Revised (WISC-R).[22] The WISC-R is based on Wechsler's view that intelligence is a person's overall capacity to understand and cope with the surrounding world and that, as a global entity, intelligence is multifaceted and multidetermined. The WISC-R is a widely used, standardized, individually administered test. There are 12 subtests which measure various factors contributing to intelligence. Five of these subtests contribute to the determination of verbal IQ and five are used to determine the performance IQ. Two tests are supplementary. Subtest raw scores are converted into scale scores with a mean of 10. Three IQ scores are thus obtained: verbal IQ, performance IQ, and full-scale IQ.

Visual motor functioning was measured by the Koppitz visual motor perceptual age score on the Bender-Gestalt Visual Motor Test, a widely used clinical test originally developed by Loretta Bender in 1938.[23] The Koppitz developmental age scoring system is based on data from over 1100 public school children aged 5 to 10 years. This score was expressed in percentiles in our study.

Academic achievement was measured by the Peabody Individual Achievement Test (PIAT). The mathematics and word reading recognition tests were administered. The PIAT is a wide-range academic screening measure. It gives an overview of scholastic attainment and measures academic ability from kindergarten through 12th grade. A total of 2800 students were included in its standardization. Scores in this study were expressed in percentiles of normative scores.

A Personality Inventory for Children (PIC) was used as a measure of social and emotional adjustment. This scale requires that parents rate their children's behavior by responding to a total of 600 questions. The responses are transformed to provide a 16-scale clinical profile. The empirical scales were devised using the method of contrasting groups as in the construction of the Minnesota Multiphasic Personality Inventory, and other scales were devised using a content-oriented strategy. Seven scales most highly correlated with neurological impairment were used: hyperactivity, withdrawal, social skills, achievement, adjustment, and intellectual screening and development. Scores over 70 were considered pathological.

Socioeconomic status was determined by Hollingshead's[24] two-factor index on all subjects. This method incorporated the level of education and the profession of the parents into a formula. A score was derived that was equal to social classes ranging from I to V. Lower numbers indicate higher socioeconomic status.

Since it was demonstrated that socioeconomic status was significantly correlated with dependent and independent measures, results were analyzed by one-way analysis of covariance, using socioeconomic status as the covariate. In addition, the actual numbers of children with abnormal results in both the ritodrine and control groups were compared by a chi-square with Yates modification when applicable. A value of $p \leq 0.05$ was considered significant.

III. RESULTS

Socioeconomic status was found to be significantly higher in the control group (2.85 = middle class) as compared to the ritodrine group (3.75 = working class); $p = 0.25$ and was significantly related to 7 of the 13 dependent measures. Socioeconomic status, therefore, was used as a covariate in all the analyses.

TABLE 2
Means, Standard Deviations, F Ratios for Growth, and Intellectual Measures

	Experimental		Control			
	Adjusted mean	SD	Adjusted mean	SD	F	p
Height (percentile)	40.66	34.67	57.40	32.40	1.82	0.187 (NS)
Weight (percentile)	38.94	32.28	57.78	29.37	2.71	0.110 (NS)
WISC-R						
FSIQ	107.80	14.97	116.30	18.23	1.11	0.298 (NS)
VIQ	107.84	18.19	116.10	19.82	0.52	0.475 (NS)
PIQ	106.47	11.56	113.35	16.19	1.39	0.247 (NS)
VMI	41.37	22.96	40.83	24.70	0.01	0.945 (NS)
PIAT						
Reading (percentile)	52.84	29.62	64.25	24.01	0.39	0.538 (NS)
Mathematics (percentile)	50.39	30.70	53.81	30.26	0.19	0.664 (NS)

Note: NS = not significant; SD = standard deviation; FSIQ = full-scale intelligence quotient; VIQ = verbal intelligence quotient; PIQ = performance intelligence quotient; VMI = visual-motor integration; PIAT = Peabody Individual Achievement Test; F = one-way analysis of covariance with socioeconomic status as covariate.

TABLE 3
Deviation of Subjects from the Norm

	Ritodrine (20) no.	Control (20) no.	p^{a}
FSIQ[b]	2	1	NS
VIQ[b]	3	0	NS
PIQ[b]	0	0	NS
VMI (20th percentile)	5	8	NS
PIAT (20th percentile)			
Reading	2	1	NS
Mathematics	4	2	NS
PIC (70T)	2	0	NS

Note: NS = not significant; FSIQ = full-scale intelligence quotient; VIQ = verbal intelligence quotient; PIQ = performance intelligence quotient; VMI = Visual-Motor Integration; PIAT = Peabody Individual Achievement Test; PIC = Personality Inventory for Children.

[a] χ^{2} test.
[b] 90 IQ.

Although the test scores were generally higher in the control group, there were no statistically significant differences between the ritodrine and control groups in height, weight, intelligence, visual-motor coordination, and academic achievement after correction for socioeconomic class (Table 2). Additionally, there were no differences in the numbers of cases that deviated from generally accepted norms (Table 3).

Similarly, there were no significant differences between the two groups in any of the personality factors assessed, although most measures showed higher mean scores (indicating greater pathology) in the ritodrine group (Table 4).

There was one child in the ritodrine-exposed group who showed mild spastic diplegia with inward deviation of the toes upon walking. No other subject in either group had any

TABLE 4
Means, Standard Deviations, F Ratios for Personality Measures[a]

	Experimental		Control			
	Adjusted mean	SD	Adjusted mean	SD	F[b]	p
Hyperactivity	47.17	7.67	51.99	11.36	1.03	0.322 (NS)
Withdrawal	52.88	12.37	53.45	7.18	0.02	0.890 (NS)
Social skills	51.33	9.44	49.33	7.52	0.05	0.818 (NS)
Achievement	48.95	13.24	45.39	6.66	0.583	0.454 (NS)
Intellectual screening	46.83	10.06	45.33	7.06	2.22	0.152 (NS)
Development	48.05	10.00	42.53	8.73	1.47	0.239 (NS)
Adjustment	64.16	19.61	50.42	8.84	3.69	0.068 (NS)

Note: NS = not significant; SD = standard deviation.

[a] Scores over 70 are considered to be in the pathological range.
[b] F = one-way analysis of covariance with socioeconomic status as covariate.

neurologic deficit. One ritodrine experimental subject showed delayed growth and development for his age. He was twin B in a set of successfully delivered twins. In contrast to his twin brother, who was well from birth, twin B spent 3 months in treatment for RDS.

IV. DISCUSSION

There were no significant differences between the experimental and control groups in any category of testing when the effects of socioeconomic status were taken into account. Some aspects and limitations of our study, however, need to be discussed. Of concern are the significantly higher socioeconomic status scores in the control group. This may reflect the fact that premature labor is more common in lower social classes. Additionally, it may be an artifact in the study reflecting the process by which control subjects were recruited. Control subjects of higher socioeconomic levels were easier to locate than their poorer counterparts, since they more frequently maintained the same residence and telephone number several years after discharge from the hospital than those in the lower socioeconomic status groups. In this way, a disproportionate number of upper- and middle-class children may have become members of the control groups.

While our ritodrine children seem to be a well-functioning group (an IQ of 104 is slightly above the expected for a working-class population), there were insignificantly but consistently poorer scores in the ritodrine group, even after correction for socioeconomic status. Additionally, large standard deviations were found in many measures, indicating considerable within-group variation. In such cases, significance is hard to obtain. For example, there was a difference of 8.5 points between the experimental and control groups in full-scale IQs. A difference of this magnitude is frequently considered significant; however, with an SD of 17.57 and a small sample size, significance was not found.

In measuring subtle differences between groups, as when measuring central nervous system functioning, large sample sizes may be needed to demonstrate an effect, and admittedly our sample size was small. In this connection, it is interesting to look at a larger study by Hadders-Algra et al.[25] These authors studied 78 6-year-old children exposed to ritodrine treatment prenatally and compared them with matched controls. No significant differences were found in urinalysis, body length, body weight, head circumference, neurological findings, and general behavior as perceived by parents and teachers. School performance, however, as rated by their teachers, was poorer in the ritodrine group, and the authors noted a remarkably smaller number of bright students in the ritodrine group.

Interpretation of poorer findings in ritodrine-exposed children as opposed to matched controls requires consideration of other factors. For example, it might be argued that there were factors causing some women to go into premature labor which were absent from the matched controls' mothers. It may be that these factors (poorer nutrition, greater stress, etc.) contributed to the poorer performance of the offspring.

V. CONCLUSION

While our study found no significant differences between ritodrine-exposed children and matched controls, the need for ongoing studies of this nature remains, since it cannot be said with certainty that there are no untoward effects of ritodrine on the neurological development of children exposed to this drug *in utero* until larger populations of such children have been evaluated.

REFERENCES

1. **Wesselius-deCasparis, A., Theiry, M., Yo Le Sian, A., et al.,** Results of a double-blind, multicentre study with ritodrine premature labour, *Br. Med. J.,* 3, 144, 1971.
2. **Lauersen, N. H., Merkatz, I. R., Tejani, N., Wilson, K. H., Roberson, A., Mann, L. I., and Fuchs, R.,** Inhibition of premature labor: a multicenter comparison of ritodrine and ethanol, *Am. J. Obstet. Gynecol.,* 127, 837, 1977.
3. **Thiery, M., Baumgarten, K., Brosesn, I., et al.,** A multicentre trial with ritodrine in the treatment of premature labour in patients with intact membranes, in *Proceedings of the International Symposium on the Treatment of Foetal Risks,* Baumgarten, K. and Wesselius-deCasparis, A., Eds., Vienna, 1973, 61.
4. **Seidel, A., Baumgarten, K., Eisner, R., Frohlich, H., Gruber, W., and Urban, G.,** Auswirkung der Ritodrine behandlung auf das Kindesgewicht, in *Proceedings of the International Symposium on the Treatment of Foetal Risks,* Baumgarten, K. and Wesselius-deCasparis, A., Eds., Vienna, 1973, 61.
5. **Karlsson, K., Krantz, M., and Hamberger, L.,** Comparison of various betamimetics on preterm labor, survival and development of the child, *J. Perinat. Med.,* 8, 19, 1980.
6. **Huisjes, H. J. and Touwen, B. C. L.,** Neonatal outcome after treatment with ritodrine, *Am. J. Obstet. Gynecol.,* 147, 250, 1983.
7. **Kristoffersen, K. and Hansen, M. K.,** The condition of the foetus and infant in cases treated with ritodrine, *Dan. Med. Bull.,* 26, 121, 1979.
8. **Larsen, J. F., Hansen, M. K., Hesseldahl, H., Kristoffersen, K., Larsen, P. K., Osler, M., Weber, J., Eldon, K., and Lange, A.,** Ritodrine in the treatment of premature labor, *Br. J. Obstet. Gynaecol.,* 87, 949, 1980.
9. **Boog, G., Grahim, M. B., and Gandar, R.,** Betamimetic drugs and possible prevention of respiratory distress syndrome, *Br. J. Obstet. Gynaecol.,* 82, 285, 1975.
10. **Lauersen, N. H.,** Managing premature labor, *Perinat. Care,* 1(2), 15, 1977.
11. **Rosanelli, K., Lichtenegger, W., and Werb, P.,** The effect of tocolysis by means of betamimetics on fetuses and neonates, *Z. Geburtschilfe Perinatol.,* 186, 93, 1982.
12. **Freyz, H., Willard, D., Lehr, A., et al.,** A long-term evaluation of infants who received a betamimetic *in utero, J. Perinat. Med.,* 5, 94, 1977.
13. **Lauersen, N. H.,** Tocolytic drugs and the cardiac patient, in *Cardiac Problems in Pregnancy,* Elkayam, U. and Gleicher, N., Eds., Alan R. Liss, New York, 1979, 273.
14. **Spellacy, W. N., Cruz, A. C., Buhi, W. C., and Birk, S. A.,** The acute effects of ritodrine infusion on maternal metabolism: measurement of levels of glucose, insulin, glucagon, triglycerides, cholesterol, placental lactogen and chorionic gonadotrophin, *Am. J. Obstet. Gynecol.,* 131(6), 637, 1978.
15. **Kirkpatrick, C., Quenon, M., and Desir, D.,** Blood anions and electrolytes during ritodrine infusion in preterm labor, *Am. J. Obstet. Gynecol.,* 138, 523, 1980.
16. **Schreyer, O., Caspi, E., Arieli, S., Maor, J., and Modai, D.,** Metabolic effects of intravenous ritodrine infusion in pregnancy, *Acta Obstet. Gynecol. Scand.,* 59, 1997, 1980.
17. **Osler, M.,** Side effects of metabolic changes during treatment with betamimetics (Ritodrine), *Dan. Med. Bull.,* 26, 119, 1979.
18. **Dobbins, J. and Sands, J.,** Quantitative growth and development of the human brain, *Arch. Dis. Child.,* 48, 757, 1973.

19. **Barlow, S. M. and Sullivan, F. M.,** Behavioral teratology, in *Teratology, Trends and Applications,* Berry, C. L. and Poswillo, D. E., Eds., Springer-Verlag, New York, 1975.

20. **Dobbins, J.,** in *Teratology, Trends and Applications,* Berry, C. L. and Poswillo, D. E., Eds., Springer-Verlag, New York, 1975, 107.

21. **Vaughan, V. C., McKay, R. J., and Nelson, W. E., Eds.,** *Textbook of Pediatrics,* W.B. Saunders, Philadelphia, 1975.

22. **Wechsler, D.,** Manual for the Wechsler Intelligence Scale for Children, Revised, Psychological Corporation, New York, 1974.

23. **Koppitz, E. M.,** *The Bender-Gestalt Test for Young Children,* Grune & Stratton, New York, 1963.

24. **Hollingshead, A. B. and Redlich, F. C.,** *Social Class and Mental Illness, a Community Study,* John Wiley & Sons, New York, 1958.

25. **Hadders-Algra, M., Touwen, B. C. H., and Huisjes, H. J.,** Long-term follow-up of children prenatally exposed to ritodrine, *Br. J. Obstet. Gynaecol.,* 93, 156, 1986.

Chapter 4

FOLLOW-UP OF ETHANOL-EXPOSED CHILDREN

Florence E. Sisenwein and Nergesh Tejani

TABLE OF CONTENTS

I. INTRODUCTION

Over the past 20 years, the concern of the medical profession has shifted somewhat from the mother during pregnancy and childbirth to her offspring.[1] While maternal mortality has reached an unprecedented low, the number of perinatal deaths, although decreasing, is still relatively high.[2]

A significant cause of perinatal death is prematurity, accounting for about 75% of all infant mortality.[3] Additionally, the low birth weight neonate is at risk for abnormal neurological and psychological development.[4] Major emphasis has, therefore, been placed on identifying both the causes of preterm labor and the means to control it.

As recently as 1980, however, no drug had been approved by the Food and Drug Administration (FDA) for this purpose. In the absence of FDA approval, a number of pharmacological agents were used with relative effectiveness.[5] The potential complications in the use of these medications are generally agreed to be less of a threat than the problem of prematurity itself. The goal, of course, is to develop a treatment that will inhibit uterine activity without side effects for either mother or fetus. A completely benign treatment, however, does not now and may never exist.

In the late 1960s, maternal intravenous infusion of ethyl alcohol was found to be effective in arresting preterm labor. In a controlled study, Zlatnick and Fuchs[6] found that this procedure successfully postponed delivery in 80% of the women treated. With the availability of beta agonists, magnesium sulfate, and other tocolytic agents, the use of ethyl alcohol was discontinued in 1980.

A. HISTORICAL USE OF ETHANOL IN OBSTETRICS

The use of alcohol for the relief of pain, both physical and psychic, is as old as man's discovery of the euphoria-inducing and analgesic properties of the fermented products of grape and grain. Similarly, we must suppose that the use of alcohol as a home remedy for the pain of childbirth stretches back into the mists of prehistory.

Belinkoff and Hall[7] pointed to the frequent use of intravenous alcohol to relieve postoperative pain as an indication for its obstetric use as an analgesic. In a study of 20 deliveries, good analgesia was obtained in 80% of the cases, although some difficulty was experienced in selecting the proper dosage for various subjects.

Chapman and Williams[8] studied 100 cases in which intravenous alcohol was used alone and in combination with Demerol® as an analgesic in labor. As with the Belinkoff and Hall[7] study, it was found effective as an analgesic, and, apart from nausea and vomiting in the mother, side effects for both mother and infant were found to be negligible.

Both Belinkoff and Hall[7] and Chapman and Williams[8] made reference to the fact that when alcohol was administered too early in labor, uterine contractions stopped or were slowed. The significance of this observation for the problem of premature labor did not appear to have been grasped until Fuchs et al.[9,10] set it in the context of research by Fuchs and Wagner[11,12] which had demonstrated that normal parturition in the rabbit is initiated by the release of oxytocin and that this release (and resultant labor) was inhibited by infusion of ethyl alcohol. The juxtaposition of observations made during the use of alcohol as an obstetric analgesic with research on the role of oxytocin in parturition led Fuchs et al.[9] to investigate the effect of alcohol on threatened preterm labor.

B. MODE OF ACTION OF ETHANOL IN PRETERM LABOR

It is not clear how the tocolytic effect of ethanol is mediated. Beginning with the studies of Fuchs and Wagner[11] on the effect of alcohol on the release of oxytocin by the neurohypophysis in rabbits, a number of investigations have pointed to alcohol having an inhibitory effect on labor, predominantly through suppressing the release of oxytocin from the posterior pituitary into the maternal blood stream.[11] This mode of action was further emphasized because of a failure to observe a direct effect of ethanol on the myometrium in either rabbits or humans.[9,12] However, Bueno-Montano et al.[13] did report a depressant effect of ethanol on the isolated pregnant and nonpregnant myometrium. Wilson et al.[14] further investigated the effect of ethanol on specimens of human myometrium *in vitro*. Their findings indicated that concentrations of ethanol equivalent to the blood levels used to arrest preterm labor or to inhibit the activity of the nonpregnant uterus *in vivo* do not have any effect on the activity of the human myometrium *in vitro*. Much higher concentrations of ethanol were required in order to achieve a sustained effect *in vitro*.

C. USE OF ETHANOL INFUSION TO ARREST PRETERM LABOR

Fuchs et al.[9] provided the first comprehensive report on the use of ethanol to control uterine activity in the second half of pregnancy. A total of 68 patients were treated for threatened preterm labor between the 21st and 36th weeks of pregnancy. Labor was considered imminent when regular, frequent, mild-to-strong contractions were observed for ≥ 1 h.

Two parameters were used to evaluate the effects of alcohol on threatened preterm labor: the initial effect on uterine contractions and the prevention of preterm delivery for ≥ 72 h. An inhibitory effect on uterine contractions was observed in all 68 patients: in 43 cases, contractions ceased completely, and in the remainder there was a clear reduction in intensity and frequency. Delivery was postponed for ≥ 72 h in 35 of the 52 patients with intact membranes, but in none of 16 cases with ruptured membranes. Of the 35 successful cases, 30 carried their pregnancy to the 37th week or beyond. In ten patients with intact membranes and seven with ruptured membranes, labor was arrested initially, but recurred and resulted in delivery within 48 h or in the termination of pregnancy, and these cases were considered equivocal successes. In seven patients with intact membranes and nine with ruptured membranes, delivery took place within 24 h and the result was considered unsuccessful. The 68 pregnancies resulted in the delivery of 74 infants, 4 of which were stillborn and 10 of which died in the neonatal period. Of these deaths, all occurred in infants with a birth weight of ≤ 2100 g. Relevant to the present consideration, the 60 surviving infants were reported to show no immediate adverse effect of the treatment, although each one born during therapy had a blood alcohol concentration at the same level as the mother.

A number of methodological criticisms arise when evaluating this most important study. There is no detailed account of the condition of the newborn infants, which makes it impossible to evaluate the claim that ethanol treatment had no effect on them. No reference is made to the possible effects of variables such as gestational age at the time of therapy. Most importantly, the absence of control cases left in doubt a placebo effect and failed to provide a basis for the comparison of newborn status.

Zlatnick and Fuchs[6] attempted to answer these questions in a randomized study comparing the effects of ethanol with a placebo consisting of 5% glucose in water. A total of 42 patients presenting at a New York hospital with threatened preterm labor were included in the study. Patient selection was more uniform in that women in whom delivery seemed imminent, those whose membranes were ruptured, and those who were actively bleeding or had some other problem which contraindicated the continuation of the pregnancy were excluded. The 42 subjects were randomly assigned to ethanol and placebo groups. They received 15 ml/kg body weight of the assigned solution intravenously over a 2-h period as the loading dose. They then received 1.5 ml/kg/h as a maintenance dose for 6 to 10 h. If labor progressed and delivery seemed imminent, ethanol treatment was stopped. If labor ceased and then recurred, the assigned solution was again administered. Labor was regarded as successfully postponed if delivery did not occur within 72 h.

Randomization ensured that no difference was found between the two groups with regard to age, marital status, race, parity, weeks of gestation, or cervical dilation at the start of the treatment. Of the 21 patients who received ethanol, 81% had delivery postponed for at least 72 h, compared with 38% in the glucose and water group (difference significant at $p < 0.02$). The median postponement gained in the ethanol group was 19 days compared with <1 day in the control group. Excluding multiple births, the median birth weight in the ethanol group was 2490 g, compared with 2000 g in the control group. It is suggested that "successes" in the placebo group were due to false labor. No serious maternal or infant side effects were noted. The Zlatnick and Fuchs study[6] offered clear evidence of the effectiveness of ethanol infusion in the arrest of preterm labor with patients in the early stages of labor. However, its effectiveness in comparison to other pharmacologic agents, specifically ritodrine, was still to be demonstrated.

In response to this question, a randomized, controlled study was carried out at three participating medical centers by Lauersen.[15] He and his co-investigators randomly assigned 135 women to one of two groups, ethanol or ritodrine. Success in this study was defined as postponement of delivery for >72 h and was achieved in 73% of the ethanol group and in 90% of the ritodrine group (difference significant at $p < 0.05$). The initial intravenous infusion of both ethanol and ritodrine resulted in a reduction or complete cessation of labor in all subjects. Among all successfully treated patients, ritodrine administration resulted in a significantly longer gain in days (48.9 vs. 36.5).

With regard to perinatal outcome, there were no stillbirths in either group. Of the singletons, 88% survived in the ethanol group and 95% in the ritodrine group. Among singleton pregnancies, 45% of the ethanol-treated group and 72% of the ritodrine-treated group had birth weights in excess of 2500 g ($p < 0.01$). Seven infants died in the ethanol group and three in the ritodrine group. Of the 76 infants born to ethanol-treated mothers, 15 developed respiratory distress syndrome and 5 died. Of the 73 infants born to ritodrine-treated mothers, 6 developed respiratory distress syndrome and 1 died. No comparative long-term information was available on the children.

D. EFFECTS ON FETUS AND NEWBORN

In a study of the placental transfer of ethanol and its elimination in 23 normal pregnant patients,[16] it was found that ethanol in small doses (1.2 to 4 g) injected intravenously into the mother from 1 to 2 min before delivery traverses the placenta and is present in the neonate's bloodstream in 1 min or less. Traces of ethanol were still present 24 h after delivery in serum samples from 5 of 17 mothers and from 1 of 17 infants. In 22 of 23 patients, serum ethanol levels in the umbilical vein and artery were consistently lower than or equal to those in simultaneously drawn maternal venous blood. With the dose of ethanol employed, no ill effects were observed in the newborn, as judged by 1- and 5-min Apgar scores and their later clinical course.

After infusing ethanol in six mothers from 90 min to $3^1/_2$ h prior to delivery, Indanpaan-Heikkila et al.[17] studied placental transfer and elimination as well as the clinical and metabolic effects of ethanol on the mother, fetus, and neonate. After 30 min of infusion a lower blood alcohol level was present in the fetus than the mother, but after 1 h this difference had disappeared. It was found that elimination in the neonate was about twice as slow as in the mother. Acid-base balance, blood glucose levels, and serum insulin concentrations in the fetus and newborn did not show any conclusive changes. It should be noted, however, that in this study, as well as that of Waltman and Iniquez,[16] the intent was not to prevent delivery, so lower concentrations of ethanol were used than for tocolysis.

Zervoudakis et al.[18] presented a retrospective study of 165 infants whose deliveries followed pregnancies in which ethanol was used to inhibit preterm labor. Only infants deemed appropriate for gestational age were studied. A control case was selected for each infant and matched for intactness of membranes, gestational age, and methods of anesthesia and delivery; they were not, however, matched for maternal socioeconomic status (SES) and race. With regard to neonatal mortality, there was no statistical difference between study and control infants or with respect to 5-min Apgar scores. Study patients had a higher incidence of respiratory distress syndrome than controls, and it was concluded by the authors that ethanol administration carried a significant risk to the immature fetus if delivery took place <12 h after the infusion was completed.

It appears, therefore, that if the ethanol therapy does not seem to be successful, it must be terminated immediately to allow as much time as possible to elapse before delivery so that the burden of metabolizing the alcohol can be assumed by the mother. Since the enzyme alcohol dehydrogenase is present in very small amounts in the preterm fetus, sustained effects of central nervous system depression, respiratory distress, hypoglycemia, and excessive loss of body heat have been described.[17,19] Others have noted additional sequelae in the immediate neonatal period in areas as diverse as cardiac and respiratory performance,[20] abnormal bone morphology,[21] elevated bilirubin levels.[22] glucose metabolism,[23] and acid-base balance.[24]

Despite widespread use of this technique with potentially negative outcomes, the research literature reveals only a few studies of short-term effects and no follow-up studies of older children whose mothers were given therapeutic doses of alcohol during pregnancy. The literature is replete with studies on the fetal effects of chronic alcohol abuse in mothers, but this issue constitutes a separate problem. Chronic maternal alcohol ingestion during pregnancy has resulted in effects that range from growth problems to "fetal alcohol syndrome"[25] and increased morbidity and mortality. Little is known, however, about the effects of single, large doses.[26-28]

II. ETHANOL TREATMENT PROTOCOL

A. SELECTION OF CANDIDATES

Candidates for the procedure are women in the 24th to 34th week of gestation with a diagnosis of true progressive labor, as judged by uterine contractions at regular intervals of at least once every 10 min with or without progressive cervical dilation and effacement.

Ethanol was not used where there was evidence of (1) intrauterine growth retardation, (2) third-trimester bleeding, (3) ruptured membranes, (4) fetal abnormality or demise, (5) cervix 5 cm or more dilated, or (6) fetal distress. Generally, if preterm delivery was thought to be protective to a fetus in a comprised intrauterine environment, pharmacological intervention was avoided.

B. TREATMENT PROCEDURE

A loading dose consisting of 15 ml of ethanol per kilogram of body weight in a 9.5% solution of dextrose in water was administered over the first 2 h. A maintenance dose of 1.5 ml of ethanol per kilogram of body weight in a 9.5% solution was administered over the next 10 h. These doses maintained a blood level of about 100 mg%. If labor recurred during therapy, the patient was given modified loading dose followed by a maintenance dose (as described) up to three times, if necessary. Patients were carefully observed, and medication (primarily compazine) was administered to control restlessness, nausea, vomiting, and other associated symptoms of intoxication. If the procedure was successful, the patient was discharged 48 to 72 h after termination of treatment. The entire process might be instituted again if labor recurred before the 34th week of gestation.

C. CURRENT RESEARCH

Our study[29] was undertaken because developmental outcomes of the ethanol infusion treatment had not been systematically explored. The study looked at various parameters of the procedure — maternal blood alcohol levels during treatment, gestational age at time of treatment, number of discrete treatments, degree of intoxication of the fetus (if any) at time of delivery — and attempted to assess their individual impact on subsequent development.

The study assessed the intellectual functioning, academic achievement, perceptual motor skills, personality, and physical status (height, weight, and head circumference) of 4- to 7-year-old children whose mothers received at least one alcohol infusion during gestation to arrest preterm labor.

D. HYPOTHESES

It was hypothesized that when the factors of birth weight, chronological age, gestational age at birth, age at testing, sex, race, socioeconomic status, comparable method of delivery, and anesthesia are controlled for

1. Children born to mothers who were treated with ethanol during pregnancy (Group A) will score lower than children who were not exposed to this treatment (Group B) on measures of intelligence, academic performance, visual-motor skills, personal adjustment, height, weight, and head circumference.
2. Within Group A, children will score lower on tested measures under the following conditions:
    A. Higher maternal blood alcohol levels
    B. Lower gestational age at time of treatment
    C. More than one discrete treatment
    D. Greater degree of intoxication at birth
    E. Lower 1- and 5-min Apgar scores
    F. Smaller physical size at birth (height, weight, and head circumference)
3. A positive correlation between dependent measures and SES will be demonstrated.

III. METHOD

A. SUBJECTS

The subjects for this study were drawn from a population of 4- to 7-year-old children, whose birth weights were appropriate for gestational age, born between the years 1973 and 1977 at the Nassau County Medical Center, East Meadow, New York. A review of the records indicated that 97 infants whose mothers received at least one ethanol infusion to arrest preterm labor were born during these years. Of the 97 live births, there were 87 survivors.

Of the 87 families, 29 responded and agreed to participate in the study. However, four children were not included because they did not meet the "appropriate-for-gestational-age" criterion; four were small for gestational age, and one fell into the large-for-gestational-age category.

A control group of infants whose mothers did not receive ethanol infusions during pregnancy was also identified. They were matched with the 25 ethanol-exposed children for birth weight (± 200 g), gestational age (± 2 weeks), sex, race, SES, age at testing (± 6 months), route of delivery (vaginal vs. cesarean), and type of anesthesia (regional vs. general).

Each of the 25 children in the ethanol group was placed in one of three groups: those children who were exposed to only one ethanol treatment as a result of which labor was successfully arrested and delivery postponed (group A1; $n = 14$), those children for whom the ethanol infusion was unsuccessful and who were born within 15 h of termination of treatment in a condition of intoxication (group A2; $n = 7$), and those children who were exposed to more than one infusion after which labor was arrested and delivery postponed (group A3; $n = 4$). Each member of an ethanol group (A1, A2, or A3) was matched with a control on the variables cited above. The control groups were labeled B1, B2, and B3 to correspond to their ethanol counterparts.

TABLE 1
Patient Characteristics in Groups A and B

Characteristic	Group A Mean	SD	Group B Mean	SD	p Value
Birth weight (g)	2308.6	526.43	2372.88	570.81	NS
Birth height (percentile)	58.68	28.08	61.16	22.69	NS
Birth weight (percentile)	60.92	25.79	55.16	21.20	NS
Birth head circumference (percentile)	59.56	21.02	59.76	21.49	NS
Gestational age at birth	34.6	2.01	35.2	2.67	NS
Apgar score					
1 min	7.60	1.68	8.32	1.08	NS
5 min	9.40	1.00	9.72	0.68	NS
Socioeconomic status score	55.12	3.20	55.56	4.06	NS
Moderate/severe neonatal idiopathic respiratory distress syndrome	4/25		1/25		NS

Note: NS = not significant.

From Sisenwein, F. E., Tejani, N., Boxer, H., and DiGuiseppe, R., *Am. J. Obstet. Gynecol.*, 145, 52, 1983. With permission.

One-way analyses of variance compared each experimental group with its controls on the factors of birth weight, gestational age at birth, age at resting, and SES. No significant differences were found between the experimental groups (A1, 2, and 3) and their controls (B1, 2, and 3). These groups can be considered drawn from the same population for these matching variables (Table 1).

One-way ANOVAs were also used to compare within experimental conditions. Significantly lower birth weights were found both for those children born intoxicated (A2) and those exposed to multiple infusions (A3). The children exposed to a single successful infusion (A1) were born at significantly higher birth weights and spent a longer time *in utero* (increased gestational age at birth).

A question can be raised at this point. If the group exposed to multiple infusions (A3) spent as much time *in utero* as the single infusion group (A1), why were its members born at lower birth weights? The answer may lie in a statistical artifact because of the small sample size of the multiply infused group ($n = 4$) or in the other factors that have a depressant effect on fetal growth. This issue will be discussed later in greater detail.

B. PROCEDURE

All testing was done "blind" to group membership. The independent variables for this study were all taken from hospital records:

1. Physical size at birth (weight, length, and head circumference) — These measures are expressed in percentiles taken from standard charts for the classification of newborns based on maturity and intrauterine growth.
2. Gestational age at the time of ethanol treatment — Gestational age was calculated from the first day of the mother's last menstrual period and was confirmed by clinical examination. Only those children whose intrauterine growth patterns appeared to be appropriate for gestational age were included.
3. The number of discrete times the ethanol procedure was used during the pregnancy
4. Degree of intoxication expressed as the elapsed time between termination of treatment and delivery (≤ 15 h)

The dependent variables being measured for this study were as follows:

1. Intellectual functioning — The Wechsler Intelligence Scale for Children — Revised (WISC-R) was administered to those children who were 6 years of age or older. The downward extension of this test, the Wechsler Preschool and Primary Scales of Intelligence (WPPSI), was given to those children under 6 years of age.
2. Perceptual-motor skills — The Beery-Buktenika Developmental Test of Visual-Motor Integration was administered.
3. Academic performance — The arithmetic and reading (word recognition) subtests of the Wide-Range Achievement Test were used.
4. Personality adjustment — The Personality Inventory for Children was given to the mother. She was asked to rate her child on various dimensions of personality.
5. Physical status — Measurements of height, weight, and head circumference were taken and converted to percentiles on standard growth charts for males and females.

C. DESIGN

The design involved an *ex post facto* experiment first introduced by Chapin and Queen[30] and elaborated on by Greenwood.[31] Typically, *ex post facto* experiments study the effects of a given variable on subsequent outcomes using the original population. Difficulties with this type of research center around control factors. The "solution" to this problem is usually to examine control subjects matched on as many relevant factors as possible and differing only in the original experimental variable. The addition of each matching factor reduces the post-test discrepancy between the x (ethanol) and no-x (nonethanol) groups. If all the matching is effective, significant differences should be related to the original experimental variable.

A final confounding problem in this type of research can be called experimental mortality, or the production of differences between treatment and outcome due to differential drop-out rates of individuals from the original group.[32] Standard practice in this type of research considers at least one third of the original group an acceptable number for experimentation. Exactly one third of the original population agreed to participate in this study.

D. DATA ANALYSIS

Analysis of variance was used to determine the effect of the presence or absence of prenatal exposure to maternal ethanol infusion on the dependent variables. Comparisons were made between the experimental and control groups as well as within the experimental group on the dependent measures.

Stepwise multiple regression analyses were used to sequentially enter the independent variables (physical size at birth, gestational age at time of treatment, maternal blood alcohol levels, etc.) into the computer to determine their contribution to the variance in the dependent variables.[33]

The 0.05 level of significance was adopted in accordance with common convention.[34]

IV. RESULTS

In comparing developmental testing on groups A and B, no significant differences were seen (Table 2), except in visual-motor integration ($p < 0.05$). No significant differences were encountered in any facet of personality testing.

When subgroup A2 was compared with B2, there were no differences in physical factors. However, several problems were encountered in the developmental and personality testing (Table 3). Group A2 functioned at a significantly lower level than group B2 in the categories of performance intelligence quotient ($p < 0.01$), Wide-Range Achievement Test in arithmetic ($p < 0.01$), and visual-motor integration ($p < 0.001$). In addition, personality problems (most significantly, hyperactivity) were noted; the mean score for group A2 was 69.27 (SD = 8.79), as compared to a mean score of 50.00 (SD = 9.24; $p < 0.001$) for group B2. Note that a higher score signifies more pathology.

TABLE 2
Means, Standard Deviations, and Analysis of Variance Comparisons for All Variables: Total Ethanol Group by Total Control Group

Variable	Ethanol (n = 25)		Control (n = 25)		F	p
	Mean	SD	Mean	SD	df (1,48)	
Physical						
At present						
Height[a]	65.00	26.82	69.32	23.98	0.36	NS
Weight[a]	53.36	25.48	65.08	24.54	2.74	NS
Head circumference[a]	53.56	25.58	67.16	26.17	3.45	NS
Performance						
Intellectual ability						
Intelligence quotient						
Verbal	90.68	13.06	92.20	10.99	0.20	NS
Performance	81.83	13.95	89.16	14.94	3.17	NS
Full-scale	86.44	13.54	91.44	11.60	1.97	NS
Academic ability						
Wide-range achievement tests						
Reading[b]	93.24	20.25	102.56	18.13	2.90	NS
Arithmetic[b]	95.16	14.94	104.12	17.80	3.42	NS
Visual-motor integration						
Beery intelligence quotient ratios	85.92	10.70	94.16	13.52	5.71	<0.05
Personality inventory	—	—	—	—	—	NS

Note: NS = not significant.

[a]   Percentiles.
[b]   Standard scores.

From Sisenwein, F. E., Tejani, N., Boxer, H., and DiGuiseppe, R., *Am. J. Obstet. Gynecol.*, 145, 52, 1983. With permission.

Four of seven children with obvious behavior problems had already been identified in school and were in special classes. This result appeared to be unrelated to the incidence of neonatal idiopathic respiratory distress syndrome. There were two cases of severe idiopathic respiratory distress syndrome in group A2, one of which resulted in a child with abnormal developmental testing. There was one severe case of neonatal idiopathic respiratory distress syndrome in control group B2 with a normal outcome. When group A3 was compared with B3, no significant differences were encountered in any category.

V. COMMENT

Animal and human experience has established that there is a theoretical basis for fetal detriment when ethanol is administered to the mother.

The transfer of ethanol across the placenta takes place through a process of simple diffusion.[23,35] There is a direct correlation between maternal and fetal alcohol levels, with fetal levels often exceeding those of the mother within 120 min into the infusion.[23] Indeed, because of inadequate levels of alcohol dehydrogenase in the premature fetal liver, high fetal levels usually persist for several hours after infusion is terminated.[36]

In primate studies, a reduction of umbilical blood flow, fetal hypoxemia, and acidosis as a result of acute ethanol infusion were demonstrated.[37] This finding, however, was not substantiated in the sheep model, in which Dilts[35] found significant changes only in fetal acid-base status. In an acute sheep model, Mann and associates[24] demonstrated significant lactic acidosis, probably as a result of the increased diphosphopyridine nucleotide and reduced

TABLE 3
Means, Standard Deviations, and Analysis of Variance Comparisons for All Variables: Unsuccessful Infusion (Intoxicated) and Control Group

Variable	Intoxicated (A2; $n = 7$)		Intoxicated control (B2; $n = 7$)		F	
	Mean	SD	Mean	SD	df (1,12)	p
Physical						
At present						
Height[a]	66.14	31.32	68.43	27.50	0.02	NS
Weight[a]	60.00	32.48	67.71	33.54	0.16	NS
Head circumference[a]	59.14	32.15	68.86	39.23	0.22	NS
Performance						
Intellectual ability						
Intelligence quotient						
Verbal	91.14	15.94	94.43	11.60	0.17	NS
Performance	75.14	16.69	100.43	11.65	10.81	0.01
Full-scale	83.57	15.67	98.29	11.43	0.09	NS
Academic ability						
Wide-range achievement tests						
Reading[b]	92.29	21.57	109.86	16.23	1.75	NS
Arithmetic[b]	87.57	16.91	106.86	9.97	7.45	0.01
Visual-motor integration						
Beery intelligence quotient ratios	83.29	13.38	105.00	6.66	14.78	0.001
Personality inventory						
Hyperactivity[c]	69.57	8.79	50.00	9.24	16.49	0.001

Note: NS = not significant.

[a]   Percentiles.
[b]   Standard scores.
[c]   A higher score indicates greater pathology.

From Sisenwein, F. E., Tejani, N., Boxer, H., and DiGuiseppe, R., *Am. J. Obstet. Gynecol.,* 145, 52, 1983. With permission.

diphosphopyridine/nucleotide ratio associated with the reduction of ethanol in the liver. No changes were observed in the fetal oxygen tension; however, oxygen content probably decreased because of the shift of the oxygen dissociation curve to the right due to the more acidotic pH. Furthermore, the fetal electroencephalogram showed a reduction and slowing of the record when pharmacological levels were reached.[23]

In another study, isolated helical preparations of the human umbilical artery showed a shift to the left of the log dose response curve to a standard serotonin solution when bathed in dilute ethanol solutions,[38] but not in higher concentrations.[23] All of the above factors may contribute to the compromised long-term outcome in those children born within 15 h of the termination of treatment (group A2).

In humans, it is currently recognized that fetal exposure to chronic maternal ingestion of about 3 oz of absolute alcohol increases the risk of alcohol teratogenicity associated with fetal alcohol syndrome.

The fetal effects of maternal binge drinking in the third trimester are unknown. It is not unreasonable to extrapolate the findings in our study to binge drinking in pregnancy, which therapeutically administered ethanol mimics. One may therefore suspect that if delivery occurs while the mother is still intoxicated, behavioral problems may ensue. If delivery occurs at some time remote from the binge, no alcohol-related fetal effects are to be expected.

All of the above factors may contribute to the compromised long-term outcome in those children born within 15 h of the termination of treatment (group A2).

This is further substantiated in immediate neonatal effects[18] where infants born within 12 h of termination of maternal ethanol infusion demonstrated the most depression of vital signs, leading the authors to conclude that if labor progresses and cannot be arrested, ethanol should be discontinued as soon as possible to allow the maximum amount of time to elapse between termination of treatment and birth.

In the interpretation of the long-term effects of tocolysis with ethanol, severe confounding variables may influence the results. Of greatest significance are the environmental influences on these early years. Maternal SES is a powerful influence on the psychometric performance of the child and should be matched for in control subjects. This is especially important in this study, as it has been shown that mothers of low SES show a higher incidence of low birth weight infants.[39] In addition to SES, our study patients were controlled for factors of gestational age, birth weight, birth weight percentile, sex, race, route of delivery, anesthesia used, and age at testing. In successful cases, one factor that may be of significance and cannot be controlled for is the very fact that the study patient showed signs of preterm labor. Whether this in some way signifies an existent problem is not known; however, since group A1 did not differ from group B1, we feel that this effect was not evident.

In our follow-up of 4- to 7-year-old children, no apparent problems were manifested in children born 15 h or more after termination of ethanol infusion. This finding also held true for children exposed to multiple infusions, implying that no dose-related effects were seen.

However, when the group of seven children born within 15 h of termination of treatment was examined, major pathology was encountered. Four of these children were manifestly disinhibited and hyperactive. They also scored significantly lower in performance IQ, tests of visual-motor integration, and mathematical computation. All seven had already been identified by their schools and had been placed in modified educational programs. The results clearly represent a disturbing continuum of morbidity noted by Zervoudakis and associates.[18]

Comparable results have been reported by other authors. In similar studies that assessed children over the age of 4 who had been exposed to varying amounts of ethanol *in utero*, deficits were found in neurophysiological development (e.g., visual-motor coordination),[40] scores on all intelligence test subscales,[41] and speed and accuracy of information processing.[42]

For all practical purposes, the implications of this study indicate that while single or even multiple binges in the late second and early third trimesters are ill-advised, they seem to cause no discernible effect on the fetus if sufficiently remote from delivery (i.e., >15 h). Most significantly, however, when ethanol is used in the management of preterm labor, patients must be carefully monitored during infusion to assess the progress of labor. If, during the process of infusion, it appears that the ethanol therapy is unsuccessful and labor continues to progress, the treatment should be discontinued immediately to allow the maximum alcohol-free interval between termination of therapy and delivery.

In conclusion, the use of ethanol infusion for the management of preterm labor appeared to have no immediate or long-term adverse effects in cases where labor was successfully postponed. In cases where therapy was unsuccessful and the baby was born intoxicated, immediate and long-term problems were identified.

REFERENCES

1. **Pritchard, J. A. and MacDonald, P. C.,** *Williams Obstetrics,* 16th ed., Appleton-Century-Crafts, New York, 1980.
2. National Center for Health Statistics, Vital Statics, Final Mortality Statistics, 1978, PHS 80-1120, Department of Health and Human Services, Washington, D.C., 1980, 29.
3. **Chez, R. A.,** Management of preterm labor: an overview, in Ritodrine in the Management of Preterm Labor: A Symposium, Merrell National Laboratories, New Orleans, LA, 1980.

4. **Caputo, D. V., Taub, H. B., Goldstein, K. M., Smith, N., Dalack, J. D., Gursner, J. D., and Silbertsein, R. M.,** An evaluation of various parameters of maturity at birth as predictors of development at one year of life, *Percept. Mot. Skills,* 39, 621, 1974.

5. **Niebyl, J., Blake, D., Johnson, J., and King, T.,** The pharmacological inhibition of premature labor, *Obstet. Gynecol. Surv.,* 33, 507, 1978.

6. **Zlatnick, F. J. and Fuchs, F.,** A controlled study of ethanol in threatened premature labor, *Am. J. Obstet. Gynecol.,* 112, 610, 1972.

7. **Belinkoff, S. and Hall, O. W.,** Intravenous alcohol during labor, *Am. J. Obstet. Gynecol.,* 59, 429, 1950.

8. **Chapman, E. R. and Williams, P. T.,** Intravenous alcohol as an obstetrical analgesia, *Am. J. Obstet. Gynecol.,* 61, 676, 1951.

9. **Fuchs, F., Fuchs, A. R., Poblete, V. F., and Risk, A.,** Effect of alcohol on threatened premature labor, *Am. J. Obstet. Gynecol.,* 99, 627, 1967.

10. **Fuchs, F.,** Treatment of threatened labour with alcohol, *J. Obstet. Gynaecol. Br. Commonw.,* 72, 1011, 1964.

11. **Fuchs, A. and Wagner, G.,** The effect of ethyl alcohol on the release of oxytocin in rabbits, *Acta Endocrinol. (Copenhagen),* 44, 593, 1963.

12. **Fuchs, A. and Wagner, G.,** Effect of alcohol on release of oxytocin, *Nature (London),* 198, 92, 1963.

13. **Bueno-Montano, M., McGaughey, H. S., Harbert, G. M., Jr., and Thornton, W. M., Jr.,** Drug preservatives and uterine contractility, *Am. J. Obstet. Gynecol.,* 94, 1, 1966.

14. **Wilson, K. H., Landesman, R., Fuchs, A. R., and Fuchs, F.,** The effect of ethyl alcohol on isolated human myometrium, *Am. J. Obstet. Gynecol.,* 104, 436, 1969.

15. **Lauersen, N. H.,** Managing premature labor, *Perinat. Care,* 1, 15, 1977.

16. **Waltman, R. and Iniquez, F.,** Placental transfer of ethanol and its elimination at term, *Obstet. Gynecol.,* 40, 180, 1972.

17. **Indanpaan-Heikkila, J., Jouppila, P., Akerblom, H., Isoaho, R., Kawppila, E., and Koivisto, M.,** Elimination and metabolic effects of ethanol in mother, fetus, and newborn infant, *Am. J. Obstet. Gynecol.,* 112, 387, 1972.

18. **Zervoudakis, I. A., Krauss, A., and Fuchs, F.,** Infants of mothers treated with ethanol for premature labor, *Am. J. Obstet. Gynecol.,* 137, 713, 1980.

19. **Cook, L. N., Shott, R. J., and Andrews, B. F.,** Acute transplacental ethanol intoxication, *Am. J. Dis. Child.,* 129, 1075, 1978.

20. **Kirkpatrick, S. E., Pitlick, P. L., Hirschklau, M. J., and Friedman, W. F.,** Acute effects of maternal ethanol infusion on fetal cardiac performance, *Am. J. Obstet. Gynecol.,* 126, 1034, 1976.

21. **Lopez, R. and Montoya, M. F.,** Abnormal bone marrow morphology in the premature infant associated with maternal alcohol infusion, *J. Pediatr.,* 76, 1008, 1971.

22. **Waltman, R., Bonura, F., Nigrin, G., and Pipat, C.,** Ethanol and neonatal bilirubin levels, *Lancet,* 2, 108, 1969.

23. **Mann, L. I., Bhakthavathsalan, A., Liu, M., and Makowski, P.,** Effect of alcohol on fetal cerebral function and metabolism, *Am. J. Obstet. Gynecol.,* 122, 845, 1975.

24. **Mann, L. I., Bhakthavathsalan, A., Liu, M., and Makowski, P.,** Placental transport of alcohol and its effect on maternal and fetal acid-base balance, *Am. J. Obstet. Gynecol.,* 122, 837, 1975.

25. **Abel, E. L.,** Fetal alcohol syndrome, *Psychol. Bull.,* 87, 29, 1980.

26. **Streissguth, A. P., Landesman-Dwyer, S., Martin, J. C., and Smith, D. W.,** Teratogenic effects of alcohol in humans and laboratory animals, *Science,* 209, 353, 1980.

27. **Hanson, J. W., Streissguth, A. P., and Smith, D. W.,** The effects of moderate alcohol consumption during pregnancy on fetal growth and morphogenesis, *J. Pediatr.,* 92, 457, 1978.

28. **Ouellette, E. M., Rosett, H. L., Rosman, N. P., and Weiner, L.,** Adverse effects on offspring of maternal alcohol abuse during pregnancy, *N. Engl. J. Med.,* 297, 528, 1977.

29. **Sisenwein, F. E., Tejani, N., Boxer, H., and DiGiuseppe, R.,** Effects of maternal ethanol infusion during pregnancy on the growth and development of children at four to seven years of age, *Am. J. Obstet. Gynecol.,* 147, 52, 1983.

30. **Chapin, F. and Queen, S. A.,** Research Memorandum on Social Work in the Depression, Bull. 39, Social Science Research Council, New York, 1937.

31. **Greenwood, E.,** *Experimental Sociology: A Study in Method,* King's Crown Press, New York, 1945.

32. **Campbell, D. and Stanley, J.,** *Experimental and Quasiexperimental Designs for Research,* Rand McNally, Chicago, 1963.

33. **Nie, N. H., Hull, C. H., Jenkins, J. G., Steinbrenner, K., and Bent, D. H.,** *Statistical Package for the Social Sciences,* 2nd ed., McGraw-Hill, New York, 1975.

34. **Ferguson, G.,** *Statistical Analysis in Psychology and Education,* 4th ed., McGraw-Hill, New York, 1976.

35. **Dilts, V. P.,** Placental transfer of alcohol, *Am. J. Obstet. Gynecol.,* 107, 1195, 1970.

36. **Horiguchi, T., Suzuki, K., Comas-Urrutia, A., Mueller-Heubach, E., Boyer-Milic, A., Baratz, R., Morishim, H., James, L. I., and Adamsons, K.,** Effect of ethanol upon uterine activity and fetal acid-base state of the rhesus monkey, *Am. J. Obstet. Gynecol.,* 109, 910, 1971.

37. **Mukherjee, A. B. and Hodgen, G. D.,** Maternal ethanol exposure induces transient impairment of umbilical circulation fetal hypoxia in monkeys, *Science,* 218, 700, 1982.

38. **Altura, B. M., Altura, B. T., Carella, A., Chatterjee, M., Halevy, S., and Tejani, N.,** Alcohol produces spasms of human umbilial vessels: relationship to fetal alcohol syndrome (FAS), *Eur. J. Pharmacol.,* 83, 2, 1982.

39. **Schwartz, J. and Schwartz, L.,** *Vulnerable Infants: A Psychosocial Dilemma,* McGraw-Hill, New York, 1977.

40. **Rosett, H. and Weiner, L.,** Alcohol and pregnancy: the clinical perspective, *Annu. Rev. Med.,* 36, 73, 1985.

41. **Aronson, M., Kyllerman, M., Sabel, K., and Olegard, R.,** Children of alcoholic mothers, *Acta Paediatr. Scand.,* 74, 27, 1985.

42. **Streissguth, A. P., Barr, M., and Martin, D.,** Alcohol exposure *in utero* and functional deficits in children during the first four years of life, in *1984 Mechanisms of Alcohol Damage in Utero,* Ciba Found. Symp. 105, Elsevier/North-Holland, Amsterdam, 1984, 176.

Chapter 5

LONG-TERM FOLLOW-UP OF CHILDREN EXPOSED TO BETAMETHASONE *IN UTERO*

Barton MacArthur, Ross N. Howie, Anne DeZoete, John Elkins, and Allen Y. L. Liang

TABLE OF CONTENTS

I. INTRODUCTION

Respiratory distress syndrome (RDS) and hyaline membrane disease have been described as the most common causes of neonatal death in the U.S.[1]

After the publication of research by Liggins and Howie[2] demonstrating the possible preventive effect against RDS of betamethasone therapy to mothers in preterm labor, the method came into widespread use in cases of threatened premature delivery.[3] Although this study promised an increased chance of survival and a lower risk of RDS for the premature infant, and despite the confirmation of the effectiveness of the therapy by other workers,[4] reservations concerning its employment were raised by some researchers who still had doubts about possible adverse effects arising from maternal steroid administration.

Caveats were based mainly on the paucity of knowledge concerning the effects of steroids on organs other than the lungs — in particular, the possible modification of brain development.[5] Effects on organ cellular growth[6] and somatic growth[7] were also of concern. There is evidence in animal experiments that cortisol has a detrimental influence on fetal growth, resulting in a decreased cell number (particularly in the lung) and impaired myelination and cellular development in the central nervous system.[8,9] While the effects (at least on the lung) might only be temporary, there remained the question of the long-term safety of glucocorticoid therapy for the human fetus.

Toward identification of possible risks inherent in the therapy, an investigation was begun of children born to mothers with unplanned premature labor studied in the original double-blind and controlled Auckland trial.[2] The aim of the follow-up was to ascertain whether the glucocorticoid therapy was associated with any lasting effect on the children with respect to physical growth, neurological and psychological development, and lung function.[10,11] Cases had been originally assigned to betamethasone or placebo therapy, and neither the team of experienced investigators nor the mothers of the children were aware of the group membership of the children.

II. DEVELOPMENT AT 4 YEARS

Follow-up evaluation was carried out at two stages, 4 and 6 years of age. The first interviews and assessments were undertaken in the subjects' homes at approximately 4 years and 3 months of age, and the second after the children had been in school for 1 year.

Data gathered in the preschool phase of the study included

1. Measures of intelligence (Stanford-Binet Intelligence Scale and Peabody Picture Vocabulary Test)
2. A measure of visual perception (Frostig Developmental Test of Visual Perception)
3. A measure of social maturity (Vineland Social Maturity Scale)
4. Speech assessment (evaluation of a tape recording of speech samples by a speech therapist)
5. Assessment of general development (medical and developmental history from birth)
6. Assessment of environment by parental interview and questionnaire (family background, socioeconomic status, aspects of child's rearing and development)

A. RESULTS

Included in this phase were 177 betamethasone and 141 control children from the 318 who survived 28 days. Seven betamethasone children (4.0%) and six control children (4.3%) had died before the age of 4 years, leaving 305 survivors. Of these, 85% (258) were fully assessed, with 14% (15% betamethasone and 14% controls) not located for evaluation. The remaining 144 bethamethasone and 114 control patients were evaluated.

TABLE 1
Frequencies and Percentages of Subjects
Included in Treatment and Control Group at 4
Years

Sex	Treatment group		Control group		p
	No.	%	No.	%	
Male	87	60.4	62	54.4	
Female	57	39.6	52	45.6	NS
	144	100.0	114	100.0	

Note: NS = not significant.

TABLE 2
Mean and Standard Deviation for Birth Weight and
Gestation at 4 Years

Birth weight (g)	Betamethasone		Control		p
	Mean	SD	Mean	SD	
Males	2231	689	2584	696	<0.01
Females	2233	723	2219	594	NS
Males and females	2232	700	2401	670	<0.05
Gestation (weeks)					
Males	34.9	3.4	36.1	3.0	<0.05
Females	35.1	4.0	35.1	3.0	NS
Males and females	35.0	3.6	35.6	3.0	NS

Note: NS = not significant.

The proportion of boys in the betamethasone group was slightly higher than in the control group, and the proportion of girls was higher in the controls (Table 1), but these differences were not statistically significant.

Differences were also not significant in the number of multiple births (16.0 and 11.4%, respectively) in the betamethasone and control groups and the number of those who were non-European in origin (22.9 and 20.2%, respectively).

Members of the betamethasone group were both lighter and of shorter gestation than the control group (Table 2), with the difference in weight achieving significance at $p < 0.05$. Mean weight and gestational age for the boys in the betamethasone group were significantly lower than in the control boys. The differences for girls were not statistically significant.

The numbers of cases in the betamethasone and control groups who were breast fed (24.3 and 27.2%, respectively) and the reported duration of breast feeding (14.4 and 15.0 weeks, respectively) were similar in the two groups.

No significant differences between the groups were obtained for number of children in the family, position of the subject in the family, occupation of both mother and father, and family mobility.

B. STANDARDIZED TESTS

Two measures of intelligence were employed: the Stanford-Binet and the Peabody Picture Vocabulary Test. A measure of social maturity (Vineland) was also included. In no instance did the difference between betamethasone and control groups prove to be significant either for the groups as a whole or when the sexes were compared separately (Table 3).

TABLE 3
Results of Standardized Tests at 4 Years

Test	Betamethasone			Control			
	n	X	SD	*n*	X	SD	*p*
Stanford-Binet							
Males	87	101.4	17.3	62	102.4	20.9	NS
Females	57	106.9	20.4	52	107.6	20.9	NS
Males and females	144	103.6	18.6	114	104.8	20.9	NS
Peabody Picture Vocabulary							
Males	87	89.9	18.9	62	93.9	18.6	NS
Females	57	93.1	19.4	52	92.0	20.8	NS
Males and females	144	91.9	19.1	114	93.1	19.5	NS
Frostig							
Males	87	92.8	15.9	62	96.3	14.9	NS
Females	57	95.7	15.7	52	95.3	17.8	NS
Males and females	144	94.0	15.8	114	95.8	16.2	NS
Vineland Social Maturity Scale							
Males	87	56.9	7.1	62	56.9	5.8	NS
Females	57	58.2	6.1	52	55.9	7.9	NS
Males and females	144	57.4	6.7	114	56.5	6.9	NS

Note: NS = not significant.

TABLE 4
Mental Development (Stanford-Binet IQ) at 4 Years
for Different Gestational Age Groupings[10]

Gestational age (weeks)	Betamethasone		Control		
	Mean	SD	Mean	SD	*p*
<32	97.0	18.4	91.4	25.9	NS
32—<34	106.5	20.4	116.2	18.6	NS
34—<36	98.8	18.5	101.9	21.5	NS
≥36	109.0	16.3	106.5	18.2	NS

Note: NS = not significant.

As interest has been expressed in the benefits of antenatally administered steroid for children born at different gestational ages, this issue was considered in relation to the Stanford-Binet results. As may be seen from Table 4, there were no significant differences between the betamethasone and control groups when comparisons were made within the gestational age groups selected.

The higher perinatal survival rate of infants in the betamethasone category resulted in an over-representation of boys and children of low birth weight in this group. To correct for possible bias resulting from this, two groups (betamethasone and control) were formed of singleton children matched for sex, gestational age, and birth weight.

From Table 5 it may be seen that none of the differences between these matched groups reached significance.

C. DEVELOPMENTAL MILESTONES AND SPEECH

There were no significant differences between the groups in the mean age at which solid foods were started, the proportion of children who were walking by 18 months, or any of the measures of health or development included in a checklist used during parental interviews.

TABLE 5
**Results of Cognitive Tests at 4 Years for Groups Matched for Sex,
Gestational Age, and Birth Weight[10]**

	Betamethasone		Control		
	Mean	SD	Mean	SD	*p*
Stanford-Binet	105.6	18.6	104.2	20.5	NS
Peabody Picture Test	93.3	18.6	91.9	19.6	NS
Frostig Developmental Test of Visual Perception	95.3	15.6	95.6	15.8	NS
Vineland Social Maturity Scale	57.4	6.1	56.1	6.8	NS

Note: NS = not significant.

However, there were three questions raised during discussions with mothers which did produce marked differences in response between the two groups. More mothers of control girls than betamethasone reported feeding problems with their infants ($p < 0.01$), and they also regarded these girls as more vulnerable to illness ($p < 0.02$). In fact, more mothers of control subjects than of the betamethasone group expressed this concern regarding vulnerability to illness ($p < 0.02$).

The proportion of children in each group using at least two-word sentences was not significantly different, nor were the numbers exhibiting normal speech development, from two samples of the groups as assessed by a speech therapist.

D. ADDITIONAL VARIABLES

No effect was found for additional variables, including time of administration of betamethasone, use of ethanol and salbutamol in labor, mode of delivery, Apgar scores at birth, presence or absence of respiratory distress, hypoglycemia, and jaundice.

E. CONCLUSIONS FROM THE STUDY ON 4-YEAR-OLDS

There was no evidence in the findings from the areas assessed in the 4-year-old group that the prenatal betamethasone therapy used in the original trial[2] was detrimental to development. Although the betamethasone group had a greater representation of boys and preterm infants, the results were not depressed by the presence of these less mature subjects. In fact, the betamethasone group appears to have produced even better results than would have been expected given the disadvantages frequently cited in the literature for immature male infants.

III. DEVELOPMENT AT 6 YEARS

After the subjects had been at school for approximately 1 year (school entry is at 5 years, 0 months in New Zealand), the second evaluation phase was completed.

Assessment at this stage was carried out in the schools attended by the subjects as close as possible to the age of 6 years, 2 months.

Data gathered at this school-age phase of the study included

1. School progress
2. Speech and language development
3. Measures of cognitive development (Illinois Test of Psycholinguistic Abilities, Peabody Picture Vocabulary Test, Raven's Progressive Matrices, and Bender Visual Motor Gestalt Test)
4. General development and physical measurements

A. RESULTS

One child died between the two stages of the study, leaving 304 survivors, and a full second assessment was completed for 250 of the 304 survivors (82%), 139 of the 170 in the betamethasome group (82%), and 111 of the 134 in the control group (83%).

B. SCHOOL VARIABLES

Mean school attendance was similar for the treatment and control groups (92 and 93%, respectively), providing no evidence of significant differences in amount of illness as reflected in absences from school.

Problems related to adjustment to school, as reported by both mothers and teachers, and classroom behavior (as scored by teachers) did not produce any significant differences between the groups. However, when subgroups were formed of the sexes, a significant difference emerged. The proportion of betamethasone group girls (1.8%) rated as below average for classroom behavior was lower than the percentage for the control girls (13.7%), a difference which proved to be significant ($p = 0.02$, Fisher exact test).

While there was no significant difference between the groups so far as teachers' ratings of motor coordination were concerned, control girls were significantly more often recorded as below average than betamethasone-treated girls. In neither general progress in school nor specifically in reading was there a significant difference between the two groups. Quality of language, quantity, and intelligibility of speech showed no significant differences, nor was there any difference in incidence of speech problems reported by teachers.

C. COGNITIVE DEVELOPMENT

There were no significant differences between the groups for the results of the Peabody Picture Vocabulary Test and the Bender-Gestalt Test. However, the other two tests employed in this area produced significant differences for the groups in one instance and for two subtests in the other.

In the Raven's Colored Progressive Matrices, the betamethasone group obtained a mean score which was significantly lower than that of the control group ($p < 0.05$). Most of this difference resulted from lower scores obtained by betamethasone-treated boys. Visual Memory and Visual Closure subtests of the Illinois Test of Psycholinguistic Abilities produced lower scores for the betamethasone group ($p < 0.05$). The eight other subtests and the mean scaled score for the Illinois Test showed no significant differences.

D. HEALTH AND GROWTH DEVELOPMENT

When mothers were questioned concerning the health and general development of the subjects over the period (20 months) since the previous interview, one significant difference between the groups emerged. More subjects ($p < 0.05$) were reported to have had health problems in the control group (59.5%) than in the betamethasone group (46.8%). This difference was brought about largely by a higher incidence of reported respiratory problems in the control group. There were no significant differences between the groups when measures of height, weight, and head circumference were taken.

E. MATCHED GROUPS

Again, as in the case of the results from the 4-year-olds, subjects from the two groups were matched for sex, gestational age, and birth weight. This resulted in the formation of two groups of 90 subjects. Comparisons were then made between these groups on the variables which had produced significant differences when the unmatched groups were compared. The result of this adjustment was that two differences were no longer significant (Visual Closure and Visual Memory), and one difference proved to still be significant (Raven).

F. LUNG FUNCTION

During this phase of the study, lung function tests were carried out on 40 children from each of the groups (betamethasone and control). Subjects were matched for sex, gestational age, birth weight, and other important perinatal variables. No significant differences were found.

There was also no significant difference between two groups made up of 20 matched pairs when lasting depression of lymphocyte function was investigated.[12]

G. CONCLUSIONS FROM THE STUDY ON 6-YEAR-OLDS

The composition of the school-age follow-up study differed little from the 4-year-old phase, with only 3.1% of that cohort being lost.

As with the earlier research, differences could well have been anticipated, with the betamethasone group at a disadvantage, irrespective of any treatment effects, because of its higher perinatal survival rate and greater proportion of males and more immature infants. Contrary to this expectation, no differences between betamethasone and control groups were revealed on the majority of measures employed.

After the first year at school, measures which showed no significant treatment differences were school attendance and adjustment, academic progress, motor coordination, speech and language, physical measurements, Peabody Picture Vocabulary Test, Illinois Test of Psycholinguistic Abilities total score, and the Bender Visual Motor Gestalt Test.

The betamethasone group obtained lower scores than the control group on Visual Sequential Memory and Visual Closure, two of the ten subtests of the Illinois Test of Psycholinguistic Abilities (but not on the total score), and on Raven's Progressive Matrices.

Before any conclusions were reached concerning possible adverse outcomes resulting from betamethasone treatment, carefully matched groups were formed, and two of the differences were no longer significant; only differences associated with the Raven's Progressive Matrices remained significant. It must also be realized that, with the large number of comparisons made in this analysis of data, it might be expected that one or two statistically significant differences would be found by chance alone.

The size of the sample employed in this study is associated with another important caution. One should give consideration to the practical importance of a difference between two means[13] as the t-test is sensitive to the sample size. In fact, Hays[14] has stated that virtually any study can be made to show significant results if enough subjects are included, and the omega-squared index (Ω^2) should be calculated to determine the proportion of total variance that can be attributed to the difference between group means. For the three measures considered, the association with betamethasone therapy explained <5% of the total variance. Therefore, it was concluded that these differences were not important.

In addition, these measures (Visual Sequential Memory, Visual Closure, and Raven's Progressive Matrices) displayed only a low correlation with each other (0.32 to 0.40), thus failing to support the conclusion that they represent an underlying difference between the groups.

There were long-term benefits associated with betamethasone therapy which may be set against these possible adverse effects, but similar cautions must again be applied. Betamethasone girls showed fewer behavioral problems and better motor coordination, and they were taller and heavier than control girls.

IV. SUMMARY

The findings of both the preschool and school-age studies supported the conclusion that no adverse effects of betamethasone treatment were apparent. Issues were raised in both phases of the research which warrant further investigation, but there was no evidence that betamethasone had any genuine effect on the tested areas of development.

From the results of the research it is possible to conclude that, in spite of the greater number of "at-risk" infants surviving in the betamethasone group, there does not appear to be an increased likelihood of developmental problems, school-related difficulties, or poor performance on standardized tests of cognitive function.

V. NOTE: STATISTICAL POWER

It has been strongly suggested[15-17] that authors should report not only the probability of stating that a treatment effect exists when the null hypothesis is true (type I error), but also the probability of failing to detect a treatment effect when it exists (type II error).

When the power of a statistical test is calculated, the probability is indicated, having established a significance level of the type I error, of avoiding the corresponding type II error.

In the present study, because most of the measures had arbitrary population standard deviations of varying magnitudes, power calculations were carried out using a common effect size of one third and one half of a standard deviation.

There was a 75% chance of detecting a real difference between the betamethasone and control groups (in either direction) of a size equal to one third of a standard deviation when the significance level chosen for type I error was $p < 0.05$. For the detection of a larger true effect equal to one half of a standard deviation, the power of the test was 97.5%.

In the case of the Stanford-Binet test, this study had a 75% chance of detecting a real difference of 6.5 IQ points between the groups and a 97.5% chance of detecting a difference of 9.8 IQ points.

REFERENCES

1. **Perelman, R. H. and Farrell, P. M.,** Analysis of causes of neonatal death in the United States with specific emphasis on fatal hyaline membrane disease, *Pediatrics,* 70, 570, 1982.
2. **Liggins, G. C. and Howie, R. N.,** A controlled trial of antepartum glucocorticoid treatment for prevention of the respiratory distress syndrome in premature infants, *Pediatrics,* 50, 515, 1972.
3. **Doyle, L. W., Williams, B. S., Kitchen, W., Ford, G. W., Rickards, A., Lissenden, J. V., and Ryan, M. M.,** Effects of antenatal steroid therapy on mortality in very low birth weight infants, *J. Pediatr.,* 108, 287, 1986.
4. **Ballard, P. L. and Ballard, R. A.,** Corticosteroids and respiratory distress syndrome: Status 1979, *Pediatrics,* 63, 163, 1979.
5. **Howard, E. and Granoff, D. M.,** Increased voluntary running and decreased motor coordination in mice after neonatal corticosterone implantation, *Ep. Neurol.,* 12, 661, 1968.
6. **Frank, L., Summerville, J. I., and Massaro, D.,** The effect of prenatal dexamethasone treatment on oxygen toxicity in the newborn rat, *Pediatrics,* 65, 287, 1980.
7. **Kotas, R. V., Mims, L. C., and Hart, L. K.,** Reversible inhibition of lung cell number after glucocorticoid injection into fetal rabbits to enhance surfactant appearance, *Pediatrics,* 53, 358, 1974.
8. **Gumbinas, M., Oda, M., and Huttenlocker, P.,** The effects of corticosteroids on myelination of the developing rat brain, *Biol. Neonate,* 22, 355, 1973.
9. **Weichsel, M. E., Jr.,** Glucocorticoid effect upon thymidine kinase in the developing cerebellum, *Pediatr. Res.,* 8, 843, 1974.
10. **MacArthur, B. A., Howie, R. N., DeZoete, J. A., and Elkins, J.,** Cognitive and psychosocial development of 4 year old children whose mothers were treated antenatally with betamethasone, *Pediatrics,* 68, 638, 1981.
11. **MacArthur, B. A., Howie, R. N., DeZoete, J. A., and Elkins, J.,** School progress and cognitive development of 6 year old children whose mothers were treated antenatally with betamethasone, *Pediatrics,* 70, 99, 1982.
12. **Howie, R. N.,** Pharmacological acceleration of lung maturation, in *Respiratory Distress Syndrome,* Raivio, K. O., Hallman, N., Kouvalainen, K., and Valimaki, I., Eds., Academic Press, London, 1984, 385.

13. **Popham, W. J.,** *Educational Evaluation,* Prentice-Hall, Englewood Cliffs, NJ, 1975, 252.
14. **Hays, W. L.,** *Statistics,* Holt, Rinehart & Winston, New York, 1963, 326.
15. **Hopkins, K. D.,** Research design and analysis clinic, *J. Spec. Educ.,* 103, 1973.
16. **Berwick, D. M.,** Experimental power: the other side of the coin, *Pediatrics,* 65, 1043, 1980.
17. **Freiman, J. A., Chalmers, T. C., Smith, H., Jr., and Kuebler, R. R.,** The importance of beta, the type II error and sample size in the design and interpretation of the randomized control trial, *N. Engl. J. Med.,* 299, 690, 1978.

Chapter 6

FOUR- TO SEVEN-YEAR EVALUATION IN TWO GROUPS OF SMALL-FOR-GESTATIONAL-AGE INFANTS

Eve K. Winer and Nergesh Tejani

TABLE OF CONTENTS

I. INTRODUCTION

Infants weighing ≤2500 g at birth have long been of concern to the medical and mental health professional. As infants, their survival rate is significantly related to the degree to which they are undersized and the causes of the low birth weight (LBW).[1] As they grow, they are at risk for abnormal intellectual, physical, and emotional development.

In making prognoses for LBW neonates, it is important not only to be aware of the actual birth weight and condition of the neonate at birth, but also the gestational age of the neonate and the condition of the mother during the pregnancy.[2] In response to this need, the American Academy of Pediatrics Committee on the Fetus and Newborn[3] introduced a classification based on the Colorado Weight Percentile curves. As a result, LBW neonates may be subclassified into appropriate (average) for gestional age (AGA), which are those newborns that fall between the 10th and 90th percentile for their gestational age; small for gestational age (SGA), which are those falling below the 10th percentile for their gestational age; and the occasional large for gestational age (LGA), where birth weight is above the 90th percentile in spite of the absolute weight being ≤2500 g. A third of all LBW neonates are SGA, while two thirds are AGA.[4]

Earlier research has had the limitation of not specifying gestational ages of LBW subjects.[5,6] Some of the more recent research on SGA neonates continues to present mixed findings. Some studies find significant effects on later development, and others find no relationship between SGA and later development of the child. A major reason for this is that SGA neonates are not a homogeneous group, and one or more subgroups of SGA children may be confounding the results of these studies.

One of the major causes of SGA has been identified as maternal vascular disease.[4,7] Fetal head growth in maternal hypertensive disease is different from that seen in SGA infants with other disorders. These babies may, therefore, have different prognoses for later development.

This chapter will review the developmental consequences and factors influencing later development of SGA babies. Additionally, our own study comparing long-term evaluation of SGA children born of hypertensive mothers to the outcome of SGA children born of mothers without hypertension will be discussed to emphasize the heterogeneity of the group.

A. DEVELOPMENTAL CONSEQUENCES OF BEING A SMALL-FOR-GESTATIONAL-AGE NEONATE

In general, SGA babies are considered to be at risk for later abnormal development.[1] They may manifest failure of growth,[10-12] reduced intellectual functioning, academic limitations, neurological impairment, and behavioral disorders.[11,12] However, some studies have found SGA children not to show any deficits and to be developing normally throughout childhood.

Cruise,[13] in a study that did not consider the causes of SGA, measured distance growth and velocity growth of 202 SGA children between the ages of 6 months and 1 year. Distance growth compares the absolute measures of a child (height, weight, and/or head circumference) with established norms for his/her age. Velocity growth compares that rate of growth of a child with norms. He found that preterm AGA infants born before 36 weeks gestation surpassed full-term SGA infants in velocity growth, particularly in head circumference.

In a South African study[14] of SGA and AGA very LBW (500 to 1500 g) infants, it was found that head circumference was normal, although the children were lighter and shorter than expected at 2 years of age. The premature termination of these pregnancies at a gestational age of ≤32 weeks may have accounted for these findings. This issue will be discussed later in this chapter.

Where the cause of SGA is congenital anomaly or major intrauterine fetal infection of the TORCH type, severe compromise in growth factors is often present due to a basic deficiency in cell numbers.

1. Growth Factors — Height, Weight, and Head Circumference

Most researchers seem to agree that SGA children tend to be shorter and lighter in early childhood than the rest of the population.[5,14,15-18] Tanner[19] adds that deficits in later size are greater for lower birth weight babies.

Gallagher and O'Brien,[7] in a sample of 487 women, point out a significant correlation between the incidence of SGA babies and mothers' height of ≤155 cm (61 in.). Westwood et al.[18] controlled for maternal height and still found SGA children to be significantly smaller in adolescence.

Davies et al.[20] studied light-for-date (LFD) infants to determine how intrauterine undernutrition influences growth during the first 6 months of postnatal life. They found that the rates of growth (weight, length, and head circumference) of these LFD babies were greater than in normal infants. They saw the first 3 months after birth as a period of ''catch-up'' growth in LFD term infants.

2. Intellectual Development

Several studies have found the intellectual functioning of SGA children to be impaired in later childhood.[11,21] Davies and Stewart[22] report that the incidence of intellectual retardation increases directly with decreasing birth weight and gestational age.

Caputo et al.[23] found gestational age alone to account for almost one fourth of the variance of Cattell Developmental Quotient scores at 1 year of age.

In a review of the literature on consequences of LBW, Caputo and Mandell[1] examined 64 studies, none of which considered gestational age and the medical condition of the mother during the pregnancy as factors affecting the later development of LBW children. They summarized the results and concluded that among heavier LBW children in adolescence, intelligence seems to be only minimally impaired, if at all. However, there was evidence of significant impairment among very LBW individuals.

Rutter et al.,[8] in their extensive study of all handicapped children on the Isle of Wight, found a significantly greater number of SGA children among retardates.

Commey and Fitzhardinge[17] studied 109 preterm SGA infants (<1500 g and <33 weeks of gestation) and found significant deficits on the Bayley Scales of Infant Development in these children. They found that 42% had scores of 80 or less and showed significant cognitive abnormalities.

Tanner[19] notes that SGA children, as compared with AGA children, fail to develop the same level of mental ability as normal children and adds that deficits in later ability are worse in LBW babies.

Several studies of SGA children have failed to find intellectual deficits among these children. In an earlier study of 96 children, Fitzhardinge and Stevens,[24] using the Stanford-Binet Test, the Metropolitan Achievement Test, the Wechsler Intelligence Scale for Children, the Draw-A-Person Test, and the Bender Test, found no significant correlation between degree of intrauterine growth retardation and intelligence test scores.

Weiner et al.[26] reexamined the data of 822 children from the Baltimore study,[27] assigning gestational age to the subjects using the report of the mothers. They found no difference between SGA and AGA LBW children in later intellectual performance. This study used the Wechsler Intelligence Scale for Children—Revised (WISC-R), the Wide Range Achievement Test (WRAT), and the Bender Test. A report of the mother, however, cannot be accepted as completely reliable.

Westwood et al.[18] found no significant cognitive deficits in their study of 33 adolescents born small for gestational age (13 to 19 years).

3. Academic Achievement

Academic limitations of SGA children may be inferred when limited intellectual capabilities are reported. Most studies of SGA children do not include achievement testing in their data collection. Caputo and Mandell,[1] in reviewing previous research on LBW children, have found that scores in academic areas such as reading, spelling, and arithmetic are often retarded in LBW children. The earlier studies included AGA as well as SGA children in their sample and did not consider causative factors.

Fitzhardinge and Stevens[24] gave the Metropolitan Achievement Test as part of their battery to 96 children and found no difference in performance between SGA babies and controls on test performance.

Harvey et al.[27] looked specifically at school achievement in 45 SGA children between the ages of 5 and 9 years, using linear analogues since these children were of diverse ages and attended different schools. They found that SGA children might have difficulties at school and that the severity of these problems was determined by the sex of the child, social class, and the stage of pregnancy at which slow head growth began. Those most likely to exhibit poor school achievement and behavioral problems were males from the more depressed social class whose rate of head growth slowed before 34 weeks gestation.

4. Neurological Functioning

Neurological impairment seems to be found to a greater degree among SGA children. Davies and Stewart[22] studied the neurological sequelae of very low birth weight (VLBW) preterm infants (<1500 g). They report that better management of VLBW children born in the last decade has greatly reduced the incidence of severe neurological disturbance, cerebral palsy, and visual and hearing defects, although these children are still at greater risk for neurological impairment than AGA children.

Westwood et al.[18] gave a good prognosis for neurological development of children born SGA.

5. Behavioral Disorders

Few studies of LBW children consider their emotional development. Caputo and Mandell,[1] in a review of the literature on the consequences of LBW, indicated that these children manifested a variety of behavior disorders, including hyperkinesis and disorganization. None of the studies they reviewed took into account the gestational age of the subjects or the cause of LBW.

Koops[28] studied SGA children at ages 8 to 23 months. She found a high incidence of sleep and eating disturbances and said that these symptoms are good predictors of subsequent handicaps, suggesting future behavioral disorders in these children. To date, no studies seem to have been undertaken to evaluate the behavioral development of SGA children born to mothers with vascular disease.

6. Summary

According to the research to date, the SGA neonate is at some risk for later development, but the degree and nature of the deficit are not clear. Further research must subdivide the group of LBW neonates according to actual weight at birth, gestational age, head circumference at birth, and head growth pattern *in utero*. The cause of intrapartum growth failure, particularly the presence or nonpresence of vascular disease, should be taken into account if more accurate prognoses are to be made.

B. FACTORS INFLUENCING THE LATER DEVELOPMENT OF SMALL-FOR-GESTATIONAL-AGE BABIES

SGA infants are not a homogeneous group. In a study of these children, it is important to attempt to determine why the neonate is undersized before a prognosis can be made.[2]

1. Etiology of Growth Retardation

Tejani and Mann[4] examined all SGA neonates born at their institution during the years 1973 to 1975. There were 154 cases, representing an incidence of 4%. They found that the single most prevalent medical condition associated with SGA neonates was maternal vascular disease (25%). Gallagher and O'Brien,[7] in a study conducted in Dublin, Ireland, noted that 26% of the SGA infants that they studied had mothers with hypertensive vascular disease. In the general discussion at a Ciba Foundation symposium,[29] it was stated that 30 to 40% of LBW children have been suspected of having an etiology associated with some form of vascular disease in the mother during the pregnancy. Resnick[30] states that hypertensive disease is by far the most common identifiable cause of fetal intrauterine growth retardation (IUGR) attributable to a maternal disease entity.

Hypertensive disorders of pregnancy that have been associated with fetal growth problems include persistant chronic hypertension which then continued into pregnancy, implying a chronically diseased state of the blood vessels and preeclampsia or pregnancy-induced hypertension, a disease peculiar to pregnancy and implying a more temporary state involving spasm of blood vessels. The situation may coexist in either circumstance due to fetal redistribution of circulation to its own vital organs, typically head growth which proceeds at a normal or near normal rate. Retardation of the rate of growth, which occurs beyond 37 weeks in normal pregnancy, may occur somewhat earlier in these cases. This brain-sparing effect is presumably the basis for these cases doing intellectually (and otherwise) better than where head growth is more severely affected.

If the causative factor of SGA is congenital anomaly or major fetal infection due to cytomegalovirus, toxoplasmosis, rubella, and other similar situations, the likelihood for growth and for intellectual and neurological pathology is extremely high due to a basic and early compromise in cell numbers, particularly in the brain.

Most cases of SGA have no obvious cause and are often vaguely thought of as "nutritional". If true, nutritional deficiencies occurred early in pregnancy. This may also compromise cell numbers and, therefore, ultimate outcome. However, some of these "unknown" cases are constitutional and would be expected to show no adverse outcome.

2. Pattern and Rate of Head Growth *In Utero*

Ultrasonic evaluation of fetal head growth recognizes differing patterns in fetal growth retardation which are of importance in the ultimate prognosis of the child.

In mothers with vascular disease there is compromise in the uterine blood flow. The fetus makes readjustments in its own circulation with redistribution in favor of its vital organs, particularly the brain. With the "brain-sparing effect",[31] the sonographically measured cephalic growth keeps pace with expected growth for gestational age until a point is reached, usually at 34 to 36 weeks gestation, at which time compensation breaks down and the rate of growth is slowed. Campbell[32] refers to this type of growth as a "late-flattening" growth retardation pattern.

In growth-retarded fetuses of mothers who do not show vascular disease, the type of fetal head growth is typically different and has been termed "low profile" by Campbell.[32] These fetuses show compromise in head growth from early in the second trimester of gestation and maintain a persistently low rate of growth throughout the remainder of the pregnancy.

Rosso and Winick[9] also differentiate between two types of IUGR infants, with the head growth pattern distinguishing between Type I and Type II IUGR. A Type I is a small infant with a proportionally small head who would probably resemble Campbell's "low-profile" infant. A Type II is a small infant whose head is disproportionately larger than the rest of the infant. This child would be like Campbell's "late-flattening" child. They state that Type I children are born to mothers suffering from undernutrition and other as yet unknown factors. Type II children are typically the product of a vascularly deprived uterine environment as a result of the mother having vascular disease during the pregnancy. In experimentally induced vascular insufficiency in pregnant rats, the offspring are born with a normal brain weight, although they are otherwise undersized. Lowrey[33] confirms the finding that vascular deficiency to the pregnant uterus, although resulting in undersized human neonates, allows the brain to be completely spared, with resulting normal later development.

The study of Fancourt et al.[15] is unique in that they followed 60 SGA children who had been monitored by serial ultrasonic cephalometry *in utero*. Those children who had shown head growth failure by the 26th week had a significantly lower developmental quotient at 4 years of age (93.3 ± 8.05) on Griffith's Extended Scales than all other groups (102.0 ± 10.86).

3. Head Circumference Percentile at Birth

A head circumference below the tenth percentile for gestational age is the product of "low-profile" head growth seen in the symmetrically growth-retarded newborn where there has been no preferential growth of the brain. The etiology of this situation is often indeterminate; however, the prognosis is compromised. In its extreme form, microcephaly occurring as part of a congenital anomaly or infection syndrome, or idiopathically, carries a very poor prognosis for long-term development.

4. Gestational Age

It is at present unclear if an SGA neonate delivered at an early gestational age is at an advantage because it has been removed from its hostile environment.

Several researchers have found no relationship between gestational age and later development of LBW neonates. Moltens et al.,[14] in a study of 86 children, claim no difference between SGA and AGA VLBW surviving children. However, they do not comment on their statistics that show that 40% of VLBW AGA children (prematures) die, and only 20% of the VLBW SGA children died in infancy.

Vohr et al.[34] studied 29 VLBW AGA (29 ± 2 weeks gestational age) children and 28 VLBW SGA (33 ± 2 weeks gestational age) children at 2 years of age and found no difference between these two groups on the Bayley Scales.

Cruise[13] compared 202 preterm LBW AGA children with 113 full-term SGA LBW children. She found at ages 1, 2, and 3 years that the full-term SGA children showed less growth in height than the preterm AGA children. Velocity growth (rate) of preterm AGA infants of each sex surpassed that of SGA infants, particularly in head circumference from birth to 6 months.

Several authors find the prolonged gestational age to term of slow-growing fetuses to be harmful. Tanner[19] states that the prognosis for a small child born after a normal gestation period is very different from the prognosis for an equally small child born after a shortened gestation. Leaving the uterus early is not in itself harmful, whereas growing less than normal during a full uterine stay implies pathology of the fetus, placenta, or mother.

Davies[35] points out that most SFD babies are underfed *in utero*. Birth can, therefore, be seen to release many SFD babies from a nutritionally inadequate intrauterine environment, with the postnatal period providing the necessary opportunity to recover any growth deficit. Koops[28] states that an unfavorable *in utero* environment, if allowed to persist, will result in a fetus with IUGR. She goes on to suggest that the current obstetric practice of attempting to stop premature labor may need to be reexamined where growth retardation has not been excluded. These babies may do better outside of an insufficient uterus.

The question of the risks vs. benefits of advancing gestational age is unlikely to be easily resolved, since the cases delivered earlier are usually due to severity of growth problems or maternal disorders and are therefore more compromised than milder cases (when delivery is usually effected later). Whether such cases would be better off delivered to release them from a growth-restricting environment is presently unknown.

5. Absolute Birth Weight

It is generally felt that long-term compromise is directly related to lower birth weights in the AGA situation. However, this matter is unresolved in SGA neonates. As in the case of gestational age, the very light neonates are often delivered because of severe *in utero* compromise. Additionally, cases of congenital anomaly and fetal infection often fall into this group. Whether milder cases would benefit from early delivery and elimination of a hostile intrauterine environment is at present not known.

6. Socioeconomic Status

Socioeconomic status (SES) has been found to be highly correlated with IQ in studies by Broman et al.,[11] Fitzhardinge and Ramsey,[36] Davies and Stewart,[22] and Birch and Gussow.[37] Of the prenatal variables used in the Broman study to predict IQ in early childhood, SES, together with maternal education, contributed by far the largest proportion of explained variance in IQ.

Other researchers have found similar relationships between SES and IQ scores. A recent study by Rubin and Barlow[38] found that SES was a better single predictor of outcome variables than the Bayley Infant Scales of Mental Development. Their results also suggested that high SES may obscure cognitive deficits associated with early developmental impairment.

In studying school achievement, Parkinson et al.[39] found that social class was a strong factor in the success of SGA children.

Vane,[40] in evaluating the effects of compensatory education on preschoolers, noted the importance of SES. She used the Index of Status Characteristics[41] and found significant differences between lower-lower and upper-lower SES groups in performance on the Boehm Test of Basic Concepts.

McCall et al.[42] found that SES predicted IQ better for children under 12 months than it did for 12- to 24-month-old children. On the other hand, Beckwith and Cohen[43] found that social class was not related to the developmental measures in the first year of life, but was significantly related to 2-year performance. They qualified these findings by adding that social class is not a variable that works in a simple way; rather, it interacts with other demographic variables.

The effect of social class was also noted by Francis-Williams and Davies[44] and by Davies and Tizard,[45] who found a significantly poorer outcome in SGA vs. AGA infants of <1500 g at birth. Ounsted et al.[46] found social class to be a powerful influence on intellectual ability in all of the 7-year-old children they compared, irrespective of birth weight percentile.

In view of the evidence that SES has a strong impact on the intellectual development and attainment of a child, any data analysis examination must take into account the influence of this important variable.

7. Summary

Although researchers are concerned about SGA babies, there is little agreement among them regarding the degree of influence of various antepartum variables on later development. Among the variables studied have been gestational age, absolute birth weight, head circumference at birth, and, to a lesser extent, intrauterine head growth patterns. The causative factor(s) and the effect of vascular disease in the pregnant mother on the later development of the child have not been examined.

C. RATIONALE FOR THIS STUDY

SGA children do not constitute a homogeneous group, thus explaining divergent results on follow-up. If one is to study prognosis in SGA neonates, it is necessary to differentiate among the various causes of IUGR. Vascular disease in the mother during pregnancy is known to retard the birth weight of the baby, but may not adversely affect the growth of the fetal head. SGA babies born to mothers with vascular disease are believed to be at lesser risk for later neurological, intellectual, behavioral, and physical development problems than cases where SGA is caused by other factors.

In comparing serial sonograms of fetal head growth *in utero*, it has been noted that fetuses of mothers who have hypertensive disorders do not show compromise of intrauterine head growth until about the 34th week of gestation, when the critical period of brain hyperplasia has passed. This suggests that these children, although born small, may not be at risk for impaired later intellectual or emotional development. However, if they are extremely small at birth (<1500 g), they may show later developmental difficulties regardless of the medical condition of the mother during the pregnancy.

A follow-up study of 55 out of 166 SGA infants, 20 born to mothers with vascular disease and 35 to mothers without vascular disease, was undertaken to note their intellectual, academic, perceptual-motor, psychological, and physical growth and development at 4 to 7 years of age. The areas tested include

1.   Intelligence, using the Wechsler Intelligence Scale for Children—Revised (WISC-R) or the Wechsler Preschool and Primary Scales of Intelligence (WPPSI) and the Raven's Coloured Progressive Matrices (CPM)
2.   Perceptual motor skills, using the Bender Test or the Test of Visual Motor Integration (VMI)
3.   Achievement, using the Wide Range Achievement Test (WRAT), reading recognition and arithmetic subtests
4.   Personality, using the Personality Inventory for Children (PIC)
5.   Height
6.   Weight
7.   Head circumference
8.   Socioeconomic status

II. METHOD

A. SUBJECTS

The subjects for this study came from an original population of 180 SGA children born at the Nassau County Medical Center in East Meadow, New York between the years 1973 and 1976. These children's weights were at the tenth percentile or less for their gestational ages at birth on Colorado weight-gestational age curves. Gestational age was confirmed by physical and neurological examination of the baby at birth. Since mean birth weights in Colorado are lower than those on the East Coast, the tenth percentile on the Colorado curves corresponds to about the fifth percentile for the New York area. Therefore, the study population represented the more severely growth-retarded cases for this area.

Of the 180 SGA babies, 53 (29.5%) were born to mothers with vascular disease and constituted Group A. Group B consisted of 127 (70.5%) children born to mothers who had no evidence of vascular disease. These mothers exhibited a variety of problems, including narcotic addiction, nutritional disorders, asthma, and seizure disorders. A majority of these women had no obvious medical problems.

Of the original sample of 180 SGA children, there were 14 perinatal deaths, of which 11 were stillbirths and 3 neonatal deaths. Of these 14 perinatal deaths, 11 occurred in Group B and the remaining cases (3) occurred in Group A.

Each of the remaining families received a letter informing them of this study and requesting participation. About half of the letters were returned as undeliverable, and others did not wish to participate.

The final sample in the study consisted of 55 boys and girls between the ages of 4 and 7 years. Of these 55 children, 20 were born to mothers with vascular disease (Group A) and 35 to mothers who did not have vascular disease (Group B).

B. PROCEDURE

The women who gave birth to SGA children were identified in the Perinatal Unit of the Nassau County Medical Center. All available children were brought into the Nassau County Medical Center for evaluation. The testing included measures of intelligence, perceptual-motor ability, and academic ability. This testing was carried out by one of the authors (E.W.), a certified school psychologist, and five other testers with similar credentials. Evaluation was done without the testers knowing the perinatal background of the neonate or the status of the mother during pregnancy. Physical measurements were taken by a trained research assistant.

Parents were interviewed to determine SES. A questionnaire (PIC) that was designed to evaluate the personality adjustment of the child was completed by the parents. The significant findings were shared with the parents.

C. VARIABLES

The independent variables of this study were

1. The presence or absence of maternal vascular disease
2. Head circumference of the neonate
3. Gestational age
4. Birth weight
5. SES of the families

The dependent variables being measured at 5 to 7 years of age were

1. Intellectual functioning — WPPSI or WISC-R, and CPM (Wechsler scores broken down into verbal, performance, and full-scale IQ scores)
2. Perceptual-motor functioning — Bender Visual Motor Gestalt Test or VMI
3. Academic ability — WRAT
4. Personality adjustment — PIC
5. Physical measurements, including
   A. Height
   B. Weight
   C. Head circumference

D. DATA ANALYSIS

Stepwise multiple regression techniques were employed using the five criterion variables listed above, allowing the variables to be introduced into the computation sequentially depending on their explanatory power.

Analysis of variance was performed to assess the effect of the independent variables on the dependent variables. Pearson product moment correlations were calculated to obtain zero-order correlations between criterion and predictor variables. Discriminant analyses were made on the differences between the two groups being compared, Groups A and B.

SES was expected to be a confounding factor in the study. Therefore, analysis of the data included partial-order correlations which controlled for SES and analysis of covariance with SES as a covariate. This was done so that the effects of the medical condition of the mother during pregnancy and the length of the pregnancy could best be evaluated. A 0.05 level of significance was adopted in accordance with common convention.

TABLE 1

Comparison of Group A and Group B on Intellectual and Physical Variables

	Whole group (n = 45—55)		Group A — with vascular disease (n = 18—20)		Group B — other medical problems (n = 25—35)		F[a]	F[b]
	Mean	SD	Mean	SD	Mean	SD		
Verbal IQ[c]	98.15	14.18	105.75	13.50	93.68	12.84	10.82***	5.42*
Performance IQ[c]	95.91	15.04	99.40	14.44	93.85	15.21	1.74	0.17
Full-scale IQ[c]	96.70	14.82	102.70	14.48	93.18	14.05	5.66*	1.55
Raven's CPM[d]	44.19	28.34	47.40	28.42	42.29	28.54	0.40	0.78
WRAT — reading[c]	98.15	21.16	104.70	13.60	93.30	24.49	3.52	1.62
WRAT — arithmetic[c]	96.51	16.12	101.95	10.41	92.16	18.60	4.42*	0.91
Bender or VMI[e]	89.15	21.67	94.20	16.39	86.00	24.10	1.79	0.14
Height[d]	54.82	28.40	48.78	25.45	58.32	29.81	1.29	0.18
Weight[d]	48.32	27.91	55.50	28.44	44.28	27.23	1.89	0.71
Head circumference[d]	47.10	31.48	56.28	29.67	41.94	31.74	2.46	0.36
Birthweight (g)	2162.22	363.32	2085.00	425.08	2206.34	321.19	1.43	0.12
Gestational age (weeks)	38.98	2.41	38.20	2.31	39.44	2.39	3.48	1.08
Head circumference at birth[d]	25.96	15.10	30.40	16.53	23.35	13.78	2.84	1.14
SES[f]	59.87	14.34	53.21	18.00	63.70	10.10	7.23**	

Note: * denotes $p < 0.05$, ** denotes $p < 0.01$, and *** denotes $p < 0.001$.

[a]   From one-way analysis of variance.
[b]   From analysis of covariance, controlling for SES.
[c]   Scaled score.
[d]   Percentile.
[e]   IQ equivalent.
[f]   High scores relate to low SES; low scores relate to high SES.

III. RESULTS

Our first hypothesis was that 4- to 7-year-old SGA children born to mothers with vascular disease during pregnancy (Group A) would have better scores than SGA children in the same age range born to mothers who did not have vascular disease (Group B).

A comparison of Groups A and B for intellectual and physical variables is shown in Table 1. When SES was included in the analysis, verbal IQ discriminated very well between Group A and Group B. Full-scale IQ differences were also significant, as were WRAT arithmetic scaled scores. As expected, SES also differed significantly between the two groups. When SES is controlled using partial correlation with SES as a covariate, the only significantly different scores between the two groups were on verbal IQ.

Where Groups A and B were compared on personality testing, only one of the personality variables (Table 2) demonstrated a significant difference between the groups when SES was included as a variable. This was "development", which measured a child's intellectual and physical development as perceived by his/her mother. When SES was controlled for, the personality variable that demonstrated the greatest difference between the groups was "withdrawal". This scale measures the degree of withdrawal from social contact. SGA children born to women without vascular disease tend to be more withdrawn, as described by their mothers, regardless of SES. In both of these scales, the difference between the groups was in the direction of greater pathology in Group B.

Although the rest of the measures did not show significant differences between the groups, in all but height, birth weight, and gestational age the mean scores were in the predicted direction in that Group A children had better scores than Group B children.

TABLE 2

Comparison of Group A and Group B on Personality Variables

	Whole group (n = 52)		Group A — with vascular disease (n = 19)		Group B — other medical problems (n = 33)			
	Mean	SD	Mean	SD	Mean	SD	F[a]	F[b]
Defensiveness	49.08	12.51	47.84	2.46	49.79	2.36	0.29	0.26
Adjustment	55.60	14.81	51.74	3.27	57.82	2.59	2.08	0.13
Achievement	55.71	13.70	55.00	3.49	56.12	2.26	0.08	0.42
Intelligence	57.67	12.28	58.42	3.05	57.24	2.06	0.11	0.00
Development	55.44	12.79	50.68	2.64	58.18	2.24	4.42*	0.32
Somatic concerns	66.35	18.27	61.63	3.91	69.06	3.25	2.03	0.35
Depression	59.94	14.56	62.84	3.76	58.27	2.33	1.19	2.43
Family relations	54.71	11.76	53.42	2.52	55.45	2.14	0.30	0.12
Delinquency	58.87	14.09	55.68	2.81	58.87	2.60	1.54	0.15
Withdrawal	60.83	12.91	64.15	3.25	59.91	2.08	1.03	4.48*
Anxiety	57.31	11.44	55.84	2.09	58.15	2.20	0.49	0.20
Psychosis	61.04	17.38	57.11	3.31	63.30	3.26	1.55	0.15
Hyperactivity	48.19	12.08	46.21	2.18	49.33	2.32	0.80	0.20
Social skills	54.60	10.73	51.26	1.79	56.52	2.05	3.73	0.96

Note: * denotes $p < 0.05$; df = 1, 50.

[a] From one-way analysis of variance.
[b] From analysis of covariance controlled for SES.

The second hypothesis was that the head circumference of a neonate at birth would relate to later development. Small head circumference would be associated with poorer scores on measures being made. The larger and more normal the head circumference of the neonate, the higher the probability that his/her development would be normal in early childhood.

Comparisons of the two groups of SGA children were made with regard to head circumference at birth and the measured variables. The two groups had similarly nonsignificant relationships between head circumference at birth and intellectual and academic measures. Physical measurements of height, weight, and head circumference at 4 to 7 years of age were also not significantly related to head circumference at birth in either of these groups (Table 3).

When comparing the two groups on head circumference at birth and the personality variables, Group A children born to mothers with vascular disease scored significantly higher on ''development'' and ''family relations'', and Group B scored significantly higher on ''adjustment'' (Table 4). Greater head circumference at birth was related to better development and family relations for Group A and better adjustment in Group B as defined by the PIC.

Hypothesis 3 predicted that within Group A, greater birth weight would be associated with better scores on the measures taken.

Verbal IQ, performance IQ, and full-scale IQ correlated positively with birth weight in Group B (Table 5). The heavier the neonate in this group, the better he/she performed on intelligence scales at 4 to 7 years of age. These children also performed better on the test for perceptual-motor ability (Table 5). In addition, Group B children who were heavier at birth were significantly taller and heavier in early childhood (Table 5).

Group A children demonstrated significantly negative correlations between birth weight and both verbal and full-scale IQ scores. Lighter SGA children in Group A had better scores on all IQ, achievement, and perceptual-motor tests, with significant negative correlations between greater birth weight and poorer verbal and full-scale IQ scores.

TABLE 3

Comparison of Correlations Group A and Group B on Head Circumference at Birth Percentile and Intellectual and Physical Variables

	Group A — with vascular disease			Group B — without vascular disease		
	r	r²	n	r	r²	n
Verbal IQ	−0.096	0.009	20	0.056	0.003	33
Performance IQ	0.153	0.024	20	0.277	0.078	33
Full-scale IQ	0.048	0.002	20	0.178	0.032	33
Raven's CPM	0.353	0.124	20	−0.150	0.022	33
WRAT — reading	0.052	0.003	20	0.298	0.089	26
WRAT — arithmetic	0.223	0.050	20	0.303	0.092	24
Bender or VMI	0.047	0.002	20	0.083	0.007	31
Height	0.068	0.005	18	0.075	0.006	30
Weight	0.276	0.076	18	0.063	0.004	31
Head circumference	0.131	0.017	18	0.091	0.008	31

Note: No significant relationships.

TABLE 4

Comparison of Correlations Group A and Group B on Head Circumference at Birth Percentile with Personality Variables

	Group A — with vascular disease (n = 19)		Group B — without vascular disease (n = 32)	
	r	r²	r	r²
Defensiveness	0.487	0.237	0.316	0.010*
Adjustment	0.277	0.077	0.386	0.149*
Achievement	0.036	0.001	0.057	0.003
Intelligence	0.007	0.000	−0.092	0.008
Development	0.409	0.117*	0.183	0.034
Somatic concerns	0.276	0.076	−0.113	0.013
Depression	0.126	0.016	0.096	0.009
Family relations	0.441	0.194*	0.211	0.044
Delinquency	0.134	0.018	0.150	0.023
Withdrawal	−0.026	0.008	0.077	0.006
Anxiety	−0.126	0.016	0.005	0.000
Psychosis	−0.038	0.001	0.071	0.005
Hyperactivity	−0.085	0.007	0.144	0.021
Social skills	0.152	0.023	0.187	0.035

Note: * denotes $p < 0.05$.

In the fourth hypothesis it was predicted that SGA children of greater gestational age would have poorer scores on measures taken in early childhood than SGA children of shorter gestational age.

Between-group analyses demonstrated that the Group A children's intelligence test scores correlated *negatively* with gestational age, as the hypotheses predicted (Table 6). These Group A children also showed a significant positive relationship between gestational age and perceptual-motor test scores. However, these were in the direction contrary to the

TABLE 5
Comparison of Correlations of Group A and Group B
on Birth Weight with Measured Variables

	Group A — with vascular disease		Group B — without vascular disease	
	r	r²	r	r²
Verbal IQ	−0.408	0.167*	0.566	0.321***
Performance IQ	−0.341	0.116	0.477	0.227**
Full-scale IQ	−0.387	0.150*	0.568	0.322***
Raven's matrices	0.009	0.000	0.227	0.052
WRAT — reading	−0.252	0.063	0.204	0.042
WRAT — arithmetic	−0.150	0.023	0.242	0.058
Bender or VMI	−0.220	0.048	0.448	0.201**
Height	0.039	0.001	0.357	0.127*
Weight	0.352	0.124	0.386	0.149*
Head circumference	0.035	0.001	0.142	0.020

Note: Mean = 2162 g; SD = 363.3 g; range = 1200—2620 g; * denotes
$p < 0.05$, ** denotes $p < 0.01$, *** denotes $p < 0.001$.

TABLE 6
Comparison of Correlations of Group A and Group B on
Gestational Age with Measured Variables

	Group A — with vascular disease			Group B — without vascular disease		
Variable	n	r	r²	n	r	r²
Verbal IQ	20	−0.399	0.159*	33	0.274	0.075
Performance IQ	20	−0.465	0.216*	33	0.186	0.035
Full-scale IQ	20	−0.466	0.217*	33	0.242	0.059
Raven's CPM	20	−0.016	0.000	33	0.319	0.102*
WRAT — reading	20	−0.124	0.015	27	0.274	0.075
WRAT — arithmetic	20	−0.043	0.001	25	0.319	0.101
Bender or VMI	20	0.385	0.148*	31	0.311	0.096*
Head circumference	18	0.181	0.033	31	0.137	0.019
Height	18	0.026	0.000	30	0.189	0.036
Weight	18	0.329	0.108	31	0.202	0.041

Note: * denotes $p < 0.05$.

hypothesis. The higher scores of these children on perceptual-motor tasks were related to greater gestational age.

The SGA children in Group A also showed a significant negative relationship between gestational age and both "delinquency" and "anxiety" (Table 7). SGA children born to mothers affected by vascular disease during pregnancy were more anxious and had a tendency toward delinquency, as described by their mothers on the PIC.

The Group B SGA children showed a significant positive relationship between gestational age and the Raven's CPM. These larger-at-birth SGA children also performed better on tests of visual motor perception (Table 6).

Only one of the personality scales was significantly related to greater gestational age in Group B. This was "hyperactivity". SGA Group B children born at advanced gestational age tended to be more hyperactive in early childhood, as reported by their mothers (Table 7).

TABLE 7
Comparison of Group A and Group B on
Gestational Age with Personality Variables

Variable	Group A — with vascular disease (n = 19)		Group B — without vascular disease (n = 32)	
	r	r²	r	r²
Defensiveness	−0.213	0.046	0.064	0.004
Adjustment	−0.252	0.064	0.048	0.002
Achievement	−0.293	0.086	0.176	0.031
Intelligence	−0.034	0.001	0.094	0.009
Development	−0.342	0.117	0.285	0.081
Somatic concerns	−0.343	0.118	−0.044	0.002
Depression	−0.360	0.129	−0.010	0.000
Family relations	−0.294	0.086	−0.225	0.050
Delinquency	−0.476	0.227*	−0.132	0.017
Withdrawal	−0.342	0.117	−0.081	0.007
Anxiety	−0.435	0.189*	−0.029	0.001
Psychosis	−0.269	0.073	−0.187	0.035
Hyperactivity	−0.278	0.078	−0.417	0.174**
Social skills	0.071	0.005	0.072	0.005

Note: * denotes $p < 0.05$. ** denotes $p < 0.01$.

TABLE 8
Correlation between Socioeconomic Status
and Intellectual and Physical Variables

Variables	r	r²	n
Verbal IQ	0.504	0.254***	51
Performance IQ	0.464	0.215***	51
Full-scale IQ	0.522	0.272***	51
Raven's CPM	0.451	0.203***	51
WRAT — reading	0.225	0.051	44
WRAT — arithmetic	0.326	0.106*	43
Bender or VMI	0.252	0.064*	49
Height	−0.332	0.110*	46
Weight	−0.023	0.001	47
Head circumference	0.015	0.000	47

Note: * denotes $p < 0.05$, *** denotes $p < 0.001$; other
r² values not significant.

Hypothesis 5 predicted that low SES of these SGA children's families would have a negative effect on the intellectual, academic perceptual-motor, and emotional functioning of the children tested. SES was also expected to be correlated with the physical measurements of height, weight, and head circumference of these SGA children at the time of testing in early childhood.

The results of this study showed that SES of the whole group of SGA children was positively and significantly correlated with all intelligence tests, arithmetic achievement tests, and perceptual motor tasks (Table 8). Higher SES related significantly to better intellectual scores, concurring with the hypothesis. Height in early childhood was negatively significantly correlated with SES; however, lower SES SGA children were taller than higher SES SGA children (Table 8).

TABLE 9
Correlation between Socioeconomic
Status and Personality Variables

Variables	r	r²
Defensiveness	0.033	0.001
Adjustment	−0.436	0.190***
Achievement	−0.325	0.105**
Intelligence	0.120	0.14
Development	−0.619	0.383***
Somatic concerns	−0.376	0.141**
Depression	−0.161	0.026
Family relations	−0.410	0.168***
Delinquency	−0.278	0.077*
Withdrawal	−0.207	0.043
Anxiety	−0.146	0.021
Psychosis	−0.371	0.138**
Hyperactivity	−0.193	0.037
Social skills	−0.338	0.114**

Note: $n = 51$. * denotes $p < 0.05$, ** denotes $p < 0.01$, *** denotes $p < 0.001$; other values not significant.

TABLE 10
Comparison of Group A and Group B on
Socioeconomic Status

	Group A — with vascular disease ($n = 19$)	Group B — without vascular disease ($n = 33$)
Mean SES score[a]	53.21	63.70
SD	18.10	10.10
Range	20—79	20—80

Note: $F = 7.23$; d.f. = 1, 50; $p < 0.01$ (sig. = 0.009).

[a] High scores relate to low SES; low scores relate to high SES.

Since a high score on SES reflects a lower SES and vice versa, for easier comprehension the signs in Tables 8 and 9 were reversed. In Table 10, where Groups A and B were compared, the original signs of the numbers were retained. In this table, the SES scores of Group A and Group B are significantly different. The mean SES score is lower (better) in Group A; M = 53.21, which is the lower-middle or upper-middle range as defined by Warner et al.[41] The families of Group B SGA children had higher (poorer) scores; M = 63.70, in the upper-lower or lower-lower range.

IV. DISCUSSION

All SGA and, thus, growth-retarded neonates are born as a result of some pathology during pregnancy and are therefore considered at risk for normal development. However, some of these babies may be more at risk than others. A large percentage of SGA babies are born to mothers who have had vascular disease during pregnancy (Group A). This study compared these children with SGA children born to women who had other, sometimes unknown complications during pregnancy, resulting in growth-retarded neonates (Group B).

One of the findings of this study was that SGA children born to mothers with vascular disease during pregnancy had a higher SES than SGA children born to mothers without vascular disease. When SES was controlled statistically, the differences between the two groups were significant for WISC-R or WPPSI, verbal IQ, and the "withdrawal" scale of the PIC.

The literature shows that the growth of the head *in utero* in mothers with vascular disease differs from that in mothers with nonvascular disease.[4,9] In growth-retarded fetuses of mothers with vascular disease, Campbell[32] has identified a "late-flattening" head growth pattern. The "brain-sparing effect"[31] associated with this head growth pattern results in normal head growth until 34 to 36 weeks of gestation, at which time the rate of growth is slowed. In fetuses of mothers without vascular disease, but with other medical problems during pregnancy, Campbell[32] has identified a "low-profile" head growth pattern in which the head develops more slowly throughout the pregnancy. The resulting head size of each type of baby may be smaller than average, but the child in this study whose mother had vascular disease seems to show better intellectual, academic, perceptual-motor, and emotional development in early childhood.

The PIC[48] has proved to be useful for differentiating between the two groups of children being studied. The PIC provides comprehensive and clinically relevant personality descriptions of these children, as reported by their parents. Although individual scales revealed some statistically significant differences between the groups when compared with some of the criterion variables, the composite inventory discriminated extremely well between the two groups of children. The group of children born to mothers in Group B had consistently poorer scores on the individual personality scales. In general, these children had poorer personality adjustments, as reported by their mothers on the PIC.

Sameroff[48] indicates that small-at-birth babies may be perceived by their parents as different and vulnerable. Since the PIC is a parent report of the child's emotional status, this parental view of the child whose mother has other medical problems (Group B) may be distorting the child's actual emotional functioning. That did not seem to be the case in this study. The mothers who had vascular disease during their pregnancies (Group A) also gave birth to small, seemingly vulnerable babies, but they did not perceive them as emotionally deviant. Therefore, the children born to mothers in Group B may indeed be more deviant emotionally than those born to mothers who had vascular disease during pregnancy (Group A).

There were no significant differences between Groups A and B when examining the relationship between head circumference at birth and the intellectual and physical variables. However, greater head circumference at birth in the overall group of SGA children was significantly related to better scores on several of the personality scales of the PIC. These were "defensiveness", "adjustment", "development", and "family relations". When controlling for SES, only "defensiveness" and "adjustment" remained significantly related to head circumference at birth. Better emotional adjustment was related to greater head circumference at birth in this sample of SGA children (both groups).

When comparing the two groups of SGA children on the relationship between birth weight and development, only in the children born in Group B was lower birth weight associated with poorer development at 4 to 7 years of age. Lower birth weight in Group B was associated with poorer scores in intelligence, poorer visual-motor perception, and lesser height and weight.

The personality scales of the PIC that were significantly related to birth weight in Group B were "adjustment" and "development". Lower birth weight was associated with poorer scores, and higher birth weight was associated with better scores on these scales of the PIC in Group B. These results had been predicted for the entire group of SGA children, but only occurred in Group B.

The group of children born to mothers in Group A did not have the same type of results. Instead, lower birth weight in this group was correlated with better scores and higher birth weight with poorer scores on intelligence measures. The PIC scales that were significantly correlated with birth weight were "depression", "delinquency", "withdrawal", and "anxiety". These results were also contrary to what we had hypothesized. For children born to mothers with vascular disease during pregnancy (Group A), greater birth weight was related to poorer scores on these PIC scales.

In examining the effects of gestational age on the groups, the findings are similar to those on birth weight. Greater gestational age of babies in Group A seems to be a negative factor in the development of these children.

The baby whose mother is affected by vascular disease seems to have a less favorable later intrauterine environment. The longer gestational time of this fetus seems to result in some poorer later development. On the other hand, the children whose mothers had non-vascular medical problems during pregnancy seem to have derived some benefit from the greater gestational age.

These findings indicate that in growth retardation due to maternal vascular disease there may be an optimal and earlier time for delivery beyond which *in utero* residence may be debilitating from the long-term point of view.

Low SES of these children's families was significantly related to poor performance on intelligence tests and perceptual-motor tasks and to lesser academic ability and emotional development at 4 to 7 years of age. These findings agree with those of Vane,[40,49] Broman et al.,[11] Ounsted et al.,[46] and Rubin and Barlow,[38] that SES adversely affects later development. However, SES did not play a significant role in all of the results of this study. Advanced gestational age of SGA babies had some negative consequences regardless of SES. A significant number of greater gestational age SGA children are described as "hyperactive" in early childhood regardless of SES. Intelligence is lower among advanced gestational age children of mothers with vascular disease during pregnancy (and of higher SES) than lower gestational age SGA children whose mothers had vascular disease.

It was found unexpectedly that among the two groups of SGA children studied, those in Group B were significantly different in SES. One explanation for this may be that vascular disease is a medical condition that does not occur as a result of a poor or inadequate environment. The various medical problems of the nonvascular disease group included such conditions as addictions, nutritional deficiencies, asthma, kidney disease, sickle cell trait, and epilepsy. Many of these disorders are exacerbated as a result of a disadvantaged environment.

Thus, the relationship between SES and later development has several dimensions. The SGA fetus within the lower SES mother has a less favorable environment during the gestational period. In addition, this child is born into, and grows up in, a poorer, more barren environment.

SES of the families of these SGA children is probably the strongest single influence on their later development. Sameroff[48] suggests that the effects of social status tend to reduce or amplify intellectual deficits, and, as mentioned earlier, Rubin and Barlow[38] found that higher SES seems to be able to counteract the potential deficits of a less than optimal intrauterine environment. The lower SES child is at greater risk during later development.

Socioeconomic status strongly and positively correlated with intellectual and emotional variables, but did not correlate with weight and, surprisingly, had a negative correlation with height in this sample.

The effect of SES on development of children is not a new finding. What emerged from this study that had not been reported in the literature was that intrauterine growth-retarded babies born to mothers exhibiting vascular disease during pregnancy showed greater deficits in early childhood if they were born at an advanced gestational age. The last 4 to 6 weeks of pregnancy seem to adversely affect the fetus, and in spite of an enriched home environment these children have lower intelligence in early childhood. The entire group of SGA children ($n = 55$) of greater gestational age were also found to be more hyperactive than those SGA children of lesser gestational age.

In view of this finding, we can begin monitoring the pregnancies of women suspected of carrying a growth-retarded fetus, and who have vascular disease, earlier to identify the optimal time for delivery.

REFERENCES

1. **Caputo, D. V. and Mandell, W.,** Consequences of low birth weight, *Dev. Psychol.,* 3, 363, 1970.
2. **Lentz, G. A.,** Infants small-for-age should be differentiated before prognosis, *Pediatr. News,* 14, 55, 1980.
3. American Academy of Pediatrics Committee on the Fetus and Newborn, Nomenclature for duration of gestation, birth weight and intrauterine growth, *Pediatrics,* 39, 935, 1967.
4. **Tejani, N. and Mann, L.,** Diagnosis and management of the small-for-gestational-age fetus, *Clin. Obstet. Gynecol.,* 20, 943, 1977.
5. **Drillien, C. E.,** *The Growth and Development of Prematurely Born Infants,* Williams & Wilkins, Baltimore, 1964.
6. **McDonald, A. D.,** Retarded fetal growth, in *Gestational Age, Size and Maturity,* Dawkings, M. and MacGregor, W. G., Eds., Spastics Society Medical Education and Information Unit, 1965.
7. **Gallagher, M. and O'Brien, N.,** The small for date infant, *Ir. Med. Assoc.,* Suppl. 1, 13, 1976.
8. **Rutter, M., Tizard, J., and Whitmore, K.,** *Education, Health and Behavior,* John Wiley & Sons, New York, 1975.
9. **Rosso, P. and Winick, M.,** Intrauterine growth retardation. A new systematic approach based on clinical and biochemical characteristics of this condition, *J. Perinat. Med.,* 2, 147, 1974.
10. **Fitzhardinge, P. M.,** Early growth and development in low birth weight infants following treatment in an intensive care nursery, *Pediatrics,* 56(2), 162, 1975.
11. **Broman, S. H., Nichols, P. L., and Kennedy, W. A.,** *Preschool IQ, Prenatal and Early Developmental Correlates,* Lawrence Erlbaum Associates, Hillsdale, NJ, 1975.
12. **Silva, P. A., McGee, R., and Williams, S.,** A longitudinal study of the intelligence and behavior of preterm and small for gestational age children, *Dev. Behav. Pediatr.,* 5(1), 1, 1984.
13. **Cruise, M. O.,** A longitudinal study of the growth of low birth weight infants, *Pediatrics,* 51(4), 620, 1973.
14. **Moltens, C. D., Ahrens, W., Higgs, S. C., Malan, A. F., and Heese, H. DeV.,** Infants of very low birth weight, *S. Afr. Med. J.,* 50, 955, 1976.
15. **Fancourt, R., Campbell, S., Harvey, D., and Norman, A. P.,** Follow-up study of small-for-date babies, *Br. Med. J.,* 1, 1435, 1976.
16. **Mercer, H. P., Lancaster, A. L., Weiner, T., and Gupta, J. M.,** Very low birth weight infants: a follow-up study, *Med. J. Aust.,* 2, 581, 1978.
17. **Commey, J. O. and Fitzhardinge, P. M.,** Handicap in preterm small-for-gestational age infant, *J. Pediatr.,* 5(94), 779, 1979.
18. **Westwood, M., Kramer, M. S., Munz, D., Lovett, J. M., and Walters, G. V.,** Growth and development of full-term nonasphyxiated small-for-gestional-age newborns: follow-up through adolescence, *Pediatrics,* 71(3), 376, 1983.
19. **Tanner, J. M.,** *Foetus Into Man,* Harvard University Press, Cambridge, MA, 1978.
20. **Davies, D. P., Platt, P., Pritchard, J. M., and Wilkinson, P. W.,** Nutritional status of light-for-date infants at birth and its influence on early postnatal growth, *Arch. Dis. Child.,* 54, 703, 1979.
21. **Bjirre, I. and Hansen, E.,** Psychomotor development and school adjustment of seven year old children with low birth weight, *Acta. Paediatr. Scand.,* 65, 88, 1976.
22. **Davies, P. S. and Stewart, A. L.,** Low birth weight infants: neurological sequelae and later intelligence, *Br. Med. J.,* 31(1), 85, 1975.
23. **Caputo, D. V., Taub, H. B., Goldstein, K. M., Smith, N., Dalack, J. D., Pursner, J. P., and Dilberstein, R. M.,** An evaluation of various parameters of maturity at birth as predictors of development of one year of life, *Percept. Mot. Skills,* 39, 631, 1974.

24. **Fitzhardinge, P. M. and Stevens, E. M.,** The small-for-date infant. II. Neurological and intellectual sequelae, *Pediatrics,* 50(1), 50, 1972.
25. **Weiner, G.,** The relationship of birth weight and length of gestation to intellectual development at eight to ten years, *J. Pediatr.,* 76(5), 694, 1970.
26. **Weiner, G., Rider, R. V., Oppel, W. C., and Harper, P. A.,** Correlates of low birth weight: psychological status of eight to ten years of age, *Pediatr. Res.,* 2, 110, 1968.
27. **Harvey, D., Prince, J., Bunton, J., Parkinson, C., and Campbell, S.,** Abilities of children who were small-for-gestational-age babies, *Pediatrics,* 69, 296, 1982.
28. **Koops, B. L.,** Neurologic sequelae of infants with intrauterine growth retardation, *J. Reprod. Med.,* 21(6), 343, 1978.
29. **Anon.,** General discussions, in *Size at Birth,* Ciba Found. Symp. 27, Elliott, K. and Knight, J., Eds., Elsevier/North-Holland, Amsterdam, 1974, 383.
30. **Resnick, R.,** Maternal diseases associated with abnormal fetal growth, *J. Reprod. Med.,* 21(5), 315, 1978.
31. **Gruenwald, P.,** Chronic fetal distress and placental insufficiency, *Biol. Neonate,* 5, 215, 1963.
32. **Campbell, S.,** The assessment of fetal development by diagnostic ultrasound, *Clin. Perinatol.,* 1, 511, 1974.
33. **Lowrey, G. H.,** *Growth and Development of Children,* Year Book Medical Publishers, Chicago, 1978.
34. **Vohr, B., Oh, W., Rosenfield, A., and Cowett, R.,** The preterm small-for-gestational age infant: a two-year follow-up study, *Am. J. Obstet. Gynecol.,* 133, 425, 1979.
35. **Davies, D. P.,** Growth of small-for-date babies, *Early Hum. Dev.,* 5, 95, 1981.
36. **Fitzhardinge, P. M. and Ramsey, M.,** The improving outlook for small prematurely born infants, *Dev. Med. Child Neurol.,* 15, 447, 1973.
37. **Birch, H. and Gussow, J.,** *Disadvantaged Children, Health, Nutrition and School Failure,* Grune & Stratton, New York, 1970.
38. **Rubin, R. and Barlow, B.,** Measures of infant development and socioeconomic status as predictors of later intelligence and school achievement, *Dev. Psychol.,* 15(2), 225, 1979.
39. **Parkinson, C. E., Willis, S., and Harvey, D.,** School achievement and behavior of children who were small-for-dates at birth, *Dev. Med. Child Neurol.,* 23, 41, 1981.
40. **Vane, J.,** Intelligence and achievement test results of kindergarten age children in England, Ireland and the United States, *J. Clin. Psychol.,* 24(2), 191, 1973.
41. **Warner, W., Meeker, M., and Eels, K.,** *Social Class in America,* Harper & Row, New York, 1960.
42. **McCall, R., Hogarty, P. S., and Hurlburt, N.,** Transition in infant sensorimotor development and the prediction of childhood IQ, *Am. Psychol.,* 27(8), 728, 1972.
43. **Beckwith, L. and Cohen, S.,** Interaction of preterm infants with their caretakers and test performance at age two, in *High Risk Infants and Children,* Field, T., Ed., Academic Press, New York, 1980.
44. **Francis-Williams, J. and Davies, P. A.,** Very low birth weight and later intelligence, *Dev. Med. Child Neurol.,* 16, 709, 1974.
45. **Davies, P. A. and Tizard, J. P. M.,** Very low birth weight and subsequent neurological defects, *Dev. Med. Child Neurol.,* 17, 3, 1975.
46. **Ounsted, M. K., Moar, V. A., and Scott, A.,** Children of deviant size, and developmental status, *Early Hum. Dev.,* 9, 323, 1984.
47. **Wirt, R. D., Lachar, D., Klinedinst, J., and Seat, P.,** *Multidimensional Description of Child Personality,* Western Psychological Corporation, Los Angeles, 1977.
48. **Sameroff, A.,** Early influences in development: fact or fancy, *Merrill-Palmer Q. Behav. Dev.,* 21(4), 267, 1975.
49. **Vane, J.,** Importance of considering background factors when evaluating the effects of compensatory education programs designed for young children, *J. School Psychol.,* 9(4), 393, 1971.

Chapter 7

SEQUELAE IN CHILDREN WHO SURVIVED *IN UTERO* FETAL TRANSFUSION: A COMPARISON WITH THOSE WHO UNDERWENT POSTPARTUM EXCHANGE TRANSFUSION ONLY

Victor Halitsky

TABLE OF CONTENTS

I. INTRODUCTION

This chapter deals with the long-term effects of *in utero* fetal transfusion. A search of literature published between 1969 and 1987 yielded 24 papers dealing with this subject alone or in combination with the techniques of intra-abdominal fetal transfusion. Of the 24 papers, 22 papers are in English, 1 in Spanish, and 1 in German. Other papers in German[1-4] were not reviewed. Three studies, two by Bowman et al.[5,6] and another by Friesen,[7] were reviewed, but they are not included in this survey because a complete analysis by Bowman[8] at a later date included the findings of these studies. A total of 788 children were evaluated in the studies described by the 24 papers.

The development of these children, all of whom had *in utero* fetal transfusions and either postpartum exchange or top-up transfusions, was compared to 412 children who had post-partum exchange and top-up transfusions only.[9,10] Nearly all authors described their subjects in standard developmental terms, some briefly and others in depth. Some scored their patients; others did not. A multitude of terms, mainly neurological or neurologically related, were used.

Abnormalities associated with the mechanics of intrauterine transfusion were also described: hernias, bowel and renal injury, and cutaneous scars. Abnormalities probably associated with the transfused blood were listed: cytomegaloviremia, chimerism, leukemia, derangements of immune globulins, and patent ductus arteriosus. Finally, squints, visual acuity, myopia, hyperemmetropia, enamel defects, dental caries, and skin and respiratory allergies were described.

II. DEFINITIONS

In an attempt to more rationally compare previously reported studies, Tripp[11] and Hardyment et al.[12] regrouped the neurological findings into major and minor deficits. In this study, all neurological abnormalities were assigned major or minor status. This assessment was only occasionally at variance with the reporting authors; i.e., Whitfield et al.'s[13] assignments of mild cerebral palsy and minimal hemiparesis to the major-deficit group were downgraded to minor central nervous system (CNS) status. Similarly, the "clumsiness" of Girling et al.[14] was placed in the minor CNS category. Ellis[15] further clarified reporting by stating whether her own patients' defects were the result of hemolytic disease of the newborn, the result of *in utero* transfusion procedure, or were related to neither transfusion nor disease. Her classification clearly separated iatrogenic factors from those specifically due to hemolytic disease and from what shall be included in developmental defects described below.

In this review, long-term effects of *in utero* fetal transfusion will be designated as those derived from the disease itself (hemolytic disease of the newborn: HDN), from the transfusion procedure (significant defects related to the transfusion: SDRT), and from *in utero* and neonatal conditions not associated with either (developmental). Table 1 lists defects associated with these three categories.

In order to sharply delimit the effects of hyperbilirubinemia from developmental effects of the prematurity-hypoxia-acidosis-cerebral hemorrhage complex, the child who had HDN-related chronic postkernicteric bilirubin encephalopathy is defined as one who manifests and who continues to demonstrate either one or two (or all) of the following: athetoid cerebral palsy, upward gaze paralysis, and significant high-frequency sensorineural hearing loss (a loss of $\geqslant 30$ dB in the 1000 Hz range).[16-23] Less specific findings, but presumably related to HDN, are aphasia, some cases of mental retardation, and some unspecified minor CNS deficits.

Although the etiology of the subtle type of chronic bilirubin encephalopathy[24-30] is in doubt, its neurological, psychological, and intellectual deficits are similar to those defects

TABLE 1
Classification of Defects Due to Hemolytic Disease of the Newborn, Developmental Defects, and Significant Defects Related to Transfusion in Both Study and Control Patients

Defects Due to Hemolytic Disease of the Newborn (HDN)

Major	Minor	Other
Severe athetosis	Mild athetosis	Mental retardation
Sensorineural deafness	Questionable gaze defect	
Aphasia	Unspecified CNS deficits	

Developmental Defects

Major	Minor	Other
Spastic hemiplegia	Mild spastic diplegia	Speech handicap
Spastic paraplegia	Mild cerebral palsy	Hyperkinesia
Seizure disorder	Minimal hemiparesis	Sobbing
Coarse tremors	Minimal hemispherical dysfunction	Perceptual problems
Hydrocephalus	Minimal slight hypotonia	Language deficit
Microcephaly	Minimal postural asymmetry	Low psychological scores
Cerebral agenesis	Minimal pyramidal tract involvement	Mental retardation
	Minor neuromuscular problems	Growth retardation
	Minor unstated CNS disorders	Developmental retardation
	Minimal cerebral signs with no difficulty	Minor DQ delay
	Fine and rapid motor incoordination	Behavioral problems
	Motor retardation	Abnormal physical exam
	Hyperreflexia	Apraxia
	Drooling	Left-right confusion
	Hyperacusia	
	Clumsiness	
	Minor unstated CNS disorders	

Significant Defects Related to Transfusion (SDRT)

Major	Minor	Other
None	Lower motor neuron paralysis	Renal damage
		Malabsorption syndrome
		Persistent donor white blood cells
		Diminished IgA
		Cytomegalo viremia

described by Walker et al.[10] in the low birth weight-hypoxic group of children (impaired reading, speech, and intelligence; changes in personality and minor perceptual-motor abnormalities) and by Hugh-Jones and associates,[31] Killander et al.,[32] Mores and co-workers,[33] Shiller and Silverman,[34] Watchko and Oski,[35] and Wishingrad et al.[36] in the premature and mature infant. Because there is lack of concensus in the bilirubin etiology of these parameters and considerable agreement in the prematurity-hypoxia etiology, these conditions will be classified under developmental defects.

Although there were an unusual number of hernias (6.2% in the reviewed series) and cutaneous scars associated with *in utero* fetal transfusion, these conditions will not be considered significant from the long-range point of view. Other conditions such as organ dysfunction resulting from procedural trauma or persistent donor white cell population and depressed immune globulin will be considered as significant defects. Visual defects, defects of dental enamel, and dental caries will not be considered since none are related to either hyperbilirubinemia or to the trauma of *in utero* transfusion. Although they are developmental in origin, their occurrence seems no different from that in the nonhemolytic disease population.

III. COMPARATIVE TABLES

Table 1 lists the developmental, SDRT, and HDN defects with their major and minor (CNS and other) deficits in both study and control groups.

Table 2 lists various data associated with children: the number of defects attributable to *in utero* transfusion (SDRT), defects related to hemolytic disease (HDN), developmental defects, major or minor neurological defects, and whether the reported children were mentally retarded or had sensorineural deafness.

Table 3 compares the abnormal children in the intrauterine transfusion (IUT) group to those in the control group.

Table 4 lists the percentages of major and minor CNS deficits related to development, HDN, and SDRT in both study and control groups.

Table 5 lists the percentages of major and minor CNS deficits related to HDN (sensorineural deafness, athetosis, aphasia, and other effects) in study and control groups.

IV. STUDY PATIENTS

Gregg and Hutchinson[37] examined 15 children who had received IUT between 9 and 38 months of age whose major neonatal complaints were acidosis, respiratory distress, and hyperbilirubinemia due to inspissated bile syndrome. They studied developmental quotient, fine and gross motor development, adaptive, personal, and social behavior, as well as language skills. They felt that all children were normal except one, who manifested growth retardation and diminished intelligence at 27 months of age.

The authors state that if IUT is performed before serious intrauterine damage occurs, it is not intrinsically harmful to the neonate. They also feel that in most minimally affected children, defects present at 2 years of age disappear by age 10 when the home environment remains favorable.[38]

Although one child with growth retardation and some mental retardation was listed as the only abnormality, they described seven children with the following defects: one with a questionable upward gaze, two with hyperreflexia, one with drooling, one with hyperacusia, one exhibiting growth retardation, and one showing a language defect. Scoring these children according to the previously mentioned synopsis, Gregg and Hutchinson in effect report no major neurological deficits, five minor neurological deficits (one gaze defect, two hyperreflexia, one drooling, and one hyperacusia), six developmental defects (all of the latter less the gaze defect plus one growth retardation and one language deficit), and one defect related to hyperbilirubinenemia (gaze defect; see Table 2). The authors also reported three children with hernias and three with heavily pigmented teeth; these were not included in the synopsis.

Cochran et al.[39] studied 41 infants whose average gestational age was 34 weeks and whose follow-up was from 6 months to $4^1/_2$ years who had one to four IUTs. There were no controls. They felt that 11 of the 41 children were abnormal: 9 had developmental problems (5 with low psychological scores and 4 with abnormal physical exams) and 2 had definite evidence of renal damage. They felt that the prognosis for the 41 children was less ideal than that expected of comparable infants who had not undergone intrauterine fetal transfusion.

Corston et al.[40] reported on 23 survivors of IUT, the first of whom began school at the time the report was made. At that time all 23 children continued to thrive mentally and physically. No further long-term details were given.

TABLE 2
Aggregate Data Study and Control Children

No of children	Gestational age (weeks) or birthweight (g)	No. of exchange transfusions	Age at evaluation (months)	Controls	Major CNS[a,b]	Minor CNS[a,b]	Mental retardation[c] (related to development or HDN)	Sensorineural deafness[a] (related to HDN)	Children with problems related to SDRT[a]	Children with problems related to HDN[a]	Children with developmental problems[a]	Abnormal[d] children	Normal children	Ref.
15	32—37	All	9—38	No	0	5	0	0	0	1	6	7	8	57
41	34 av	36/41	6—56	No	0	0	5	0	2	0	9	11	30	39
23	30—34	All	Up to 60	No	0	0	0	0	0	0	0	0	23	40
38	35	36/38	1—46	No	4	2	0	3	3	3	2	8	30	41
16	33-36	Most	3—39	No	0	4	0	0	0	0	4	4	12	42
24	30—37	21/24	4—60	Yes	2	0	0	1	0	1	2	3	21	43
10	33—36	All	12—54	Yes	0	3	0	1	0	0	3	3	7	44
26	28—38	Most	At least 9	No	1	1	2	1	0	0	3	3	23	14
48	34—35?	?	12—48	No	0	0	0	0	0	0	1	1	47	13
18	31—36	All	6—60	No	0	2	0	0	0	0	8	8	10	45
44	?	Most	3—48	No	0	0	1	0	0	0	1	1	43	46
19	32—36	All	1—60	No	0	0	1	0	0	0	2	2	17	47
46	29—36?	?	48—90	No	1	0	0	0	0	0	2	2	44	11
87	?	?	>12—<18	No	3	7	0	0	0	0	13	13	74	8
44	74% <2500 g	32/44	90% >36	No	0	0	22	0	0	0	22	22	22	48
36	26—36	Most	?	No	1	0	2	0	0	0	3	3	33	49
19	31—38	All	5—91	No	0	2	0	0	0	0	3	3	16	50
18	32—36	All	24—72	No	0	5	0	0	0	0	5	5	13	51
15	31—37	Most	36—132	Yes	1	1	0	0	0	1	2	3	12	52
21	32—36	?	22—120	Yes	2	7	0	1	0	1	8	9	12	12
8	35—37	All	36—96	No	1	2	0	1	0	1	5	6	2	53
15	34.3 ± 1.4	All	36—120	Yes	0	0	0	0	1	0	0	0	15	54
81	31—40	78—81	62% >60	No	13	2	5	9	2	13	0	15	66	15
29	27—36	All	12—132	No	1	0	0	1	0	1	0	1	28	55
Total 788					30	45	38	17	8	22	103	133	655	
129	28—40?	95%	60—72	Yes	10	3	1	7	NA	7	0	7	122	9
283	Most 38—40	60%	84—168	No	14	22	8	11	NA	13	6	19	264	10
Total 412					24	25	9	18	NA	20	6	26	386	

Note: NA = not applicable.

a See Table 1.
b Related to development, HDN, or SDRT.
c IQ ≤70.
d Abnormal children are the sum of children showing developmental problems, HDN, and SDRT.

TABLE 3
Comparison of Various Parameters in Study and Controls

Source	No.	Normal	Abnormal[a]	HDN	Development	SDRT	(Related to HDN, Development or SDRT)		Mental retardation[c] (related to HDN or development)	Sensorineural deafness[b] (related to HDN)
							Major CNS[b]	Minor CNS[b]		
Total study patients	788	655 (83.1%)	133 (16.9%)[d]	22 (2.8%)[d]	103 (13.1%)[d]	8 (1.0%)	30 (3.8%)	45 (5.7%)	38 (4.8%)[d]	17 (2.2%)
Study patients less Turner et al.	744	633 (85.1%)	111 (14.9%)[d]	22 (3.0%)	81 (10.9%)[d]	8 (1.1%)	30 (4.0%)	45 (6.0%)	16 (2.2%)	17 (2.3%)
Control patients	412	386 (93.7%)	26 (6.3%)	20 (4.9%)	6 (1.5%)	NA[e]	24 (5.8%)	25 (6.1%)	9 (2.2%)	18 (4.4%)[f]

[a] Abnormal children are the sum of developmental, HDN, and SDRT problems.
[b] See Table 3.
[c] IQ ≤70.
[d] p <0.05.
[e] NA = not applicable.
[f] Significant difference when compared to study patients, with or without data of Turner et al.

TABLE 4
A Comparison of the Composition of Major and Minor CNS Deficits Related to Development, HDN, and SDRT in Study and Control Groups

	Study group		Control group	
	Major CNS deficit	Minor CNS deficit	Major CNS deficit	Minor CNS deficit
Development	8/30 (26.7%)	40/45 (88.9%)	0/24 (0%)	16/25 (64.0%)
HDN	22/30 (73.3%)	1/45 (2.2%)	24/24 (100%)	9/25 (36.0%)
SDRT	0/30 (0%)	4/45 (8.9%)	NA	NA

Note: NA = not applicable.

TABLE 5
The Distribution of HDN Sequelae in Study and Control Groups

	Study group		Control group	
	Major CNS deficit	Minor CNS deficit	Major CNS deficit	Minor CNS deficit
Sensorineural deafness	17/22 (77.3%)	0/45 (0%)	18/24 (75.0%)	0/9 (0%)
Athetosis	5/22 (22.7%)	0/45 (0%)	3/24 (12.5%)	7/9 (77.8%)
Aphasia	0/22 (0%)	0/45 (0%)	3/24 (12.5%)	0/9 (0%)
Unspecified	0/22 (0%)	0/45 (0%)	0/24 (0%)	2/9 (22.2%)

Walker[41] studied 38 survivors of *in utero* transfusion from 1 to 46 months. He stated that one third of the 38 children had no abnormality and that "many of the defects are minor and probably coincidental". He described 11 hernias and temporarily absent leg pulses after *in utero* trauma to a femoral artery. Long-term deficits were eight in number: two developmental problems (growth retardation in premature children with respiratory distress syndrome), three HDN sequelae (all sensorineural deafness, with one athetosis), and three sequelae due to trauma (one malabsorption syndrome and two lower motor neuron paralysis). There were four major deficits (three deafness and one athetosis) and two minor ones (two lower motor neuron paralysis).

Franchini et al.[42] described 16 infants who had IUT and were evaluated between the ages of 3 and 39 months. The physical examinations in all cases were normal. All had intelligence quotients (IQs) ranging from low average to normal, and four children had minimal developmental problems (hemispherical dysfunctions and postural asymmetry) and moderate EEG abnormalities, suggesting the possibility of CNS dysfunction (two had marked RDS or hyperbilirubinemia). These were considered minor deficits.

The authors felt that IUT was not intrinsically harmful to the fetus, that neurologic sequelae do not appear provided that indirect bilirubin is prevented from rising above a critical level in the neonatal period, and that a major degree of RDS should be avoided.

Phibbs et al.[43] presented 24 children who were evaluated every 4 months until 2 years of age and yearly thereafter to age 5. They felt that it was impossible to find an adequately matched control group and therefore compared their children to normal infants and children. They found that 21 out of the 24 children were normal. Of the remaining three abnormals, two were developmental (one spastic paraplegia and one speech handicap) and one was due to hemolytic disease (sensorineural deafness). There were two major deficits (one deafness and one spastic paraplegia) and no minor deficits.

They felt that acidotic infants were particularly disposed to bilirubin toxicity and that the neonatal risk factors following IUT were prematurity, birth asphyxia, cardiorespiratory distress, and hyperbilirubinemia. The authors stressed that IUT must be combined with aggressive therapy for cardiorespiratory distress and hyperbilirubinemia during the neonatal period.

Oh and associates[44] evaluated ten children between 12 and 54 months of age. Their controls were normal infants matched for birth weight, gestational age, race, sex, home environment, and age at the time of examination. Neonatal complications included RDS (five), inspissated bile syndrome (two), hypoglycemia (three), hydrops fetalis (two), and anemia-hyperbilirubinemia (ten). Acidosis, hypoxemia, hypoxia, and hypoglycemia were vigorously treated.

Neurologic testing was a five-point scale "available at the senior author's address". Psychometric testing included the following: the Stanford-Binet Intelligence Scale, the Peabody Picture Vocabulary Test, the Cattell Infant Intelligence Scale, the Vineland Social Maturity Scale, the Gessell Developmental Schedules, and the Home Environmental Scale. It should be mentioned that most of the authors discussed in this chapter utilized similar (if not the same) testing.

The authors found no difference between their children and controls, although they described three minor neurological findings: one lateral rectus paresis and two infants with abnormal reflexes implicating minimal pyramidal tract involvement. They added that one control infant had significant cranial nerve findings and another demonstrated minimal pyramidal tract involvement.

Girling and associates[14] presented 26 infants with considerable perinatal data. They considered three infants to be abnormal, but the age of evaluation was only 9 months. The authors found that one child was hyperkinetic and mentally retarded (birth weight, 2020 g; maximum unconjugated bilirubin, 18.5 mg%), one had mild spastic diplegia (birth weight, 3020 g; no asphyxia; maximum unconjugated bilirubin, 11.0 mg%), and one kernicterus and mental retardation (birth weight, 1900 g; birth asphyxia; maximum unconjugated bilirubin, 22 mg%). There were two developmental problems (one hyperkinesia-mental retardation and one mild spastic diplegia) and one hemolytic problem (kernicterus-mental retardation). The major and minor deficits included one kernicterus and one mild spastic diplegia, respectively. Also described were two cases of mental retardation.

They felt that the main problems in the neonatal period were those of prematurity, especially RDS, but also including hypoglycemia, enterocolitis, protracted jaundice, congestive heart failure, infections, and bleeding diatheses.

Whitfield et al.[13] discussed the outcome of 48 children following IUT in a paper dealing primarily with the latter. He reported ten children (all males) with hernias, three children with low normal intelligence, and one with mild cerebral palsy. In effect, 47 of 48 children were normal.

Peniche and associates[45] evaluated 18 survivors of IUT. The parameters used were neurological, electroencephalographic, audiometric, and developmental. They found seven abnormal children; if one child with hyperactive tendon reflexes was included, eight abnormal children were identified, all showing developmental problems. One child had mild cerebral palsy (minor CNS), another had the above-mentioned hyperactive reflexes (minor CNS), and six had behavioral problems such as sobbing, deficits in individual and social behavior, and language problems.

Holt et al.,[46] in a paper devoted primarily to IUT, stated that 43 of 44 infants were developing normally. One child was seriously retarded.

Richings[47] reported on 19 children, 17 of whom were considered normal. The children's neonatal problems were as follows: anemia-bilirubinemia (19), hydrops (3), birth asphyxia (7), respiratory distress (2), and hypoglycemia (3). Of the two abnormal children, one had a mild spastic diplegia (minor CNS) and the other was mentally retarded and hyperactive. The author also reported three hernias and a large popliteal scar, all without functional residua.

Tripp[11] reported on prior authors' papers and attempted to group their findings into major and minor neurological deficits. He added 46 infants, 4 of whom he felt were abnormal.

The author had no controls, since he thought that there were inherent difficulties in selecting matched pairs. Of the four abnormal children, two were classified as low normal in developmental quotient (DQ) and IQ and therefore were not included as abnormals in Table 2. Of the remaining two, one child had cerebral palsy (major CNS) and one was developmentally retarded.

Bowman[8] reported on the University of Manitoba's 10 years of experience with IUT and the follow-up of 87 infants. Portions of this paper were reported by Bowman et al.[5,6] and Friesen.[7] Of the 54 infants evaluated by a pediatric specialist at the Winnipeg Children's Center, 44 were completely normal and 10 were abnormal: 5 had minor neuromuscular problems, 3 had a minor DQ delay, 1 had a moderate spastic hemiparesis, and 1 was hydrocephalic. Of 33 children who were evaluated elsewhere, 30 were "completely" normal and 3 were abnormal: 2 had minor neuromuscular problems and 1 had cerebral agenesis. There were therefore 13 abnormal children, all with developmental problems. There were three major deficits (one moderate spastic hemiplegia, one hydrocephalus, and one cerebral agenesis), seven minor deficits (all minor neuromuscular), and three minor DQ delay problems.

Neonatal problems facing infants with Rh erythroblastosis fetalis were listed by the author as asphyxia at delivery, pulmonary edema and difficulty with ventilation immediately after delivery, secondary heart failure, thrombocytopenia with risk of intraventricular and pulmonary hemorrhage, rapidly rising bilirubin levels with risk of kernicterus, the syndrome of hepatic cellular damage, and the possibility of mechanical bowel obstructions in fetal transfusion survivors.

Turner and associates[48] briefly described 44 of 63 infants who survived IUT. About 74% of the children weighed <2500 g at birth. The examiners, who were pediatricians, psychologists, public health nurses, and social workers, evaluated the children's physical health, intelligence, and social maturity. Reflected in the latter category were parental socioeconomic status, stability, and intelligence. Factors evaluated in the childrens' physical health were the presence or absence of birth defects and deficits (not listed) and overall assessment of health status. Evaluation of intelligence was based on test performance and child behavior.

The authors stated that about 50% of the 44 children were normal or superior in the three areas measured (physical health, intelligence, and social maturity), the remainder being below normal or retarded in each category.

Because there was no description of neurological deficits, the 22 abnormal children were placed in the developmental and mental retardation columns of Table 2 only. The significance of the authors' unusual results will be discussed later.

They listed two children in whom donor white cells persisted in circulation beyond 1 year of age; one child developed acute leukemia at $4\frac{1}{2}$ years of age, and the other demonstrated hybrid cells in peripheral blood. These two children might very well have been included in the SDRT column of Table 2, but since they could not be specifically separated from the 22 abnormal children, they were retained in the developmental column.

Contrary to all other studies, the authors felt that RDS was not a major problem and that the clinical management of the neonates was relatively uncomplicated.

Palmer and Gordon[49] reported on 36 infants. Evaluation was done by pediatricians and family practitioners. They found that 33 children were normal and 3 were not. The latter included one microcephalic (major CNS), one educationally subnormal child, and one severely educationally abnormal child. They also reported one case of harelip/cleft palate and one cloacal deformity; these were not included in Table 2.

Bock and Winkel[50] studied 19 children using the revised Denver Developmental Scale, personal-social-linguistic behavior, and fine and gross motor development. He listed three children with developmental problems (two motor retardation [minor defects] and a child with growth retardation below the 10th percentile). In addition, he described two cases of squint, four hernias, three enamel defects, and one cosmetically significant scar due to contrast medium. None of the latter have been included in Table 2.

The authors feel that *in utero* transfusions are justified in the seriously affected Rhesus-sensitized fetus who is too small to survive a preterm delivery.

Schellong et al.[51] presented 18 children whose perinatal factors included asphyxia, respiratory distress, acidosis, severe anemia, and hyperbilirubinemia. Of the 18 children, 5 were considered abnormal (all in the developmental category): 2 with slight to medium spastic diplegia or hemiplegia and 3 with minimal cerebral signs, but no disability (minor CNS). They also reported one child with a 5-cm cutaneous scar.

The authors felt that both abnormal neurological signs and abnormal psychological examinations improved with age.

White and associates[52] examined 15 children between the ages of 3 and 11 years. These children were compared to two control groups. The first control group consisted of 12 siblings, 9 of whom had not been affected by erythroblastosis fetalis and 3 who had (2 had exchange transfusions and 1 did not). The second control group included 14 children without erythroblastosis fetalis, but who had either low birth weight or cesarean or breech delivery. They were matched for gestational age, birth weight, and method of delivery.

There was no difference between the cohorts and controls concerning IQ, arithmetic achievement, and reading achievement. School performance was acceptable in all IUT children, and they had no significant behavioral problems.

The authors reported seven hernias, three minor IUT scars, and five multiple dental caries. Those abnormalities included in Table 2 are one seizure disorder (major CNS), one motor retardation (minor CNS), and one child with diminished IgA associated with recurrent urticaria (SDRT). The authors felt that the two children with the seizure disorder and recurrent urticaria might be expected in the general population and that the infant who survives IUT also has an ''excellent chance for good quality of life''.

Hardyment et al.[12] described 21 children, 22 months to 10 years of age, in a paper with considerable perinatal data. They compared their study group to 314 children born at Vancouver General Hospital between 1958 and 1966, 314 of whom were followed for over $6^1/_2$ years. This control group consisted of children of low birth weight whose neurological and ophthalmic disorders were followed in a longitudinal fashion. Major and minor neurological signs in the control group were found in 14.5 and 24.4% of the children, respectively; in the IUT children, the figures were 9.5 and 28.6%. In a compilation of prior IUT studies and the authors' data, the percentages were 5.1 and 16.7, respectively.

Included in long-term defects were the major signs of two children (one coarse tremors, one minimal hemiparesis) and the minor signs of six (very brisk tendon reflexes, below average coordination, and minimal slight hypotonia). In this review, the previously mentioned minimal hemiparesis will be considered a minor neurological deficit. The authors did not include one child with unilateral high-frequency deafness, who is included in the major CNS, deafness, and HDN columns of Table 2.

The authors feel that the majority of children who received IUTs appear neurologically normal and function well in life.

Schwalb[53] described eight children post-IUT between the ages of 36 and 96 months whose major neonatal complications were acidosis, respiratory distress, and prolonged hyperbilirubinemia. He found five children with developmental defects (two with fine and rapid motor incoordination, two with significant perceptual problems, and one hyperkinetic and impulsive child). One child had high-frequency sensorineural deafness. One child had a major defect (deafness) and two children had minor defects (fine and rapid motor incoordination).

Knobbe and associates[54] reported on the psychological development of 15 children whose ages at evaluation were between 36 and 120 months. These children were compared to controls who had HDN, but whose specific treatment consisted of exchange transfusions only. The average gestational age of the controls was 2 weeks older than the study group. The children's intellectual, visual-motor integration, and physical-social developments were studied. The authors found no overall differences between the study group and the normal population. They demonstrated that the study group, when compared to the normal population, had an above average IQ and normal development in visual-motor integration and adapted behavior.

The authors described no defects related to HDN, IUT, or development. They indicated that the study group's physical development was similar to that of the controls.

Ellis and colleagues[15] studied 81 survivors of IUT, the majority of whom were over 5 years of age at the time of evaluation. The assessment included development, general health, audiometric testing, and school performance. The authors found 29 abnormal children and subdivided them according to etiology: 13 due to HDN, 10 due to the IUT, and 6 not associated with either.

Of the 13 HDN children, 1 was profoundly deaf, spastic, athetoid, had defective vision, and had marked intellectual impairment; 1 was profoundly deaf, but physically and intellectually normal; 3 had normal hearing, but were spastic with severe intellectual impairment; 7 had only high-frequency deafness; and 1 had a severe mental handicap. A total of seven were unable to benefit from a normal education, two required special educational facilities, and four were in normal schools.

Of the ten IUT problem-related children, two had paresis of an upper abdominal quadrant associated with absent abdominal reflexes, two had leg trauma, but were functionally normal, and six males had inguinal hernias.

Of the six children who had problems unassociated with either HDN or IUT, two had patent ductus arteriosus, one developed status epilepticus at 7 months of age followed by spastic quadriplegia, and three had defective vision with squints.

Exhibiting long-term defects were 13 children with major neurological problems (all spasticity and deafness due to HDN), but no developmental problems, 2 children with minor CNS problems (abdominal pareses), 13 HDN children (spasticity, sensorineural deafness, and mental retardation), and 2 SDRT children (abdominal pareses).

Skjaeraasen and Moe[55] briefly reported on 29 survivors whose parents responded to a questionnaire sent by the authors; 13 children were reported as above average in intelligence and 1 child had a hearing defect. No mental retardation or physical impairment was found.

V. CONTROL PATIENTS

Johnston and associates[9] examined 129 children, all of whom had a serum bilirubin level of over 20 mg/100 ml in the neonatal period. A total of 24, or 18.6%, were premature infants. The etiology in 92 children was Rhesus isoimmunization, in 26 ABO incompatibility, and in 11 neither of the two. None of the children had IUTs, and 95% percent of the infants had one or more exchange transfusion.

These children had neurological, psychological, and audiological examinations between the ages of 5 and 6 years (controls were audiometric studies of 95 children who had low serum bilirubin levels in the newborn period). Controls in psychometric studies when deafness was suspected in the study group were 82 older, unaffected siblings.

The authors found seven abnormal children, each of whom had a sensorineural hearing loss of more than 1000 Hz, three of whom had associated aphasia, and one who was mentally retarded. Three were mildly athetotic. Three had hearing losses alone. The average IQ of the study group was 104.8 (control = 102.8). The general physical condition of the children was normal.

There were ten major neurological defects (seven deafness and three aphasia), three minor neurological defects (three mild athetosis), one mental retardation, and seven sensorineural deafness. All conditions were in seven children who had HDN.

The authors felt that exchanges are effective in preventing long-term sequelae due to hyperbilirubinemia.

Walker and colleagues[10] studied 283 out of 1476 survivors of Rhesus hemolytic disease. As in the previous study by Johnston and associates,[9] none of the infants had IUTs; however, 60% of the infants had exchange transfusions. They had HDN ranging from mild disease (Coombs test positive, but no treatment required) to very severe disease (cord hemoglobin <7.5 g/100 ml and overtly severe clinical disease).

The children were evaluated between the ages of 7 and 14 years. The evaluation consisted of physical and psychological examinations as well as hearing, speech, and reading skills assessments. The authors described 13 children whose conditions were directly related to HDN: 11 children were either athetotic or deaf, and 2 had minor unstated CNS disorders. A total of 18 children were described who had developmental defects. Two of them had an IQ of <70; the authors thought this was not due to HDN. Of the remaining 16 children who were described as clumsy, apraxic, or had left-right confusion, 12 were already included in the HDN group. Therefore, six children might be considered to have had developmental defects. There were 11 children who had sensorineural deafness and 8 who had mental retardation (6 related to HDN and 2 in the developmental category). A total of 22 children, 6 from the HDN group (2 minor unstated CNS disorders and 4 minor athetoses) and 16 who were clumsy, were considered to have minor neurological deficits, while 11 children had 14 major deficits (all from the HDN group — 3 severe athetoses and 11 sensorineural deafness).

The above two reports (which included 412 children who were not transfused *in utero*, but who did, for the most part, undergo postpartum exchange and/or top-up transfusions) would serve as a control for the 788 children who underwent *in utero* fetal transfusion and postpartum exchange and/or top-up transfusions.

VI. DISCUSSION

The IUT group of children was compared to the control group by analyzing the incidence of the following parameters: abnormal children, abnormalities due to hemolytic disease, defects due to the IUT procedure, and developmental abnormalities. Incidences of major and minor CNS disorders, mental retardation, and sensorineural deafness were also tabulated.

Every effort was made to quantitate the neurological and psychological conditions the authors described. If, for example, five neurological deficits were described, the five were classified as major or minor and then tabulated. If no neurological problems were mentioned or discussed by the authors, none were tabulated. Although the authors reported 52 hernias (6.6%), none of these were listed in the SDRT column of Table 2 since none of the hernias had any reported long-term sequelae. In addition, neurological and psychometric (i.e., mental retardation) deficits in a particular study will not necessarily equal the number of abnormal children. These are determined by SDRT, HDN, and developmental problems. The number of abnormal children described by the authors differs from the ones listed in somewhat less than 50% of the reported cases. These differences were explained previously in the review of study and control patients.

A comparison between the IUT and non-IUT children (Table 3) indicates that there were significantly more abnormal children in the study group: 16.9 vs. 6.3% in the controls (*p* <0.0001).

There were significantly more children with sequelae of HDN in the control group: 4.9 vs. 2.8% (*p* <0.05).

There were significantly more developmental problems in the study group: 13.1 vs. 1.5% ($p < 0.0001$).

The incidence of significant defects related to transfusion was 1.0%. These were mainly lower motor neuron deficits following traumatic IUT.

There was no significant difference in major and minor CNS problems between the two groups.

There was significantly more mental retardation in the study group: 4.8 vs. 2.2% ($p < 0.02$).

There was significantly more sensorineural deafness in the controls: 4.4 vs. 2.2% ($p < 0.03$).

Except for deafness and HDN-related sequelae, the differences in incidences between the two groups, when apparent, appear to be due to the difference in gestational age. The average gestational age in the IUT and control groups numbered 34 and 38, respectively, and one would expect more neurological problems (such as minimal cerebral dysfunction, cerebral palsy, developmental delays, hypotonia, hydrocephalus, perceptual and learning problems, convulsive disorders, and behavioral problems) in the more immature IUT group, regardless of the added factors of method of delivery, severity of disease, and sophistication of neonatal care.[56] Therefore, in the IUT group there were significantly more (1) abnormal children, (2) mental retardation, and (3) developmental defects. Conversely, in the same group there was significantly less sensorineural deafness and significantly fewer overall problems related to HDN. There were no significant differences in major and minor neurological defects in the two groups.

It seems that two parameters have statistical significance when they should not: mental retardation occurs at a higher frequency in the study group (4.8 vs. 2.2%, $p < 0.02$), and HDN abnormalities occur more frequently in the controls (4.9 vs. 2.8%, $p < 0.05$). Obviously, an easy answer would be that one would expect more mental retardation in preterm neonates and that perhaps correcting intrauterine anemia with IUTs might very well diminish the rate of neonatal kernicterus. However, in all probability it is related to the paper reported by Turner et al.[48] These authors evaluated physical health, intelligence, and social maturity in 44 survivors of IUT (5.6% of the total study group) and reported that 50% of the children (22) were below normal or retarded in each of the three categories. This characterization would appear to designate 22 children as mentally retarded. The rate of mental retardation reported by the other authors in the study group ranged from 0 to 12.2%, with an average of 2.2%. Therefore, if the report of Turner et al. was not included in the study, the frequency of mental retardation in both the study and control groups would be equal: 2.2%. In a similar fashion, by reducing the study group to 744 children through exclusion of the data of Turner and co-workers, the abnormalities due to HDN become 3.0% (compared to 4.9% in the controls) without significance ($p > 0.05$; Table 3).

When the compositions of major and minor deficits are compared, the trend appears to be similar in the study and control groups (Table 4). Of 30 major CNS deficits in the study group, 26.7% were related to development and 73.3% to HDN. In the control group there were 24 major CNS problems, all related to HDN. The difference in the development incidence in the study and control groups may very well be due to prematurity in the study group; it appears clear that as far as major CNS deficits are concerned, HDN-related problems outstrip developmental problems in both groups.

Of the 45 minor CNS deficits in the study group, 88.9% were developmental, 2.2% were HDN (1 questionable gaze abnormality), and 8.9% were related to the transfusion (all lower motor neuron defects). Of 25 minor CNS deficits in the control group, 64.0% were developmental and 36.0% were related to HDN. In both groups, minor CNS deficits occurred much more frequently in the developmental category and more so in the study group; this possibly was related to prematurity.

VII. CONCLUSIONS

1.   There were significantly more abnormal children in the study group compared to controls (14.9 vs. 6.3%). This difference was due to the greater percentage of developmental problems in the study group (10.9 vs. 1.5%; Table 3).

2.   The majority of the developmental problems in the study group were minor rather than major CNS deficits (88.9 vs. 26.7%), as they were in the controls (64.0 vs. 0%; Table 4).

3.   In both the study and control groups, problems related to HDN occupied a very high proportion of major CNS deficits (73.3 and 100%, respectively).

4.   When the distribution of HDN sequelae is tabulated, there is significantly more sensorineural deafness than athetosis in both the study and control groups (Table 5). Of 22 major HDN-related problems in the study group, 77.3% involved sensorineural deafness while 22.7% were labeled severe athetosis. Similarly, in the control group, of 24 HDN-related problems, 75.8% were found to be sensorineural deafness, 12.5% severe athetosis, and the remainder (12.5%) severe aphasia. Of 45 minor CNS deficits, none was related to HDN in the study group. Of nine minor CNS deficits in the control group, 77.8% were mild athetosis and 22.2% were unspecified minor CNS deficits related to HDN.

In summary, most survivors of IUT are without problems related to development or HDN. In the abnormal children, minor neurological deficits outweigh the major ones in the developmental category, and both deficits are probably related to prematurity. Major CNS deficits relating to HDN far outweight major CNS developmental problems in the abnormals, and sensorineural deafness occurs at a greater frequency than athetosis.

When comparing the study group to the controls there appeared to be no differences in the rates of HDN-related problems, major and minor CNS deficits, and mental retardation. There appeared to be a statistically higher rate of sensorineural deafness in the controls, perhaps related to more serious disease. The higher rate of abnormal children in the study group was correlated to the considerably higher rate of developmental problems, and the latter was related to prematurity.

REFERENCES

1. **Fischer, K., Poschmann, H., and Schultze-Mosgau, H.,** Pränatale und postnatale Behandlung der schweren Rh-Erythroblastose, *Z. Geburtshilfe Perinatol.,* 179, 319, 1975.
2. **Hofmann, D., Holländer, H-J., Mast, H., Quakernack, K., and Schellong, G.,** Erfahrungen mit der intrauterinen Transfusion bei schwerer Rhesus-Erythroblastose, *Geburtshilfe Frauenheilk.,* 31, 797, 1971.
3. **Palm, D., Schellong, G., Fischer, Ch., Jochmus, I., and Klinghammer, D.,** Nachuntersuchungen von 6 jährigen Kindern nach Erythroblastose. Die bedeutung verschiedener Belastungsfaktoren für die entstehung cerebraler Spatfolgen, in *Perinatale Medizin Bild. II,* Saling, E. and Schulte, F.-J., Eds., Georg Thieme–Verlag, Stuttgart, Federal Republic of Germany, 1972.
4. **Palm, D., Schellong, G., and Maier-Becker, E. M.,** Entwicklung von Kindern nach pränataler transfusions-Therapie wegen schwerer Rh-Erythroblastose, *Monatsschr. Kinderheilk.,* 123, 234, 1975.
5. **Bowman, J., Friesen, R. F., Bowman, W. D., McInnis, A. C., Barnes, P. H., and Grewar, D.,** Fetal transfusion in severe Rh isoimmunization, *JAMA,* 207, 1101, 1969.
6. **Bowman, J. M., Friesen, R. F., McInnis, A. C., and Shah, C. M.,** Fetal transfusion 1970, presented at the Annual Meeting of the Midwest Society for Pediatric Research, Chicago, November 4 to 5, 1970, Abstr. 59.
7. **Friesen, R. F.,** Complications of intrauterine transfusion, *Clin. Obstet. Gynecol.,* 14, 572, 1971.
8. **Bowman, J. M.,** Rh erythroblastosis fetalis 1975, *Semin. Hematol.,* 12, 189, 1975.

9. **Johnston, W. H., Angara, V., Baumal, R., Hawke, W. A., Johnson, R. H., Keet, S., and Wood, M.,** Erythroblastosis fetalis and hyperbilirubinemia, *Pediatrics,* 39, 88, 1967.

10. **Walker, W., Ellis, M. I., Ellis, E., Curry, A., Savage, R. D., and Sawyer, R.,** A follow-up study of survivors of Rh-haemolytic disease, *Dev. Med. Child Neurol.,* 16, 592, 1974.

11. **Tripp, J.,** Intrauterine transfusion, *Dev. Med. Child Neurol.,* 16, 528, 1974.

12. **Hardyment, A. F., Salvador, H. S., Towell, M. F., Carpenter, C. W., Jan, J. E., and Tingle, A. J.,** Follow-up of intrauterine transfused surviving children, *Am. J. Obstet. Gynecol.,* 133, 235, 1979.

13. **Whitfield, C. R., Thompson, W., Armstrong, M. J., and Reid, M. McC.,** Intrauterine fetal transfusion for severe Rhesus haemolytic disease, *J. Obstet. Gynaecol. Br. Commonw.,* 79, 931, 1972.

14. **Girling, D. J., Scopes, J. W., and Wigglesworth, J. S.,** Babies born alive after intrauterine transfusions for severe Rhesus haemolytic disease, *J. Obstet. Gynaecol. Br. Commonw.,* 79, 565, 1972.

15. **Ellis, M. I.,** Follow-up study of survivors after intrauterine transfusion, *Dev. Med. Child Neurol.,* 22, 48, 1980.

16. **Byers, P. K., Paine, R. S., and Crothers, B.,** Extrapyramidal cerebral palsy with hearing loss following erythroblastosis, *Pediatrics,* 15, 248, 1955.

17. **Perlstein, M. A.,** The late clinical syndrome of posticteric encephalopathy, *Pediatr. Clin. North Am.,* 7, 665, 1960.

18. **Hoyt, C. S., Billson, F. A., and Alpins, N.,** The supranuclear disturbances of gaze in kernicterus, *Ann. Ophthalmol.,* 10, 1487, 1978.

19. **Gerrard, J.,** Nuclear jaundice and deafness, *J. Laryngol. Otol.,* 66, 39, 1952.

20. **Keaster, J., Hyman, C. B., and Harris, I.,** Hearing problems subsequent to neonatal hemolytic disease or hyperbilirubinemia, *Am. J. Dis. Child.,* 117, 406, 1969.

21. **Hyman, C. B., Keaster, J., Hanson, V., Harris, I., Sedgwick, R., Wursten, H., and Wright, A. R.,** CNS abnormalities after neonatal hemolytic disease or hyperbilirubinemia, *Am. J. Dis. Child.,* 117, 395, 1969.

22. **Chisin, R., Perlman, M., and Sohmer, H.,** Cochlear and brainstem responses in hearing loss following neonatal hyperbilirubinemia, *Ann. Otol. Rhinol. Laryngol.,* 88, 352, 1979.

23. **Volpe, J. J.,** *Neurology of the Newborn,* W.B. Saunders, Philadelphia, 1981, 336.

24. **Bergman, I., Hirsch, R. P., Fria, T. J., Shapiro, S., Holzman, I., and Painter, M.,** Cause of hearing loss in the high-risk premature infant, *J. Pediatr.,* 106, 95, 1985.

25. **Devries, L. S., Lary, S., and Dubowitz, L. M. S.,** Relationship of serum bilirubin levels to ototoxicity and deafness in high-risk low-birth-weight infants, *Pediatrics,* 76, 351, 1985.

26. **Johnson, L. and Boggs, T. R.,** Bilirubin-dependent brain damage: incidence and indication for treatment, in *Phototherapy in the Newborn: An Overview,* Odell, G. B., Schaffer, R., and Simopoulous, A. P., Eds., National Academy of Sciences, Washington, D.C., 1974, 122.

27. **Naeye, R. L.,** The role of congenital bacterial infections in low serum bilirubin brain damge, *Pediatrics,* 62, 497, 1978.

28. **Odell, G. B., Storey, G. N. B., and Rosenberg, L. A.,** Studies in kernicterus. III. The saturation of serum proteins with bilirubin during neonatal life and its relationship to brain damage at five years, *J. Pediatr.,* 76, 12, 1970.

29. **Rubin, R. A., Balow, B., and Fisch, R. O.,** Neonatal serum bilirubin levels related to cognitive development at ages 4 through 7 years, *J. Pediatr.,* 94, 601, 1979.

30. **Scheidt, P. C., Mellits, E. D., Hardy, J. B., Draje, J. S., and Boggs, T. R.,** Toxicity to bilirubin in neonates. Infant development during first year in relation to maximum neonatal serum bilirubin concentration, *J. Pediatr.,* 91, 292, 1977.

31. **Hugh-Jones, K., Slack, J., Simpson, K., Grossman, A., and Hsia, D. Y.,** Clinical course of hyperbilirubinemia in premature infant, *N. Engl. J. Med.,* 263, 1223, 1960.

32. **Killander, A., Michaelsson, M., Muller-Eberhard, U., and Sjolin, S.,** Hyperbilirubinemia in full term newborn infants: a follow-up study, *Acta Paediatr. Scand.,* 52, 481, 1963.

33. **Mores, A., Fargasova, I., and Minarikova, E.,** The relation of hyperbilirubinemia in newborns without isoimmunization to kernicterus, *Acta Paediatr. Scand.,* 48, 590, 1959.

34. **Schiller, J. G. and Silverman, W. A.,** Uncomplicated hyperbilirubinemia of prematurity, *Am. J. Dis. Child.,* 101, 587, 1961.

35. **Watchko, J. E. and Oski, F. A.,** Bilirubin [20 mg/dl] = vigintiphobia, *Pediatrics,* 71, 660, 1983.

36. **Wishingrad, L., Cornblath, M., Takakuwa, P., Rozenfeld, I. M., Elegant, L. D., Kaufman, A., Lassers, E., and Klein, R.,** Studies of non-hemolytic hyperbilirubinemia in premature infants. Prospective randomized selection for exchange transfusion with observations on the levels of serum bilirubin with and without exchange transfusion and neurologic evaluations one year after birth, *Pediatrics,* 36, 162, 1965.

37. **Gregg, G. S. and Hutchinson, D. L.,** Developmental characteristics of infants surviving fetal transfusion, *JAMA,* 209, 1059, 1969.

38. **Werner, E., Bierman, J. M., French, F., Simonian, K., Connor, A., Smith, R., and Campbell, M.,** Reproductive and environmental casualties: a report on the ten-year follow-up of the children of the Kauai Pregnancy Study, *Pediatrics,* 42, 112, 1968.

39. **Cochran, W., Stark, A., and Schulhoff, C.,** Prognosis of live infants who have had intrauterine transfusions, *Pediatr. Res.,* 4, 373, 1970.

40. **Corston, J. McD., Pereira, E., Cudmore, D. W., and Morton, B. S.,** Five years' experience with intrauterine transfusion, *J. Can. Med. Assoc.,* 103, 594, 1970.

41. **Walker, W.,** Pediatric aspects of intrauterine transfusion, *Ann. Ostet. Ginecol.,* 92, 602, 1971.

42. **Franchini, A. M., Cattaneo, F., Marini, A., Dambrosio, F., and Caccamo, M. L.,** Follow-up study of intrauterine transfused infants, *Ann. Ostet. Ginecol.,* 92, 617, 1971.

43. **Phibbs, H., Harvin, D., Jones, G., Talbot, C., Cohen, M., Crowther, D., and Tooley, W. H.,** Development of children who had received intrauterine transfusions, *Pediatrics,* 47, 689, 1971.

44. **Oh, W., Arbit, J., Blonsky, E. R., and Cassell, S.,** Neurologic and psychometric follow-up study of Rh-erythroblastotic infants requiring intrauterine blood transfusion, *Am. J. Obstet. Gynecol.,* 110, 330, 1971.

45. **Peniche, F. A., Roblero, E. J., Gutiérrez, L. S., and Aguayo de la Peña, A. M.,** Evaluacíon a largo plazo de niños transfundidos *in utero, Ginecol. Obstet. Mex.,* 33, 157, 1973.

46. **Holt, E. M., Boyd, I. E., Dewhurst, C. J., Murray, J., Naylor, C. H., and Smithham, J. H.,** Intrauterine transfusion: 101 consecutive cases treated at Queen Charlotte's Maternity Hospital, *Br. Med. J.,* 3, 39, 1973.

47. **Richings, J.,** Later progress of infants who received transfusions *in utero* for severe Rhesus haemolytic disease, *Lancet,* 1, 1220, 1973.

48. **Turner, J. H., Hutchinson, D. L., Hayashi, T. T., Petricciani, I. C., and Germanowski, J.,** Fetal and maternal risks associated with intrauterine transfusion procedures, *Am. J. Obstet. Gynecol.,* 123, 251, 1975.

49. **Palmer, A. and Gordon, R. R.,** A critical review of intrauterine fetal transfusion, *Br. J. Obstet. Gynaecol.,* 83, 688, 1976.

50. **Bock, J. E. and Winkel, S.,** A follow-up study on infants who received intra-uterine transfusions because of severe Rhesus haemolytic disease, *Acta Obstet. Gynecol. Scand.,* Suppl. 53, 37, 1976.

51. **Schellong, G., Palm, D., Maier-Becker, E. M., and Quakernack, K.,** Zur Entwicklung von Kindern nach intrauterinen Transfusionen bei schwerer Rh-Erythroblastose, *Z. Geburtshilfe Perinatol.,* 181, 36, 1977.

52. **White, C., Goplerud, C. P., Kisker, C. T., Stehbens, J. A., Kitchell, M., and Taylor, J. C.,** Intrauterine fetal transfusion, 1965—1976, with an assessment of the surviving children, *Am. J. Obstet. Gynecol.,* 130, 933, 1978.

53. **Schwalb, E.,** personal communication, 1979.

54. **Knobbe, T., Meier, P., Wenar, C., and Cordero, L.,** Psychological development of children who received intrauterine transfusions, *Am. J. Obstet. Gynecol.,* 133, 877, 1979.

55. **Skjaeraasen, J. and Moe, N.,** Intra-uterine transfusions to the Rhesus-immunized fetus in the Department of Obstetrics, National Hospital, Oslo, 1968—1979, *Acta Obstet. Gynecol. Scand.,* 62, 349, 1983.

56. **Lubchenco, L. O.,** *The High Risk Infant,* Vol. 14, W.B. Saunders, Philadelphia, 1976, 249.

Chapter 8

THE EFFECT OF CHORIOAMNIONITIS ON THE DEVELOPMENT OF PRETERM INFANTS

Walter J. Morales

TABLE OF CONTENTS

I. INTRODUCTION

Premature rupture of membranes, defined as rupture of fetal membranes prior to the onset of labor, complicates about 10% of all pregnancies.[1] Of these patients with premature rupture of membranes, approximately one third involve preterm pregnancies.[2] Similarly, one third of low birth weight babies are the result of pregnancies complicated by premature rupture of membranes. Furthermore, premature rupture of membranes has been reported to have a 20% rate of recurrence.[3]

The etiology of premature rupture of membranes has received a great deal of attention. Although at this point a definitive cause has not been fully accepted, numerous clinical, microbiological, and *in vitro* studies have established a definite relationship between premature rupture of membranes and infection.[4-6] This subclinical infection is primarily the result of bacterial contamination of the lower genital tract ascending through the cervix, resulting in the colonization of the fetal membranes. Longitudinal studies have identified a higher risk for preterm rupture of membranes in patients colonized with Group B streptococcus,[7] *Chlamydia trachomatis*,[8] and bacterial vaginosis.[9] Furthermore, histopathological studies of the placenta have revealed a significantly higher incidence of chorioamnionitis in those pregnancies complicated by premature rupture of membranes.[10]

Despite this association between infection and premature rupture of membranes, in managing the preterm patient with premature rupture of membranes the clinician must decide between immediate delivery (to avoid maternal and neonatal morbidity and mortality associated with infection) and conservative management (to extend intrauterine life in order to minimize the serious neonatal complications of prematurity, particularly respiratory distress syndrome [RDS] and intraventricular hemorrhage). Currently, widely accepted protocols are based on the assumption that RDS and other neonatal complications could be reduced by adopting a conservative approach.[11-13] Unfortunately, spontaneous labor and delivery occur in about 80% of these patients within 7 days of the onset of rupture of membranes,[14,15] minimizing the potential benefits of expectant management. Moreover, while awaiting the onset of labor, 10 to 40% of patients with premature rupture of membranes will develop clinically significant chorioamnionitis,[14-16] characterized by oral temperature of at least 100.4°F persistent over 4 h with no identifiable source, uterine tenderness, fetal tachycardia, and foul-smelling lochia. Therefore, in order to establish the most rational approach in managing the patient with premature rupture of membranes, the clinician must understand the effect of chorioamnionitis on neonatal morbidity as well as long-term infant developmental handicaps.

II. EFFECT OF CHORIOAMNIONITIS ON NEONATAL OUTCOME

Published data on the effect of maternal intra-amnionic infection on neonatal outcome have resulted in conflicting conclusions. While some authors[17,18] have reported increased perinatal mortality following the clinical diagnosis of chorioamnionitis, others[19,20] have failed to observe an association. These studies, however, failed to correct their data for gestational age.

Two recent studies[14,21] addressed the question of the neonatal effects of maternal chorioamnionitis by restricting the analysis to the preterm gestation. Both studies concluded that chorioamnionitis places the neonate at a significantly increased risk of mortality, RDS, and neonatal sepsis. In addition, both studies concluded that although chorioamnionitis does place the unborn preterm baby at a significantly increased risk for serious neonatal complication and mortality and although steps should be taken to achieve delivery, neither labor itself nor its length worsens the prognosis for the neonate (Table 1).

TABLE 1
The Effect of Chorioamnionitis and Length of Diagnosis-To-Delivery Period on Neonatal Outcome[21]

Chorioamnionitis	Gestation age (weeks)	Time[a] (h)	Mortality (no.)	RDS[b] (no.)	IVH[c] Total	IVH[c] Severe	Sepsis
No	31.17	—	39	212	131	51	70
(n = 606)			(6)	(35)	(22)	(8)	(11)
Yes	30.18	—	23[d]	57[d]	52[d]	22[d]	26[d]
(n = 92)			(25)	(62)	(56)	(24)	(28)
n = 48	30.22	<6	11	32	28	13	24
			(25)	(67)	(58)	(27)	(50)
n = 44	30.13	>6	11	25	24	10	13
			(25)	(57)	(55)	(23)	(30)

Note: Numbers represent numbers of patients; values in parentheses are percentages.

a   Time from diagnosis of chorioamnionitis to delivery.
b   RDS = respiratory distress syndrome.
c   IVH = intraventricular hemorrhage (severe = grade 3 or 4).
d $p < 0.001$.

From Morales, W. J., Washington, S. R., and Lazar, A. J., *J. Perinatol.*, 7, 105, 1987. With permission.

III. EFFECT OF CHORIOAMNIONITIS ON THE DEVELOPMENTAL OUTCOMES OF PRETERM INFANTS

A recent publication[22] studied 127 mother-infant pairs of pregnancies involving a neonate under 2000 g. Of these pregnancies, 42 were complicated by chorioamnionitis. The mental and psychomotor development of these neonates was determined by Bayley's Scales[23] at corrected 1 year of life and compared to that of a group of 31 infants born to mothers with premature rupture of membranes without evidence of chorioamnionitis.

Infants were categorized as normal if the mental and psychomotor development indices were ≥85, at risk of developmental delays if either the mental or psychomotor index was between 70 and 84, and developmentally delayed if the mental or psychomotor index was ≤69. Based on this criterion, the chorioamnionitis group compared to the nonchorioamnionitis group had a worse outcome, with 64 vs. 80% diagnosed as normal, 24 vs. 10% as infants at risk for developmental delays, and 12 vs. 10% as having developmental delays (Table 2).

A major problem with the conclusions from this study starts from the definition of chorioamnionitis, which was based on a complex scoring system consisting of a number of parameters described in Table 3. Moreover, 14 of the 42 patients of the chorioamnionitis group were diagnosed retrospectively, with 3 of these 14 neonates showing developmental delays. Overall, the chorioamnionitis group consisted of patients of lesser birth weight and gestational age. Furthermore, although the incidences of RDS and of intraventricular hemorrhage were similar in both groups, the weight, incidence, and severity of RDS and intraventricular hemorrage of the group with developmental delays were not reported compared to the group without developmental delays (regardless of the diagnosis of chorioamnionitis).

A number of studies have established a very strong correlation between severity of RDS and intraventricular hemorrhage and increased risk for developmental delays.[24-26] Moreover, a study[27] recently suggested that while the long-term outcome of infants with severe intraventricular hemorrhage (grade 3 or 4) was significantly worse than those with minor hemorrhages (grade 1 or 2), patients with minor hemorrhages had Bayley mental and psychomotor development indices significantly lower than those without documented intraventricular

TABLE 2
Effect of Chorioamnionitis on Infant
Developmental Outcome[22]

| | Chorioamnionitis | |
	Yes (n = 42)	No (n = 33)
Birth weight (g)	1266 ± 267	1438 ± 339
Gestational age (weeks)	28.8 ± 2.1	30.1 ± 1.8
MDI	104.1 ± 18	111.8 ± 14
PDI	92.3 ± 21	100.0 ± 21
Normal (MDI and PDI ≥85)	64%	80%
At risk for delay (%) (MDI or PDI 70—84)	24%	10%
Developmental delay (MDI or PDI <70)	12%	10%

Note: MDI = Bayley Mental Development Index and PDI = Bayley Psychomotor Development Index.

From Hardt, N. S., Kostenbauder, M., Ogburn, M., Behnke, M., Resnick, M., and Cruz, A., *Obstet. Gynecol.,* 65, 5, 1985. With permission.

TABLE 3
Events Associated with Diagnosis of
Chorioamnionitis[22]

Events	Points[a]
Maternal temperature ≥38°C	2
Spontaneous premature rupture of membranes	2
Maternal pulse ≥100 BPM	1
Baseline fetal heart rate >160 BPM	1
Uterine tenderness to palpation	1
Spontaneous premature labor	1
Maternal white blood cell count ≥18,000/mm³	1
Positive maternal blood, endocervical culture, or endometrial culture	1
Histological confirmation by placental examination	2
Foul-smelling amniotic fluid or infant	1

Note: BPM = beats per minute.

[a]   Six or more points required for diagnosis of chorioamnionitis.

From Hardt, N. S., Kostenbauder, M., Ogburn, M., Behnke, M., Resnick, M., and Cruz, A., *Obstet. Gynecol.,* 65, 5, 1985. With permission.

hemorrhage. Therefore, in order to establish the effect of chorioamnionitis on developmental handicaps, a study[28] was conducted comparing the outcomes of a group of 43 surviving infants weighing <1500 g born to mothers with chorioamnionitis to those of a control group from mothers with premature rupture of membranes matched for birth weight and severity of RDS and intraventricular hemorrhage. The data, summarized in Table 4, failed to detect a difference between the two groups in terms of Bayley developmental indices, incidence of neurological sequelae, hearing deficits, or retinopathy of prematurity. Therefore, this

TABLE 4
Effect of Chorioamnionitis on Infant Developmental
Outcome[28]

	Chorioamnionitis (n = 43)	Control (n = 43)	p
Birth weight (g)[a]	1218 ± 256	1137 ± 185	NS
Gestational age (weeks)[a]	29.3 ± 1.8	29.1 ± 1.7	NS
Apgar scores[a]			
1 min	3.47 ± 1.9	4.61 ± 2.1	NS
5 min	5.97 ± 2.2	6.78 ± 1.6	NS
RDS[b] (%)			
Total	42	37	NS
Severe	28	26	NS
IVH[c] (%)			
Total	37	37	NS
Severe	12	12	NS
Bayley score[a]			
MDI[d]	99.4 ± 19	103.1 ± 20	NS
PDI[e]	92.0 ± 18	98.0 ± 21	NS
ROP[f] (%)	16	19	NS
Hearing deficit (%)	7	7	NS
Neurological sequelae (%)	21	19	NS

Note: NS = not significant.

[a] Mean ± SD.
[b] RDS = respiratory distress syndrome (severe ≥72 h intermittent positive pressure ventilatory support).
[c] IVH = intraventricular hemorrhage (severe = grade 3 or 4).
[d] MDI = mental development index.
[e] PDI = psychomotor development index.
[f] ROP = retinopathy of prematurity.

From Morales, W. J., *Obstet. Gynecol.*, 70, 183, 1987. With permission.

study failed to demonstrate any long-term developmental handicaps strictly attributable to chorioamnionitis.

IV. SUMMARY

The management of preterm gestation complicated by premature rupture of membranes continues to be a subject of controversy. While most investigators recommend expectant management in the hope of significantly extending *in utero* life, delivery is delayed by more than 7 days in only approximately 20% of these pregnancies. Furthermore, the potential benefit from expectant management is offset by about a 16% risk of chorioamnionitis in pregnancies under 33 weeks. Once chorioamnionitis occurs, there is a significant increase in risk of mortality and in the incidence of RDS and intraventricular hemorrhage. However, when the data is controlled for birth weight and severity of RDS and intraventricular hemorrhage, chorioamnionitis by itself does not appear to result in an increased risk for long-term developmental handicaps or neurological sequelae. Nevertheless, expectant management of preterm pregnancies with premature rupture of membranes appears to have a limited impact on improving the neonatal and long-term infant outcome. Thus, alternative or complementary approaches should be investigated.

REFERENCES

1. **Mead, P. B.,** Management of the patient with premature rupture of membranes, *Clin. Perinatol.,* 7, 243, 1980.
2. **Kaltreider, D. F. and Kohl, S.,** Epidemiology of preterm delivery, *Clin. Obstet. Gynecol.,* 60, 93, 1982.
3. **Naeye, R. L.,** Factors that predispose to premature rupture of membranes, *Obstet. Gynecol.,* 60, 93, 1982.
4. **Minkoff, H.,** Prematurity: infection as an etiologic factor, *Obstet. Gynecol.,* 62, 137, 1983.
5. **Creatsas, G., Pavlatos, M., Lolis, D., Aravantinos, D., and Kaskarelis, D.,** Bacterial contamination of the cervix and premature rupture of membranes, *Am. J. Obstet. Gynecol.,* 139, 522, 1981.
6. **Evaldson, G. R., Malmborg, A. S., and Nord, C. E.,** Premature rupture of membranes and ascending infection, *Br. J. Obstet. Gynaecol.,* 89, 793, 1982.
7. **Regan, J. A., Chaos, S., and James, L. S.,** Premature rupture of membranes, preterm delivery and group B streptococcal colonization of mothers, *Am. J. Obstet. Gynecol.,* 141, p. 1984, 1981.
8. **Martin, D. H., Koutsky, L., Eschenbach, D. A., Daling, J. R., Alexander, E. R, Benedetti, J. K., and Holmes, K. K.,** Prematurity and perinatal mortality in pregnancies complicated by maternal *Chlamydia trachomatis* infections, *JAMA,* 247, 1585, 1982.
9. **Martius, J., Krohn, M. A., Hillier, S. L., Stamm, W. E., Holmes, K. K., and Eschenbach, D. A.,** Relationships of vaginal lactobacillus species, cervical *Chlamydia trachomatis* and bacterial vaginosis to preterm birth, *Obstet. Gynecol.,* 71, 89, 1988.
10. **Naeye, R. L. and Peters, E. C.,** Causes and consequence of premature rupture of membranes, *Lancet,* 1, 192, 1980.
11. **Johnson, J. W., Daikoku, N. H., Niebyl, J. R., Johnson, T. R. B., Jr., Khouzami, V. A., and Witter, F. R.,** Premature rupture of the membranes and prolonged latency, *Obstet. Gynecol.,* 57, 547, 1981.
12. **Miller, J. M., Pupkin, M. J., and Crenshaw, C.,** Premature labor and premature rupture of the membranes, *Am. J. Obstet. Gynecol.,* 140, 39, 1981.
13. **Varner, M. W. and Galask, R. P.,** Conservative management of premature rupture of the membranes, *Am. J. Obstet. Gynecol.,* 140, 39, 1981.
14. **Garite, T. J. and Freeman, R. K.,** Chorioamnionitis in the preterm gestation, *Obstet. Gynecol.,* 59, 539, 1982.
15. **Gibbs, R. S. and Blanco, J. D.,** Premature rupture of the membranes, *Obstet. Gynecol.,* 60, 671, 1982.
16. **Taylor, J. and Garite, T. J.,** Premature rupture of membranes before fetal viability, *Obstet. Gynecol.,* 64, 615, 1984.
17. **Gibbs, R. S., Castillo, M. S., and Rodgers, P. J.,** Management of acute chorioamnionitis, *Am. J. Obstet. Gynecol.,* 136, 709, 1980.
18. **Pryles, C. V., Steg, N. L., Nair, S., Gellis, S. S., and Tenney, B.,** A controlled study on the influence on the newborn of prolonged rupture of the amniotic membranes and/or infection in the mother, *Pediatrics,* 31, 608, 1963.
19. **Schreiber, J. and Benedetti, T.,** Conservative management of preterm rupture of the fetal membranes in a low socioeconomic population, *Am. J. Obstet. Gynecol.,* 136, 92, 1980.
20. **Koh, K. S., Chan, F. H., Monfared, A. H., Ledger, W. J., and Paul, R. H.,** The changing perinatal and maternal outcome in chorioamnionitis, *Obstet. Gynecol.,* 53, 730, 1979.
21. **Morales, W. J., Washington, S. R., and Lazar, A. J.,** The effect of chorioamnionitis on perinatal outcome in preterm gestation, *J. Perinatol.,* 7, 105, 1987.
22. **Hardt, N. S., Kostenbauder, M., Ogburn, M., Behnke, M., Resnick, M., and Cruz, A.,** Influence of chorioamnionitis on long-term prognosis in low birth weight infants, *Obstet. Gynecol.,* 65, 5, 1985.
23. **Bayley, N.,** *Bayley Scales of Mental and Motor Development,* Psychological Corporation, New York, 1969.
24. **Rothberg, A. D., Maisels, J., Bagnato, S., Murphy, J., Gifford, D., McKinley, K., Palmer, E. A., and Vannucci, R. C.,** Outcome for survivors of mechanical ventilation weighing less than 1250 grams at birth, *J. Pediatr.,* 98, 106, 1981.
25. **Gaiter, J. L.,** The effect of intraventricular hemorrhage on Bayley developmental performance in preterm infants, *Semin. Perinatol.,* 6, 305, 1982.
26. **Papile, L., Munsick-Bruno, G., and Schafer, A.,** Relationship of cerebral intraventricular hemorrhage and early childhood neurological handicaps, *J. Pediatr.,* 103, 273, 1983.
27. **Morales, W. J.,** Effect of intraventricular hemorrhage on the one-year mental and neurologic handicaps of the very low birth weight infants, *Obstet. Gynecol.,* 70, 111, 1987.
28. **Morales, W. J.,** The effect of chorioamnionitis on the developmental outcome of preterm infants at one year, *Obstet. Gynecol.,* 70, 183, 1987.

Chapter 9

FETAL HEART RATE PATTERNS DURING LABOR: IS THEIR PLACE IN OBSTETRICS OVEREMPHASIZED?

Michael J. Painter, Patricia O'Donoghue, and Richard Depp

TABLE OF CONTENTS

I. INTRODUCTION

The obstetrician is limited by the inability to obtain a history of the fetal patient as well as the lack of opportunity to perform a simple physical examination of the fetus.[1] The development of fetal heart rate monitoring and its application in 1958 by Hon represented a logical attempt to assess the status of the fetus during the intrapartum period. The classification of fetal heart rate pattern characteristics and their mechanism of production defined benign and ominous patterns and allowed for apparent reassurance of the well-being of the fetus during labor and delivery.

II. DIAGNOSIS AND PATHOPHYSIOLOGY

A. EARLY DECELERATIONS

Early decelerations, characterized as small v-shaped decreases in heart rate of approximately 10 to 30 beats per minute, occur early in association with the onset of each uterine contraction; maximum heart rate deceleration is reached at the peak of the contraction, and it returns to baseline before the end of the contraction. These decelerations are caused by fetal head compression stimulating vagal reflexes mediated through the brain stem and resulting in fetal heart rate slowing. The decelerations do not appear to be a cause for concern regarding fetal well-being, nor are they reassuring regarding fetal health.[1]

B. VARIABLE DECELERATIONS

Of the periodic changes in fetal heart rate seen during labor, variable decelerations are those most frequently encountered. These decelerations are typically u-shaped declines in heart rate which occur during a uterine contraction and which usually vary in duration, intensity, and timing between contractions. Not infrequently they are preceded and followed by accelerations of the fetal heart rate. Variable fetal heart rate decelerations are caused by compression of the umbilical cord during a uterine contraction. During cord compression, the fetal blood pressure rises, and baroreceptors[3] present in the aortic arch and carotid bodies of the fetus respond to this change in blood pressure with a brain-stem-mediated reflex resulting in a decrease in fetal heart rate.[1,2] Fetal compromise may occur if the duration and degree of cord compression are sufficient and are associated with decreased fetal reserve.

Patterns that last longer than 60 s, associated with a drop in fetal heart rate to <70 beats per minute and with loss of beat-to-beat variability, are accompanied by a slow return to baseline after the deceleration; they are also associated with an overshoot pattern in which a gradual acceleration occurs after the variable deceleration, and variable accelerations associated with tachycardia are of concern. Evaluating the significance of variable decelerations is perhaps the most difficult of clinical decisions regarding fetal monitoring.[1]

C. LATE DECELERATIONS

Late decelerations cause the most concern among the periodic fetal heart rate changes noted during the intrapartum period. These decelerations usually begin more than 15 s after the onset of a contraction and continue following cessation of the uterine contraction. Animal studies have demonstrated that fetal hypoxemia results in a slowing of the heart rate, and the typical form that such slowing takes is that of a late deceleration. Late decelerations are associated with hypoxemia, acidemia, and hypotension, but hypoxemia appears to be the only component essential for the production of late decelerations.[3] Hypotension and fetal acidemia alone do not cause late decelerations. If hypoxemia is corrected by administration of oxygen to the mother, late decelerations are abolished without affecting the coexisting acidemia. With increasing hypoxemia, the interval between the onset of the contraction and the onset of the deceleration shortens and the severity of the deceleration increases.

In the human, late decelerations are uncommon when the partial pressure of oxygen is >19 mmHg and oxygen saturation is >31%, while in baboons, late decelerations are seen when the partial pressure of oxygen reaches 15 mmHg and arterial saturation of hemoglobin is decreased to 15%.[3]

Continuous and prolonged hypoxemia results in prolonged bradycardia rather than late decelerations, and a number of studies have shown that human fetuses demonstrating recurrent late decelerations in labor are depressed and asphyxiated at birth. In the Rhesus monkey model of Myers, repetitive late decelerations are associated with brain lesions that are similar to those seen in children with cerebral palsy. Hypoxemia may affect the fetal heart rate by stimulating chemoreceptors at the aortic arch or brain stem, as well as by releasing catecholamines from the adrenal glands, depressing the myocardium directly or affecting fetal breathing. It would appear that the mechanism of late deceleration involves a combination of these possibilities. Clearly, a reflex mechanism is operative, since atropine has been found to reduce or abolish late decelerations. Severe hypoxia, however, results in a slowing of fetal heart rate despite parasympathetic blockade, demonstrating a direct myocardial defect.[3] While it is quite clear that hypoxemia will result in ominous late deceleration patterns by a direct effect on the myocardium when the hypoxemia is of sufficient duration and intensity, it would appear that its mechanism of action in producing late decelerations is in large part mediated through central nervous system (CNS) pathways.

It is clear that the CNS plays an important role in the second-to-second regulation of cardiac activity and vasomotor tone.[4] Preganglionic sympathetic and parasympathetic neurons are the primary effector units of central cardiovascular regulation. The majority of preganglionic sympathetic neurons are found in the intermediolateral gray columns of the spinal cord, and 10% are found in the adjacent spinal structures.

The parasympathetic preganglionic neurons involved in cardiovascular regulation are found largely in the dorsal motor nucleus of the vagus and in the nucleus ambiguus, at the level of the medulla oblongata. These sympathetic and parasympathetic neurons, however, receive extensive connections from other CNS structures, which in turn receive afferents from both peripheral mechanoreceptors and chemoreceptors as well as innervation from other central nuclei. The majority of afferent fibers from peripheral receptors terminate in the nucleus tractus solitarius, which is also located in the medulla oblongata. Efferent pathways from the nucleus tractus solitarius project to the dorsal motor nucleus of the vagus, the nucleus ambiguus, and the intermediolateral column, as well as to serotonergic raphenuclei and the ventrolateral medullary reticular formation. These two nuclear regions and the nucleus of the tractus solitarius provide the primary supersegmental connections to the intermediolateral gray column, which also receives projections from parabranchial nuclei, vasopressor and oxytocic cells of the hypothalamus, and neuroadrenergic cells of the brain stem. The intermediolateral column does not receive direct projections from the cerebral cortex. There is, however, an anatomical substrate for cortical influences on sympathetic neurons. These influences may occur via the cortical nucleus tractus solitarius projections, projections from the limbic system, the hypothalamus, and parabrancheal nuclei. In turn, the amygdala has important relationships with the cortex, the lateral hypothalamus, and the periventricular nuclei, as well as the nucleus tractus solitarius.[4]

III. SIGNIFICANCE OF FETAL HEART RATE PATTERNS

Arrhythmias, hypertension, and hypotension are well described in adults exhibiting neurological disease. One might logically ask the question, "What role do CNS abnormalities in the fetus, both developmental and acquired, have in the production of fetal heart rate patterns during the intrapartum period?" Ayodeji and Kuhn[5], in describing a 10-year experience with antepartum cardiotocography, noted that major fetal malformations were found in 19% of infants demonstrating critical reserve patterns.

Critical reserve patterns were defined as having beat-to-beat variation of <5 beats per minute, having less than five accelerations of more than 15 beats per minute within a 20-min time frame, and entailing late decelerations. Although detailed CNS anatomical studies were not performed in this population, a number of infants (including those with trisomies 13, 18, and 21, as well as infants with anencephaly) had associated CNS anomalies. Another question that might logically be asked is, "Does the fetus with CNS abnormalities have the capability of reflex cardiovascular responses to stress during labor and delivery to ensure proper fetal and placental perfusion?"

A. IMMEDIATE OUTCOME

A number of studies have shown a decline in perinatal mortality from earlier time periods in which no monitoring was available compared to later time frames when fetal heart rate monitoring was virtually universal.[6] Controlled studies have shown improvement in the outcome of selected high-risk obstetric populations. Is fetal heart rate monitoring, however, of value in the care of the low-risk fetus during labor and delivery? Randomized prospective studies have failed to show any difference in perinatal mortality between monitored and unmonitored low-risk groups. Death rates, however, are so low in the controlled population that a huge number of patients would be needed before significant differences in perinatal mortality could be demonstrated. Studies in the low-risk population have also not been conducted in a double-blind fashion, and obstetric care may have been biased. Also of question is whether monitoring by avoiding minor degrees of asphyxia might result in better neurological outcome not reflected in the immediate neonatal course of the infant. Haverkamp et al., in a study of 690 high-risk obstetric patients, demonstrated no difference between those provided electronic fetal heart rate monitoring or auscultation, as determined by Apgar scores, cord blood gases, neonatal death, neonatal morbidity, or nursery course. However, the cesarean section rate was markedly increased in the electronically monitored group (18%, as compared to 6% in the auscultated group). Neurological assessment consisted of a Brazelton neonatal assessment at 2 to 3 days of age.[7] These infants were assessed at 9 months utilizing Bailey Scales of Infant Development and Milani-Comparetti tests.[8] Again, there was no difference in early development between the electronically monitored and auscultated groups.

Electronic fetal monitoring predicts the absence of asphyxia with greater accuracy than any other technique or combinations of techniques.[6] It has a lower false normal rate than fetal blood sampling or auscultation. Fetal monitoring appears to improve perinatal outcome by reducing the risks of intrapartum stillbirth and low Apgar score. Sudden, unexpected death of a fetus with a normal pattern has not been reported. Fetal monitoring does not predict neonatal distress resulting from trauma, sepsis, drugs, or congenital anomalies consistently, and a number of normal fetuses will demonstrate abnormal fetal heart rate patterns. Fetal heart rate monitoring is costly compared to the use of a stethoscope and clearly frustrates the objectives of the natural birthing process.

B. LONG-TERM OUTCOME

The number of randomized patients required to demonstrate an improvement in immediate neonatal morbidity and probably also in long-term outcome by the use of electronic fetal heart rate monitoring is massive. The eight prospective randomized studies with outcome confined to neonatal morbidity and development in the first year of life have not shown major advantages to the use of fetal heart rate monitoring. The Dublin trial, however, did demonstrate a lower neonatal seizure rate in the monitored groups.[9]

We undertook a prospective study to assess the neurological and cognitive outcome of a group of infants who had demonstrated "ominous fetal heart rate patterns" during labor in an attempt to understand the immediate and long-term significance of these patterns.

TABLE 1
Abnormal Fetal Heart Rate Pattern Criteria

Moderate-severe variable
Deceleration to between 70 and 80 beats per minute for >60 s with three contractions or to a rate of <70 beats per minute for 30 to 60 s

Severe variable
Deceleration to a rate of <70 beats per minute for ≥60 s (prior to pushing) on two or more occasions

Late deceleration
A uniform deceleration of the fetal heart rate of any magnitude which occurs consistently in the late phase of each uterine contraction

We first reported in 1978 on the developmental status of 50 children who had been fetally monitored.[10] The status of these children was again reported at 6 to 9 years of age.[11] The data supported an early difference in development in favor of children with normal fetal heart rate patterns. However, no difference was found in neurological and cognitive development at 6 to 9 years of age. This study did not demonstrate that abnormal fetal heart rate patterns are predictive of irreversible CNS injury.

The purpose of this study was to determine if fetal insult during labor, as demonstrated by abnormal fetal heart rate patterns, is indicative of irreversible CNS injury. The neurological and developmental statuses of 50 children who had experienced fetal monitoring were followed for a 6- to 9-year period. Each subject was placed in one of three groups according to the interpretation of the fetal monitoring trace: 12 children were judged to have normal traces, 16 had moderate-severe variable deceleration patterns, and 22 exhibited severe variable or late deceleration patterns. They were assessed at scheduled intervals according to neurological and developmental parameters. The results of the assessments are presented.

IV. MATERIALS AND METHODS

A total of 50 children with technically adequate intrauterine monitoring traces comprised the study sample. All of the children were characterized as high risk because of complications of pregnancy or labor. All of the children were 37 weeks gestation or greater, of normal birth weight (within 1 SD of the mean for gestational age), and had no observable congenital anomalies at birth. Children with prematurity or fetal malnutrition were excluded because the potential adverse effects of these conditions on development that were unrelated to the labor experience could not be analyzed separately.

The sample was drawn from consecutive abnormal and normal readings of fetal heart rate patterns interpreted by a perinatologist. A trace was identified by the perinatologist as technically adequate if it had been obtained by an internal fetal monitor which was continued until not <30 min before delivery. The trace was then categorized as normal, moderate-severe variable, severe variable, or late deceleration (Table 1).

The reasons for monitoring were identified. Prolonged labor occurred in 17 of the subjects. Meconium was also found in 17 mothers. The use of oxytocin resulted in the monitoring of 11 women. Other indications for monitoring included fetal distress (3), pre-eclampsia/toxemia (3), hypertension (11), abruptio placentae (2), and postmaturity (2).

The subjects were assigned to the three groups according to the interpretation of the fetal heart rate patterns. Group I consisted of 12 infants with normal fetal heart rate patterns. Based on type of abnormality, 38 infants were divided into two groups; Group II was comprised of 16 children with moderate-severe variables, while Group III consisted of 22 children with severe variables or late deceleration. Of the children in Group III, 15 had severe variables and 7 had late decelerations.

TABLE 2
Perinatal Characteristics of Fetal Heart Rate Monitoring
Subjects

Categories	Group I ($n = 12$)	Group II ($n = 16$)	Group III ($n = 22$)
Parity			
Nullipara	8	12	16
Multipara	4	4	6
Race			
Black	9	5	12
White	3	11	10
Socioeconomic status			
Private	5	8	10
Clinic	7	8	12
Anesthesia			
General	—	2	6
Spinal/epidural/caudal	8	13	13
None/local	4	1	3
Mode of delivery			
Cesarean section	3	2	5
Forceps	5	9	11
Spontaneous	2	1	3
Vacuum	2	4	2
Sex			
Male	6	7	10
Female	6	9	12
Weight (g)			
Range	2520—3515	2450—3690	2540—3825
Mean	3187.9	3018.8	3206.8
Apgar score (1 min)			
1—3	—	—	10
4—6	—	—	4
7—10	12	16	8
Apgar score (5 min)			
1—3	—	—	2
4—6	—	—	2
7—10	12	16	18

The children were examined by the neurologist, who was blinded to fetal heart rate results at 48 to 72 h postdelivery according to the criteria of Koenigsberger. Subsequent examinations were done at 2, 4, 6, 9, 12, 18, and 24 months, and yearly thereafter until 6 to 9 years of age. The children were assessed developmentally throughout the first year of life using the Denver Developmental Screening Test (DDST). At 6 to 9 years of age, a battery of psychological tests (which included the Wechsler Intelligence Scale for Children — Revised [WISC-R] or the Leiter International Performance Scale, the Wide Range Achievement Test, and the Bender Visual Motor Gestalt Test) were administered. The psychologist who administered the test was not aware of either the results of the fetal heart rate pattern or the results of the neurological assessment. Of the 50 subjects, 45 (90%) were seen at 6 to 9 years of age for neurological evaluation and 44 were psychometrically tested.

V. RESULTS

Demographic data on the subjects are summarized in Table 2. Mothers were predominantly black primiparous clinic patients. There was a statistically significant difference in the races of the mothers among the three groups. The higher incidence (6 of 22, or 27%)

TABLE 3
Apgar Score and Abnormal Neonatal Neurological
Examination

Apgar score	Group I (normal)	Group II (moderate-severe)	Group III (severe-late)
1 min			
1—3	—	—	7
4—6	—	—	3
7—10	2	10	6
5 min			
1—3	—	—	2
4—6	—	—	2
7—10	2	10	12

in the use of general anesthesia in Group III was noted. Most subjects were delivered vaginally; however, 10 of the 50 (20%) were delivered by cesarean section.

The study consisted of 23 males and 27 females. The overall weight range was from 2450 to 3825 g. The mean weight of 3201 g was highest in Group III, and the lower mean weight was 3018.8 g in Group II. The mean birth weight was not statistically different among the three groups.

We utilized the criteria described by Schifrin[6] of "low" Apgar scores being <7 at 1 or 5 min. The Apgar scores were ≥7 at 1 and 5 min for Group I and Group II. On the other hand, in those children with severe variable or late decelerations (Group III) the Apgar scores were <7 in 14 of the 22 subjects (64%) at 1 min and in 4 of the 22 subjects (18%) at 5 min.

A. NEONATAL EXAMINATION

A total of 28 infants had abnormal neonatal neurological examinations. Two of the infants (17%) were in Group I (normal monitoring traces). In Group II (infants with moderate-severe variable fetal heart rate monitoring traces), 10 of the 16 (63%) had abnormal neurological examinations. Of the 22 infants (73%) in Group III, 16 had abnormal neonatal examinations. The majority of these infants demonstrated hypotonia of the lower extremities. Of the abnormal neurological assessments, 10 of 28 (35%) were predicted by low 1-min Apgar scores and 4 of 28 (14%) by low 5-min Apgar scores (Table 3). Of 14 subjects with low Apgar scores at 1 min, 4 served as false predictors. Of the infants with abnormal neurologic assessments, 26 of 28 (92%) demonstrated abnormal fetal heart rate patterns (moderate-severe variable or severe variable late deceleration patterns).

B. NEUROLOGICAL EXAMINATION AT 1 YEAR

The number of abnormal neurological evaluations decreased over the first year. None of the 12 infants with normal fetal heart rate patterns had abnormal evaluations at 1 year of age. Infants having abnormal evaluations at 1 year included 1 of 16 infants with moderate-severe variable decelerations and 6 of 22 children who demonstrated severe variable or late decelerations (Table 4). There was a statistically significant difference in favor of those infants with normal fetal heart rate patterns in the number of infants demonstrating neurological abnormality at birth, but these differences decreased over the first year of life.

The child in Group II who was abnormal at 1 year was also neurologically abnormal at birth. Four of the six in Group III with abnormalities at 1 year of age also had abnormal neonatal examinations.

The children in Group III were further identified as to specific pattern on the monitoring trace. All seven children with late deceleration patterns had abnormal neonatal examinations.

TABLE 4
Abnormal Neurological Evaluation at Birth
and 1 Year of Age

	Birth	1 Year
Group I (normal)	2/12	0/12
Group II (moderate-severe)	10/16	1/16
Group III (severe-late)	16/22	6/22
	$p = 0.002$	$p = 0.174$

Note: Fisher's Exact Test was used for these comparisons.

Two of the six children who were abnormal at 1 year of age had severe variable or late deceleration patterns; the abnormalities in these two children included one child with severe retardation and another with a severe communication disorder. Three of the children with late decelerations who were abnormal at 1 year had low Apgar scores. Of the 15 children with severe variable patterns, 4 were abnormal at 1 year of age. The abnormalities included squint and developmental delay, hypotonia and an absent parachute response, and an absent parachute reflex. None of the four children with the severe variable late deceleration patterns who were abnormal at 1 year of age had low Apgar scores, while three of the four had abnormal newborn examinations.

At 6 to 9 years of age no statistically significant difference was found among the three groups ($p = 1.000$). One child with severe variable decelerations and one with late decelerations exhibited neurological abnormality at 6 to 9 years of age. One child had significant neurosensory hearing loss, but no other neurological abnormality. This child sustained repeated late decelerations for at least 130 min prior to delivery.

The second child with neurological abnormality is developmentally arrested. This child, who demonstrated almost 10 h of severe variable decelerations, has undescended testes, coarse features, widespread malformed teeth, and prognathism, all of which have become more evident with increasing age. A CT scan performed at his last evaluation demonstrated multiple asymmetrical low-density regions involving the cerebral hemispheres and cerebellum, a small cerebellum and brain stem, and a markedly enlarged fourth ventricle. Many gyri appeared malformed. The evaluation of this child suggests that he has an unspecified dysmorphic syndrome.

C. DEVELOPMENTAL STATUS

Developmental status in the first year was monitored with the DDST. Four children exhibited developmental delays at 1 year of age: one child from Group II (the moderate-severe variable deceleration group) and three children from the severe variable-late deceleration group (Group III). All of the children with abnormal DDST scores also had abnormal neurological examinations. Three of the children in Group III with abnormal neurological examinations had normal DDST scores.

At 6 to 9 years of age, cognitive testing (as determined by the WISC-R or Leiter test) demonstrated no significant differences in verbal-scale IQ (VSIQ), performance-scale IQ (PSIQ), or full-scale IQ (FSIQ) among the groups (Table 5). The average level of achievement within the areas of reading, spelling, and mathematics (as measured by the Wide Range Achievement Test) demonstrated no difference between the normal, moderate-severe variable, and severe variable-late deceleration groups (Table 6).

The means and standard deviations presented for the 6- to 9-year age group are based on the assessment of 44 children. The child with the dysmorphic syndrome was untestable. Five children were unavailable for follow-up and were not evaluated at 6 to 9 years of age.

TABLE 5

**Verbal- (VSIQ), Performance- (PSIQ), and Full-Scale
Intellectual Quotients (FSIQ) of Each Fetal Heart Rate
Pattern Group**

	Fetal heart rate pattern		
	Normal	**Moderate-severe**	**Severe-late**
VSIQ	97.9 ± 17.2 (p = 1.23)	105.5 ± 12.9 (0.31)	98.1 ± 14.3
PSIQ	98.6 ± 13.3 (0.72)	110.7 ± 13.0 (0.50)	98.1 ± 14.3
FSIQ	98.1 ± 16.1 (1.45)	108.6 ± 13.1 (0.25)	99.5 ± 12.5

Note: Factorial analysis of variance with interaction.

TABLE 6

**Wide Range Achievement Test Subtests among Fetal
Heart Rate Pattern Groups**

	Reading	**Spelling**	**Mathematics**
Normal	100.8 ± 8.5	104.8 ± 10	100.0 ± 10
Moderate-severe	109.6 ± 12	107.8 ± 11.3	106.8 ± 8.2
Severe variable	101.6 ± 16	103.2 ± 13.3	104.5 ± 13.4

Note: Repeated measures analysis of variance; p = 0.36.

Two of these children were assessed with Stanford Binet scales (one at 4 years, 6 months and the other at 3 years, 9 months) and were shown to have intellectual quotients (IQs) of 94 and 100, respectively. Both of these children had normal fetal heart rate patterns. One child with 70 min of severe variable decelerations is known to have normal school performance at 7 years, 10 months. Two children examined at 3 years, 6 months and 3 years, 0 months were neurologically and developmentally normal at that time. These two children had moderate-severe variable decelerations for 39 and 95 min, respectively.

The duration of fetal heart rate pattern abnormality in the moderate-severe variable deceleration group ranged from 23 to 375 min and from 17 to 975 min in the severe variable-late deceleration group.[9] The tracing percentages that were abnormal varied from 8 to 100%,[9] and the duration of monitoring varied from 28 to 1860 min. There was no correlation between the duration of fetal heart rate pattern abnormality, neurological abnormalities in the first year of life, or subsequent cognitive abnormalities within this sample. Interpretation of this data, however, is limited by the fact that not all infants were monitored for the same period of time. Additionally, beat-to-beat variability was not systematically evaluated in this sample.

VI. DISCUSSION AND CONCLUSION

The time frame in which this study was conducted offered a unique opportunity to evaluate the meaning of abnormal fetal heart rate patterns. One perinatologist (R.D.) was active at Magee Women's Hospital (Pittsburgh, PA) during that time period, and although he was able to convince the obstetrical staff to obtain fetal heart rate traces, intervention was not undertaken rapidly because of fetal heart rate pattern abnormalities. The duration of fetal heart rate pattern abnormalities in this population is considerably longer than would be tolerated in most labor and delivery situations in today's litigious atmosphere.

Our study demonstrates an increased frequency of abnormal neurological and developmental evaluations in children who have demonstrated "ominous" fetal heart rate patterns during labor. However, with the exception of the one child with neurosensory hearing loss and excluding the child with a dysmorphic syndrome, the degree of asphyxia as evidenced by these patterns and associated with this intervention is not associated with either fixed neurological deficits or long-term cognitive abnormalities. These findings are reminiscent of the children described by Nelson and Ellenberg[12] who "outgrew" cerebral palsy, but apparently these subjects differ from that population in not having developed a significant incidence of mental retardation or early school problems.

The fact that many of the infants with "ominous" fetal heart rate patterns have demonstrated reversible neurological abnormalities supports the value of fetal monitoring in detecting hypoxemia during labor, but we cannot conclude that early "rescue" would have had an effect on the neurological outcome of these infants based on our data. Perhaps the neurological abnormalities were due to the relatively long periods of hypoxemia evidenced by the relatively long duration of fetal heart rate abnormalities, and intervention presented the conversion of reversible to irreversible CNS injury. We do not know, however, that the degree of hypoxemia evidenced by these patterns would have ever resulted in fixed neurological injury or that "rescue" was ever necessary. What is evident, however, is that the term fetus can demonstrate many minutes of repetitive "ominous" fetal heart rate decelerations without sustaining irreversible CNS injury. The judgment that intrapartum asphyxia is the cause of developmental abnormality should not be made on the basis of fetal heart rate patterns alone. We think it is becoming more evident that a significant number of infants who have been injured neurologically prior to the intrapartum period or are developmentally abnormal (as judged by embryological evidence) can demonstrate abnormal fetal heart rate patterns during labor. Certainly, the anatomical organization of the CNS in its relationship to control of heart rate would permit abnormal fetal heart rate patterns on the basis of CNS maldevelopment or prepartum injury as well as intrapartum hypoxemia.

REFERENCES

1. **Polin, J. and Frangitane, W.,** Current concepts in management of obstetric problems for pediatricians. I. Monitoring the high risk fetus, *Pediatr. Clin. North Am.,* 33, 621, 1986.
2. **Gimovsky, M. and Caritis, S.,** Diagnosis and management of hypoxic fetal heart rate patterns, *Clin. Perinatol.,* 9, 313, 1982.
3. **Hutson, J. M. and Mueller-Heubach, E.,** Diagnosis and management of intrapartum reflex fetal heart rate changes, *Clin. Perinatol.,* 9, 325, 1982.
4. **Talman, W.,** Cardiovascular regulation and lesions of the central nervous system, *Ann. Neurol.,* 18, 1, 1983.
5. **Ayodeji, O. and Kuhn, R.,** Abnormal antepartum cardiotocography and major fetal abnormalities, *Aust. N.Z. J. Obstet. Gynaecol.,* 26, 120, 1986.
6. **Schifrin, B.,** The fetal monitoring polemic, *Clin. Perinatol.,* 9, 399, 1982.
7. **Haverkamp, A., Orleans, M., Langendoerfer, S., McFee, J., Murphy, J., and Thompson, H.,** The controlled trial of the differential effects of fetal monitoring, *Am. J. Obstet. Gynecol.,* 134, 399, 1979.
8. **Langendoerfer, S., Haverkamp, A., Murphy, J., Nowick, K., Orleans, M., Pacosa, F., and Van Doorninck, W.,** Pediatric follow-up of a randomized, controlled trial of intrapartum fetal monitoring techniques, *J. Pediatr.,* 97, 103, 1980.
9. **Prentice, A. and Lind, T.,** Fetal heart rate monitoring during labour — too frequent intervention, too little benefit?, *Lancet,* 1987, 1375, 1987.
10. **Painter, M. J., Depp, R., and O'Donoghue, P.,** Fetal heart rate patterns and development in the first year of life, *Am. J. Obstet. Gynecol.,* 132, 271, 1978.
11. **Painter, M. J., Scott, M., Hirsch, R., O'Donoghue, P., and Depp, R.,** Fetal heart rate patterns during labor: neurologic and cognitive development at 6—9 years of age, *Am. J. Obstet. Gynecol.,* 159, 854, 1988.
12. **Nelson, K. B. and Ellenberg, J. H.,** Children who "outgrew" cerebral palsy, *Pediatrics,* 69, 529, 1982.

Chapter 10

BREECH DELIVERY — MANAGEMENT AND LONG-TERM OUTCOME

I. Ingemarsson, S. Arulkumaran, and M. Westgren

TABLE OF CONTENTS

I. INTRODUCTION

Both laymen and professionals associate breech presentation with increased risk for the baby. Indeed, a survey of the literature provides a long list of hazards for the breech baby: a three- to fivefold increase in perinatal mortality;[1,2] the single greatest cause of perinatal mortality;[1,2] increased risk of antepartum stillbirth;[3,4] increased risk of congenital malformations;[5,6] a tenfold increased risk of neonatal morbidity;[7] increased risk of preterm delivery;[6] increased risk of intrapartum hazards such as birth anoxia,[8,9,10] cord prolapse,[11] and trauma involving brain, abdominal viscera, skin, and musculoskeletal system;[12] increased risk of low cord pH;[13] and low 1-min Apgar score.[4,14] In contrast to the large amount of data about perinatal problems associated with breech presentation is the sparse information about the long-term morbidity and neurological sequelae. Additionally, existing reports often come to divergent conclusions, particularly when older ones are compared with more recent ones.[15]

In this chapter we will attempt to answer a few questions which we consider important concerning the breech presentation:

1.   Is the adverse outcome inherent in the presentation itself and less a result of management and mode of delivery?
2.   What are the problems peculiar to the preterm breech baby?
3.   What is the role of external cephalic version?
4.   What selection criteria should be applied for a vaginal delivery, and how should this be managed?
5.   What is the outcome of breech infants with hyperextended head in labor?
6.   What is the long-term outcome of breech babies when current modern obstetric principles are adopted?

II. BREECH PRESENTATION — A SYMPTOM OF FETAL ABNORMALITY?

Most papers on breech presentation deal with technical questions concerning the mode of delivery, and only a few have addressed the question as to why the infant presents in the breech position in the first place. This question is fundamental to the understanding of the obstetric management of breech presentation, since it may be that the infant is presenting by breech because it is already damaged, and the trauma of the delivery is of less significance. Data supporting this opinion have been presented by several authors,[4,5,16,17] but have been disregarded in discussions on the management of breech presentation. The purpose of the present review is to summarize evidence indicating that the deficient function of breech-born infants may be of prenatal origin.

It has long been recognized that breech infants have a lower birth weight than infants born in cephalic presentations.[18] The difference in birth weight cannot be explained by the tendency toward earlier delivery in breech births, since the difference remains when birth weights are compared within gestational age subgroups.[4] The impaired fetal growth among breech infants is further indicated by the fact that the fetal-placental ratio is significantly less in breech births compared to nonbreech births[4] and that spontaneous cephalic version is less likely to occur in pregnancies with a fetus of low birth weight.[19] Why impaired growth should predispose a fetus to breech presentation is unclear, but it has been suggested that either the breech fetus with a proportionally lower birth weight may be less capable of vigorous movements[6] and, therefore, spontaneous rectification, or changes in the relative volume of the fetus and the amniotic fluid could make the fetus less mobile.[3]

Intrapartum asphyxia seems to occur more often in breech deliveries than in deliveries of infants in cephalic presentation. Intrapartum stillbirth from presumed asphyxia is more

TABLE 1
Incidence of Breech Presentation in Groups of
Morphological and Functional Injuries

Disorders	Percentage of breech presentation
Hydrocephalus (4)	65
Myelomeningocele (4)	48
Limb malformation (21)	60
Prader-Willi syndrome (5)	50
Trisomy syndrome (5)	43
Potter's syndrome (5)	36
Myotonic dystrophy (5)	21

common,[4] and studies of electronic fetal monitoring have revealed a significantly higher incidence of severe variable decelerations in term breech deliveries compared with cephalic presentations.[20] In addition, Dunn[21] has published data indicating that the cord blood hematocrit of breech-born infants is significantly higher than expected normal values, again suggesting prenatal hypoxia. Furthermore, following external cephalic version, breech infants who are delivered vaginally in cephalic presentations show a higher incidence of asphyxia compared to cephalic presentations.[22] A reasonable conclusion from these studies would be that the breech presentation is part of a syndrome associated with impaired placental circulation and that resultant intrapartum asphyxia may be of the same origin as the factor which causes breech presentation.

That preterm delivery is associated with a high incidence of breech presentation is well known and is explained by most authors as being reflective of the frequency of breech presentation occurring at that gestational age. However, papers on preterm delivery present rates of breech presentation which are about double those of breech presentation at corresponding gestational age.[22,23] The underlying cause of preterm labor and breech presentation in these cases may be the same and in some cases may suggest fetal compromise. It therefore does not seem surprising that outcome in this group has improved as a result of increased use of cesarean section for delivery.

Several authors have drawn attention to the fact that fetuses with a wide range of morphological and functional injuries more often present in the breech position (Table 1). This is especially the case with malformations of the lower limbs. For instance, the incidence of breech presentation in cases where the lower limbs are paralyzed is 93%,[21] suggesting that kicking movements are important in spontaneous rectification. Other authors[24] have demonstrated a 40% incidence of breech-born infants in cases of fetal alcohol syndrome and in mothers taking anticonvulsant therapy,[25] indicating a close association between fetal functional injury and breech presentation.

To summarize, breech presentation may be representative of preexisting damage. Appreciation of this fact is of value in the clinical management of the patient with a fetus in breech presentation.

III. PRETERM BREECH DELIVERY

Cesarean section has become the preferred method of delivery for preterm breech presentations over the last decade. The rationale for this policy has been that vaginal breech delivery carries an increased risk for the preterm fetus. Preterm vaginal breech delivery has been associated with a high percentage of footling presentations,[4,26] with a resultant greater likelihood of cord accidents[4,7] and higher risk for entrapment of the aftercoming head due to an incompletely dilated cervix.[27-30] Moreover, as previously discussed, breech presentation at preterm delivery may be a symptom of a preexisting compromise, since breech presentation

TABLE 2
Incidence of Breech Presentation in Relation to Gestational Age and Type of Population

	25—28 weeks (%)	29—30 weeks (%)	Ref.
Normal pregnancies	19	14	28
Unselected pregnancies	23	14	24
Infants born preterm	38	26	23

TABLE 3
Mortality for Preterm Breech Delivery in Infants Weighing <1500 g: Vaginal Delivery vs. Cesarean Section

Years of study	Mortality		Overall mortality (%)	Mortality C.S./vaginal	Ref.
	Vaginal	C.S.			
1970—75	49/64 (77%)	13/23 (57%)	(72)	0.8	29
Not given	34/44 (77%)	7/15 (47%)	(70)	0.6	30
1970—77	39/57 (68%)	3/12 (25%)	(61)	0.4	31
1970—75	10/16 (63%)	1/4 (25%)	(55)	0.4	32
1973—80	15/33 (46%)	26/60 (33%)	(45)	0.7	33
1977—81	71/123 (58%)	27/93 (29%)	(45)	0.5	34
1979—82	20/37 (54%)	37/99 (37%)	(42)	0.7	35
1976—82	22/40 (55%)	10/49 (20%)	(36)	0.4	36
1976—79	31/59 (53%)	17/89 (19%)	(32)	0.4	37
1972—77	5/9 (55%)	1/9 (11%)	(33)	0.2	38
1974—78	1929/4455 (43%)	664/3787 (17%)	(31)	0.4	39
1977—80	20/40 (50%)	2/32 (6%)	(31)	0.1	40
1971—77	5/13 (38%)	1/11 (9%)		0.2	41

is more common in preterm birth than in normal pregnancies of corresponding gestational age (Table 2).

Numerous authors report that delivery by cesarean section results in improved survival of the infant, with reduction in the prevalence of hypoxia, intracranial trauma, and intraventricular hemorrhage (Table 3).[29-41] However, more recently, these retrospective studies concerning the value of cesarean section for preterm breech delivery have been questioned,[35,42,43] the main problem being a failure to evaluate the circumstances surrounding the choice of cesarean section. As an example, in only two of the studies was the route of delivery chosen solely for the indication of preterm breech presentation.[38,41] Furthermore, in a number of studies, the results from one period in time are compared with those from another. This introduces bias in favor of the cesarean section route of delivery, since more cesarean sections were performed in the later time period, coincidental with other advances in neonatal care. Some of the studies deal only with neonatal intensive care unit admissions and not the overall obstetric population, thus excluding intrapartum deaths, which have been reported to account for a quarter of the total mortality.[35,36] Moreover, a number of studies pool data with ranges of birth weights and gestational ages in their analyses, thus obscuring any differences in gestational age and birth weight subsets.

Despite methodological problems in these studies, most obstetricians favor cesarean section for preterm breech delivery. This opinion has some support in the fact that the difference in outcome between routes of delivery is related to the overall mortality for each unit. Thus, centers with the lowest overall mortality rates demonstrate the greatest apparent beneficial effect of cesarean section (Table 3).

Cesarean section may, however, represent a potential hazard for the fetus and the mother. Newborns delivered by cesarean section have lower catecholamine levels.[44,45] The catecholamine surge during vaginal delivery has functional importance for respiratory adaptation after birth,[46,47] and increased incidence of respiratory difficulties after abdominal delivery have been reported.[48,49] Furthermore, during a cesarean section the immature neonate will be exposed to analgesic and anesthetic drugs, several of which have detrimental effects which enhance the problems of prematurity (such as respiratory depression and hypothermia).[43,49]

Additionally, a cesarean section is a major surgical procedure, with increased risk to the mother. Nielsen and Hökegård[50] reported an increased incidence of surgical complications during preterm cesarean section. An increased incidence of endometritis[51] and subsequent secondary infertility[52] has been reported. A relatively large number of cesarean sections performed for this indication involve the use of a vertical uterine incision, thus compromising the patient's future chances at vaginal delivery. Each case should therefore be individualized. The justification for performing a cesarean section where the fetus is of borderline viability should receive serious circumspection.

Has the liberal use of cesarean section for preterm breech presentation eliminated the differences in outcome between preterm infants in breech and cephalic presentation? Recently published studies reveal double the handicap rate in cases of breech compared with infants of similar weight and gestational age in cephalic presentation, despite the general use of cesarean section for this purpose.[53,54] Thus, these results support the opinion that the poor outcome of preterm breech birth is not only related to the route of delivery, but to the inherent pathophysiology of these tiny infants.

The ultimate verdict of the value of cesarean section in preterm breech deliveries must come from a prospective randomized study. To perform a randomized procedure in the ever-changing clinical setting of patients in preterm labor is a challenging and perhaps impossible proposition. If such a study should demonstrate no difference in outcome in relation to mode of delivery, the current policy favoring cesarean section must be questioned. Until then, however, it is our opinion that cesarean section is the preferred method of delivery for preterm breech presentations.

IV. EXTERNAL CEPHALIC VERSION IN CURRENT OBSTETRIC PRACTICE

In many centers, the uncomplicated breech presentation at term is considered an indication for cesarean section.[55] The National Institutes of Health (NIH) consensus report and reports from developed and developing countries[56-58] record a trend in rising cesarean section rates, with cesarean section for breech presentation a major indication. A much-reduced maternal morbidity and mortality associated with cesarean section has resulted from advances in anesthetic and surgical techniques, blood banking facilities, and new antibiotics; however, its contribution to such statistics cannot be ignored. A patient who has had a primary cesarean section is more likely to have a repeat cesarean section in her next pregnancy, thus exposing herself to the possible risks of surgery. Lethal congenital malformations and complications of prematurity are the major causes of perinatal morbidity and mortality, while birth asphyxia and birth injuries at term and in the preterm period represent relatively minor causes. Based on this, one has to question the value of routine elective cesarean sections for breech presentation, especially in the term fetus.[59]

An alternate line of management to reduce cesarean section rates for this indication would be to use external cephalic version (ECV) and convert the breech presentation to cephalic, thus allowing a better chance for vaginal delivery.[60]

It has been argued that the incidence of breech presentation at 37 weeks and beyond is the same whether ECV is practiced or not.[61] It is also claimed that perinatal morbidity and mortality due to the ECV procedure and in the days following up to the time of delivery may be significantly higher than if breech presentations are managed by a careful trial of vaginal delivery and cesarean section when indicated. The morbidity or mortality during or following a version could be due to cord accident, abruption, premature rupture of membranes, or premature labor.[62] If ECV is only performed after 36 weeks, it eliminates cases of spontaneous cephalic version and thus reduces the number of unnecessary procedures. Additionally, if a complication does occur, prompt delivery may be effected without the risks of delivery of a premature fetus.

Recent prospective studies dispute Hay's[61] claim that ECV does not alter the rate of breech presentation at term. Of the breech fetuses observed between 32 and 34 weeks gestation, 40 to 50% remained as breeches at 37 weeks, and 95% of the breech presentations at term were presenting by breech at 32 to 34 weeks gestation.[19] It was also noticed that primigravidae with frank breech presentations are less likely to undergo spontaneous version. The use of ECV with uterine tocolysis at 36 weeks for primigravidae and at 37 weeks for multiparae has met with high success rates and few complications. Some of the available studies are summarized in Table 4.

From these studies it may be concluded that ECV performed at 36 to 37 weeks would benefit 65 to 70% of cases by giving them a chance at spontaneous cephalic vaginal delivery. It should be emphasized that the success rate is dependent on the selection criteria used. Hofmeyer[60] analyzed six studies representing an experience of 477 cases; he found a 59% success rate,[60,63,64,67-69] with no fetal deaths attributable to the procedure. In conclusion, ECV at 37 weeks with tocolysis results in a 50% advantage over spontaneous version, with little fetal risk.

Although good success rates have been claimed at 32 to 34 weeks without tocolysis,[70-72] with a consequent reduction in cesarean section rate, the role of ECV at earlier gestational ages is questionable, since half of all cases will undergo spontaneous version by 37 weeks.[19] Furthermore, any fetal complications at this stage of gestation will force delivery of a preterm fetus with its attendant risks. A recent controlled trial of ECV before 36 weeks found no significant differences between the study and control groups in the incidence of vaginal breech delivery, cesarean section rates, and perinatal morbidity or mortality. Their results suggested no advantage to performing ECV prior to 36 weeks gestation.[73]

In summary, in the properly selected case, after 36 weeks, and with the help of tocolysis, ECV increases the likelihood of cephalic presentation and, therefore, vaginal delivery, with no added maternal or fetal risk.

V. MANAGEMENT OF THE TERM BREECH PRESENTATION IN LABOR

As discussed previously, long-term problems in the outcome of babies presenting as breech may be inherent in the presentation. However, poor outcome may also be related to events at delivery. For this reason, there are several centers that regard breech presentation as an indication for cesarean section. A "safe" cesarean section rate is difficult to arrive at, as the variance is considerable and is generally arrived at arbitrarily.

For our part, we feel that vaginal delivery in the properly selected case is indicated. The relative size of the pelvis and fetus[7,15,74-77] should be assessed clinically. Whether X-ray pelvimetry adds to this assessment is doubtful, but this is advocated by some.[78,79] Fetal size may be assessed directly and sonographically and fetal head extension looked for carefully. Labor progress[70,76,80-82] and monitoring in labor[7,8,14,83-85,115] are carefully observed, and delivery should be affected with an experienced obstetrician in attendance and a pediatrician and an anesthesiologist standing by so that a cesarean section may be performed immediately if necessary.

The details of labor management are outside the scope of this presentation; however, it should be realized that a perfect antepartum course may be undone by inadequate care at this crucial time.

VI. HYPEREXTENSION OF THE FETAL HEAD

Of special significance to immediate and eventual outcome is hyperextension of the fetal head in breech presentation. Extreme extension of the fetal head has been associated with spinal cord lesions, vertebral injury, and intrauterine death.[88] Caterini et al.[89] found that of 73 cases with hyperextended heads delivered vaginally, 10 died in the perinatal period, 5 showed signs of intracranial hemorrhage, and 15 showed medullary or vertebral trauma. In contrast, of 35 cases delivered by cesarean section, only 2 babies showed medullary or vertebral lesions. The authors recommended an X-ray examination of all breech presentations in early labor to assess the pelvic capacity and the attitude of the fetal head.

Problems arising in making the diagnosis, reflected in the varying prevalence (1 to 11%), are reported.[89-92] Ballas et al.[91] classified the degree of hyperextension by measuring the angle between the head and the fetal spine on the films. In 11 cases delivered vaginally where the deflexion angle was more than 90°, 8 babies showed cervical cord damage. Where the angle was assessed to be less than 90°, no fetal trauma occurred in 38 cases, 25 of which were delivered vaginally. In this study, only cases where the angle could be measured were included, and this was dependent on obtaining a truly lateral view of the fetal spine. In our experience, the deflexion angle is difficult to measure in most cases, even if frontal and lateral views[92] are obtained. A practical solution is to define hyperextension to mean extension of the fetal head beyond the neutral attitude.[90,92] This is a qualitative call that may be made reliably on a single AP flat plate in most cases. The degree of hyperextension may also be assessed ultrasonographically during early labor. In experienced hands it seems possible, in most cases, to estimate the angle between the fetal head and spine and thus avoid the need for X-ray evaluation.[92a] The method is noninvasive, simple, and may be repeated as indicated.

Several studies support the findings of adverse outcome after a vaginal delivery. In a study reported by Crothers and Putnam,[93] two out of three infants with spinal cord injuries had been delivered vaginally as breech. In a series reported by Bresnan and Abroms,[94] spinal cord transection was found in one out of four infants with hyperextended heads after a vaginal delivery. Westgren et al.[92] studied the infants of 33 women with the fetal head in varying degrees of hyperextension, half of whom showed extreme hyperextension. At 2 to 4 years follow-up, five (22%) of the vaginally born infants had neurological sequelae attributable to spinal, supraspinal, and cerebellar injuries, while all infants born by cesarean section were normal. Most studies have concluded that an abdominal delivery is the management of choice in this situation, preferably early in labor.[91,92,95,96]

Divergent opinions have been expressed by Stem and Rand[97] and Behrman.[98] Such controversy may be due to the varying reasons for the hyperextended fetal head.

A persistent hypertonicity of the extensor muscles[98] would prevent the normal mechanism of delivery of the aftercoming head and result in lesions of the spinal cord due to traction and torsion which have been described.[99,100] Vertebral artery compression jeopardizing the circulation to the cervical spinal cord and the brain stem might occur secondary to extension of the head.[101] Additional morbidity may be incidental. As an example, Down's syndrome is found more often among fetuses with hyperextended heads.[95]

It should also be emphasized that lesser degrees of spinal cord and central injuries may be overlooked, if not searched for specifically. The signs may be vague and may only manifest as feeding difficulties with pharyngeal incoordination, slightly delayed motor development, and speech difficulties of the clumsy child syndrome. Westgren et al.[92] observed such symptoms, together with transient paralysis, in four of five infants with sequelae.

In summary, hyperextension is a rare event, and infants damaged due to this condition represent a very small proportion of problems seen with breech birth. Assuming that extreme hyperextension occurs in 3.5% of all breech deliveries, in a service that delivers 2000 patients a year, 2 infants will have the condition. With an elective cesarean section rate of 50%, only one infant will participate in a trial of vaginal delivery, and with an assumed sequelae rate of 20%, only one damaged infant will be seen every fifth year. However, in a study where 639 breech infants were evaluated at 2 years of age, 5 of 18 children with neurological sequelae had been delivered vaginally where hyperextension of the fetal head had been diagnosed.[15]

VII. LONG-TERM MORBIDITY

It is not easy to relate different perinatal events to long-term neurological disorders and mental retardation with reasonable accuracy. The task is even more complex when minimal brain damage and learning disorders are included. It is generally agreed that only a small proportion of such problems originate during the perinatal period. Hagberg and Kyllerman[102] showed that severe mental retardation (IQ <50), with a prevalence of 0.3% in Swedish school-age children, could be related to the perinatal period in only 15% of cases. Comparable figures for mild mental retardation (IQ 50 to 70) were 0.4 and 18%, respectively. Several figures have also been published regarding different types of cerebral palsy. However, in a recent study, Hagberg et al.[103] showed a significant increase in the incidence of cerebral palsy during the last 8 years in a population-based series of 773 cerebral palsy patients born between 1959 and 1978. The incidence of cerebral palsy had increased in all birth weight specific groups, but was only statistically significant in the low birth weight group of 2000 to 2500 g. A second group showing an increase in the incidence of cerebral palsy was for babies born at term. For both groups the increase could be related to perinatal risk factors. It is also notable that the changing trends in incidence of cerebral palsy paralleled a progressive decline in perinatal mortality throughout the study period.

It should be borne in mind, however, that such epidemiological analyses will only give a rough estimation of the panorama of potential risk factors and can hardly be used for analyzing specific obstetric questions such as fetal presentation at the time of birth. As previously mentioned, breech presentation per se has inherent problems and may be a consequence of fetal compromise. Consideration must also be given to a lower mean gestational age at delivery[104] and a lower mean birth weight.[3,4,75] Luterkort[104] found that the mean gestational age at delivery was 270.7 ± 9.8 days for breech presentation and 280.2 ± 9.8 days for vertex babies in patients whose gestational age was confirmed by routine ultrasound dating during early pregnancy. Schutte et al.[105] compared vertex and breech groups in 57,819 singleton pregnancies from the Dutch nationwide obstetric data bank. After correction for gestational age, birth weight, and congenital malformations, the perinatal mortality was higher in the breech group than in the vertex group despite a higher cesarean section rate in the breech group.

A. FOLLOW-UP OF BREECH BIRTHS BORN IN THE 1950S AND 1960S

Due to differences in obstetric practices, the sequelae in studies performed in the 1950s and 1960s will be analyzed separately from studies performed in the 1970s and later. Manzke[106] critically reviewed the literature for this period. He found that results from these studies varied considerably, about half of the researchers predicting favorable developments for breech-born infants and the other half suggesting unfavorable outcomes. In a socio-psychiatric follow-up study of 192 breech-born young men and 192 controls, Hambert and Akesson[107] did not find any difference in either sociopsychiatric disorders or intelligence levels. In a recently published study[108] from Norway, 42 singleton males born vaginally in breech presentation in 1962 to 1963 were examined at 18 years of age. There was no statistical difference between the study group and control group with regard to mortality, morbidity, or general intelligence levels. Hohlweg-Majert and Willard[109] found the same intelligence levels for breech-born and nonbreech infants.

Neligan[110] investigated breech-born children of mothers residing in the city of New Castle upon Tyne, U.K. during the years 1960 to 1962. He related the outcome to birth weight, sex, and social class, and he found that mild neurological abnormalities were more common at 5 years of age for boys, but not for girls, when compared with infants born in vertex presentation, particularly for boys with heavy birth weight. The analyses of variance highlighted contributory factors such as parity, birth weight, and social class. However, the differences had more or less disappeared by reassessment at the age of 10 years.

At follow-up 4 to 14 years after birth, Bolte et al.[111] found 20% of the breech-born children to be neurologically abnormal, which represented a frequency double that of vertex infants with an instrumental or abdominal delivery. EEG abnormalities of the focal type were seen in 6.2% of the breech births compared to 3.7% of the nonbreech births.

Fianu[112] found significantly more visual disturbances, speech disorders, intellectual and/ or physical handicaps, and learning handicaps among breech births compared to children born in vertex presentation. However, the results were obtained from questionnaires sent to parents and teachers.

Muller et al.[113] also sent questionnaires to teachers. Learning difficulties were more common among breech births (24.5%) compared to controls (8.3%) at the follow-up at 9 years of age. Intelligence testing showed no significant differences.

Among children with spastic motor deficits, Sadowski and Staemmler[114] found a significantly increased rate of breech-born children, but not among children with learning difficulties or with mental retardation.

These older studies have been heavily criticized.[106] Most studies were retrospective, and the results were often obtained from patient records or questionnaires. The numbers of cases are often too small to allow subgrouping into different types of breech presentation or by route and mode of delivery. Adequate control groups are often lacking, and the follow-up investigations are often only performed once during infancy. These studies also represented a time when the obstetrical principles differed, most importantly involving cesarean section rates below 10% and never exceeding 20%.

B. FOLLOW-UP OF BREECH BIRTHS AFTER 1970

Hochuli et al.[115] examined early and late development of breech children born by the vaginal route compared to the abdominal route. Routine X-ray pelvimetry and fetal parameters obtained by ultrasound were used in selection for mode of delivery. The cesarean section rate was 34.3%. Follow-up data for 4 to 6 years was obtained in 86% of the infants. Long-term morbidity, including psychomotor retardation, minimal cerebral palsy, and behavior disorders, occurred in 21% of the vaginal group and was not different from that seen in the cesarean section group (18.5%).

Manzke[106] followed 58 breech-born infants at regular intervals from the neonatal period to 6 years of age. A total of 43 of the infants were born by vaginal delivery and 15 by cesarean section. The breech-born neonates were matched with control cases in cephalic presentation for sex, birth weight, and socioeconomic background. The author found no significant differences between breech and cephalic presentation.

Ingemarsson et al.,[41] in a combined prospective and retrospective investigation, studied the effect of routine cesarean section on breech infants delivered before the 37th gestational week. The policy of routine cesarean section was implemented in January 1975. All babies born after that date were prospectively followed for at least 2 years and compared with preterm breeches delivered vaginally in the period 1971 to 1974. In the vaginally delivered group 48 infants died (14.6%), compared to 2 in the cesarean section group (4.8%). Of the survivors, ten babies (24.4%) had developmental or neurological abnormalities, compared to one in the cesarean section group (2.5%). The long-term morbidity was 27% in infants with birth weight below 2500 g surviving vaginal breech delivery. The cesarean section group had 1 handicapped child among 24 long-term survivors weighing <2500 g at birth (4%). In a recent study, Frenzel et al.[116] retrospectively examined 126 low birth weight infants born in breech presentation — 65 by cesarean section and 61 by vaginal delivery. The control group involved 270 low birth weight infants born spontaneously in vertex presentation. For babies with a birth weight of 1500 to 2500 g, neonatal mortality, low Apgar score, acidosis, incidence of severe respiratory distress, and percentage of psycho-motor handicaps were lower in infants born by cesarean section than those born vaginally. In the group of infants with birth weights <1500 g, such differences could not be demonstrated. In contrast to these two studies, Cox et al.[117] reported no benefit from an increased use of cesarean section in preterm babies. They compared two different time periods (1973—1974 and 1979—1980) and found a decreased neonatal mortality rate, but also an increased incidence of neurological sequelae in survivors in the latter period. Effer et al.[33] followed very low birth weight breech infants for 3 years and found a handicap rate of 53% among the vaginally born infants compared to 30% in the cesarean section group. When analyzing the material in year-long segments, they found an association between an increased cesarean section rate and an improved prognosis for the small baby. However, they concluded that this relationship could be incidental and might not relate to the mode of delivery.

Faber-Nijholt et al.[118] studied the outcome of 348 infants born in breech presentation between 1969 and 1977 with a gestational age of at least 28 weeks and a birth weight exceeding 1000 g. The cesarean section rate in this study was 20%. The 256 surviving singleton breeches were matched with controls in cephalic presentation born during the same year. The matching criteria were sex, birth weight, gestational age, parity, and diastolic blood pressure of the mother. The matching was optimal in 60% of the population. The long-term follow-up included a standardized, age-specific neurological method aimed at discovering minor neurological dysfunction in particular. In the study material, 12.1% of the infants had a birth weight of <2500 g and 16.8% were preterm. Of the 256 infants, 217 were examined at an age of 3 to 10 years. Minor and minimal neurological signs were more common among breeches, but this could be more related to concomitant variables such as preterm births, intrauterine growth retardation, and multiple pregnancies than to the presentation. Differences obtained also vanished among pairs with optimal matching. The authors estimated that the relative risk of minor amenable neurological dysfunction of vaginal birth in breech presentation does not exceed 2.0. The authors found no reason to advocate a cesarean section rate higher than 20%.

In a recent study, Svenningsen et al.[15] reported on a 4-year follow-up of 709 term breech babies delivered between 1971 and 1977. The study was divided into two 3$^1/_2$-year periods, with period A extending from January 1, 1971 to May 31, 1974 and period B from June 1, 1974 to December 31, 1977, based on differences in obstetric management. In period A, X-ray pelvimetry was only performed in primiparae and cesarean section was done if the

TABLE 4
Neurodevelopmental Sequelae at 2 Years of Age in 639 Breech-Born Infants

	Period A (n = 300)		Period B (n = 339)	
	VD	CS	VD	CS
Number of infants	246	54	201	138
Cerebral palsy				
Tetraplegia	2		1	
Hemiplegia	2			
Diplegia	2			
Dyskinetic/ataxia	4		1	1
Erb's palsy	2		1	
Psychomotor retardation	2		1	
Total	14	0	4	1
%	5.7	0	2.0	0.7
(%) in each period		(4.6)		(1.5)

Note: VD = vaginal delivery, CS = cesarean section; p values: A vs. B not significant.

From Svenningsen, N. W., Westgren, M., and Ingemarsson, I., *J. Perinat. Med.*, 13, 117, 1985. With permission.

anteroposterior diameter of the pelvic inlet was <11 cm and/or the sum of the outlet diameters was <32 cm. In period B, pelvimetry was done routinely and cesarean section was performed if the anteroposterior diameter of the inlet was <12 cm or <2 cm greater than the fetal biparietal diameter measured with ultrasound, if the sum of the outlet measurement was <33.5 cm, or if the clinically estimated birth weight was >4000 g. Hyperextension of the fetal head became an additional indication for cesarean section at the end of period B. The cesarean section rate in period A was 16.9% and in period B, 37.1%.

At 2 years of age the children were given neurological examinations and development evaluations. At 4 years of age the children were provided with comprehensive health examinations, including screening for vision, hearing, and behavioral problems. The 4-year examination was supplemented with questionnaires to the parents regarding the child's development, previous health problems, and the family's social and educational standard. The 4-year examination was compared with a control group of 1201 vaginally born full-term singletons in cephalic presentation.

One baby died neonatally in each group, giving a neonatal death rate of 0.3%. Neurodevelopmental sequelae at 2 years of age are shown in Table 4. The risk was higher (4.6%) in period A than in period B (1.5%). Vaginally delivered babies had comparatively higher incidences of sequelae in period A (5.7%) compared to the same mode of delivery in period B (2.0%). Obstetric complications occurred in a majority of cases (14 of 18) in vaginally delivered patients, and footling presentation and hyperextended heads were overrepresented.

Table 5 shows neurodevelopmental sequelae at 4 years of age. The total incidence of neurodevelopmental disorders was higher in period A (5.3%) compared to both period B (2.4%) and vertex deliveries (1.5%), the difference being significant between breeches and vertex infants in period A. However, the incidences of visual and auditory disorders, behavioral problems, enuresis, and late speech development (Table 6) were not higher in period A than in the controls. It should be emphasized that term breech children in period B, with obstetric management giving a cesarean section rate of 37%, had a rate of neurodevelopmental disorders at 4 years of age (2.4%) comparable to that of infants born vaginally in vertex presentation (1.5%).

TABLE 5

Neurodevelopmental Sequelae at 4 Years of Age in 480 Breech-Born Infants

	Period A (n = 233)		Period B (n = 247)		Vertex (n = 1202)
	VD	CS	VD	CS	VD
Number of infants	185	48	155	92	1202
Cerebral palsy	5		2	1	3
Psychomotor retardation	2	1	1		4
MBD — syndrome	3	1	1	1	10
Epilepsy	1				1
Total	11	2	4	2	18
%	6.0	4.2	2.9	2.2	1.5
(%) in each period		(5.3)		(2.4)	(1.5)

Note: VD = vaginal delivery, CS = cesarean section, MBD = minimal brain damage;
p values: A vs. B not significant, A vs. vertex <0.05, B vs. vertex not significant.

From Svenningsen, N. W., Westgren, M., and Ingemarsson, I., *J. Perinat. Med.,* 13, 117, 1985. With permission.

TABLE 6

Visual and Auditory Disorders at 4 Years of Age in 480 Breech-Born Infants

	Period A (n = 233)		Period B (n = 247)		Vertex (n = 1202)
	VD	CS	VD	CS	VD
Number of infants	185	48	155	92	1202
Visual disorders					
Strabism	5	2	4	2	39
Refractory errors	11	2	4	6	82
Total	16	4	8	8	121
%	8.7	8.3	5.2	8.7	10.1
(%) in each period		(8.6)	(6.5)	(10.1)	
Auditory disorders					
Sensorineural	2	1	2		3
Conductive	4	2	1	2	27
Total	6	3	3	2	30
%	3.2	6.3	1.9	2.2	2.5
(%) in each period		(3.9)		(2.0)	(2.5)

Note: VD = vaginal delivery, CS = cesarean section; p values: A vs. B not significant,
A vs. vertex not significant, B vs. vertex not significant.

From Svenningsen, N. W., Westgren, M., and Ingemarsson, I., *J. Perinat. Med.,* 13, 117, 1985. With permission.

In another recent study using chart reviews, Rosen et al.[119] investigated the long-term outcome at 2 years or more of infants born in frank breech presentation. They matched four groups with 70 infants in each with respect to presentation and mode of delivery: (1) breech-vaginal, (2) breech-cesarean, (3) vertex-vaginal, and (4) vertex-cesarean. They found no increased risk of major brain damage either when breeches were compared to vertex or within the breech group when vaginal births were compared to cesarean deliveries.

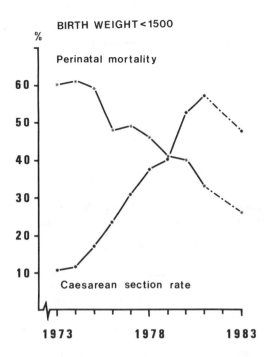

BIRTH WEIGHT < 1500

FIGURE 1.   Cesarean section rate in relation to perinatal
mortality for all babies with a birth weight of <1500 g
during the years 1973 to 1983. Data from the pregnancy
and the perinatal and neonatal periods are collected from
all births in Sweden since 1973.

VIII. CONCLUSIONS

Recent studies of long-term follow-up of cases presenting as breech seem to be in
harmony in stating that vaginal delivery in selected cases of breech presentation may be
performed with minimal risk to the infant. This is in clear contrast to some of the older
studies which indicated considerable risk for the term breech when vaginal delivery was the
routine route. A strict management protocol is necessary in order to judiciously select fetuses
for trial of vaginal delivery. The pelvic capacity should be assessed routinely; the baby's
size should be estimated clinically or, preferably, with the help of ultrasound scans. When
a patient is in labor, hyperextension of the fetal head should be excluded and obstetric
expertise should always be available to supervise labor and delivery. A neonatologist and
an anesthesiologist should be in attendance.

The ideal rate of cesarean section in term breeches is not possible to state, but if the
above–mentioned criteria for vaginal delivery are observed, at least half of all cases may
be safely delivered vaginally. Hochuli et al.,[115] Faber-Nijholt et al.,[118] and Svenningsen et
al.[15] reported cesarean section rates between 20 and 40%, with excellent results for the
children at long-term follow-up.

For the preterm breech with an estimated birth weight of <1500 to 2000 g, most studies
agree that abdominal delivery is advisable from the point of view of both immediate and
long-term outcome. It should be emphasized that this advantage for cesarean section delivery
is not applicable to all low birth weight births. Figure 1 shows the mode of delivery for all
babies, cephalic presentation included, with birth weight of <1500 g in Sweden from 1973
to 1983. The cesarean section rate rose from a little bit more than 10% in 1973 to almost
60%, but had declined to just below 50% by 1983. During the same time, the perinatal

mortality was reduced by more than 50%. Perinatal mortality rates have continued to decrease even after a decline in the cesarean section rate, indicating the importance of variables other than route of delivery.

REFERENCES

1. **Morgan, H. S. and Kane, S. H.**, An analysis of 16,327 breech births, *JAMA*, 187, 202, 1964.
2. **DeCrespigny, L. J. C. and Pepperrell, R. J.**, Perinatal mortality and morbidity in breech presentation, *Obstet. Gynecol.*, 53, 141, 1979.
3. **Schrage, R.**, Zur Atiologie der Beckenendlage, *Z. Geburtshilfe Perinatol.*, 177, 437, 1973.
4. **Brenner, W. E., Bruce, R. D., and Henricks, G. H.**, The characteristics and perils of breech presentation, *Am. J. Obstet. Gynecol.*, 118, 700, 1974.
5. **Braun, F. H. T., Jones, K. L., and Smith, D. W.**, Breech presentation as an indicator of fetal abnormality, *J. Pediatr.*, 86, 419, 1975.
6. **Kauppila, O.**, The perinatal mortality in breech deliveries and observation of affecting factors, a retrospective study of 2227 cases, *Acta Obstet. Gynecol. Scand. Suppl.*, 39, 1, 1975.
7. **Rovinsky, J. J., Miller, J. A., and Kaplan, S.**, Management of breech presentation at term, *Am. J. Obstet. Gynecol.*, 115, 497, 1973.
8. **Eliot, B. W. and Hill, J. G.**, Method of breech management incorporating use of fetal blood sampling, *Br. Med. J.*, 4, 703, 1972.
9. **Wheeler, T. and Greene, K.**, Fetal heart rate monitoring during breech labour, *Br. J. Obstet. Gynaecol.*, 82, 208, 1975.
10. **Jurado, L. and Miller, G. L.**, Breech presentation, *Am. J. Obstet. Gynecol.*, 101, 183, 1968.
11. **Alexopoulos, K. A.**, The importance of breech delivery in pathogenesis of brain damage, *Clin. Pediatr. (Philadelphia)*, 12, 248, 1973.
12. **Tank, E. S., Davis, R., Holt, J. F., and Morley, G. W.**, Mechanisms of trauma during breech delivery, *Obstet. Gynecol.*, 38, 761, 1971.
13. **Kubli, F., Boos, W., and Ruttgers, H.**, Cesarean section in the management of singleton breech presentation, in *Perinatal Medicine: 5th European Congress of Perinatal Medicine*, Rooth, G. and Bratteby, L. E., Eds., Almqvist & Wiksell, Stockholm, 1976, 69.
14. **Teteris, N. J., Botschner, A. W., Ullery, J. C., and Essig, G. F.**, Fetal heart rate during breech delivery, *Am. J. Obstet. Gynecol.*, 107, 702, 1970.
15. **Svenningsen, N. W., Westgren, M., and Ingemarsson, I.**, Modern strategy for the term breech delivery — a study with a 4 year follow-up of the infants, *J. Perinat. Med.*, 13, 117, 1985.
16. **Calvert, J. P.**, Intrinsic hazard of breech presentation, *Br. Med. J.*, 281, 1319, 1980.
17. **Hytten, F. E.**, Breech presentation; is it a bad omen?, *Br. J. Obstet. Gynaecol.*, 89, 879, 1982.
18. **Van Numers, C.**, Investigation into the etiology of breech presentation at term, *Gynaecologica*, 133, 106, 1952.
19. **Westgren, M., Edvall, H., Nordstrom, L., and Svalenius, E.**, Spontaneous cephalic version of breech presentation in the last trimester, *Br. J. Obstet. Gynaecol.*, 92, 19, 1985.
20. **Nordstrom, L., Ingemarsson, E., Ingemarsson, I., and Westgren, M.**, The significance of pronounced variable deceleration at breech deliveries, *Int. J. Feto-Maternal Med.*, in press.
21. **Dunn, P.**, Maternal and fetal aetiological factors to breech presentation, in *Perinatal Medicine: 5th European Congress of Perinatal Medicine*, Rooth, G. and Bratteby, L. E., Eds., Almqvist & Wiksell, Stockholm, 1976, 76.
22. **Phelan, J.**, personal communication, 1985.
23. **Westgren, M., Malcus, P., and Svenningsen, N.**, Intrauterine asphyxia and long-term outcome in preterm fetuses, *Obstet. Gynecol.*, 67, 512, 1986.
24. **Scheer, K. and Nubar, J.**, Variation of fetal presentation with gestational age, *Am. J. Obstet. Gynecol.*, 125, 269, 1976.
25. **Halliday, H. L., Reid, M., and McClure, G.**, Results of heavy drinking in pregnancy, *Br. J. Obstet. Gynaecol.*, 89, 892, 1982.
26. **Galloway, W. H., Bartholomew, R. A., Colvin, E. D., Grimes, W. H., Fish, J. S., and Lester, W. M.**, Premature breech delivery, *Am. J. Obstet. Gynecol.*, 99, 975, 1967.
27. **Kauppila, O.**, The perinatal mortality in breech deliveries and observations on affecting factors, *Acta Obstet. Gynaecol. Scand.*, 39, 29, 1975.
28. **Houghey, M. J.**, Fetal position during pregnancy, *Am. J. Obstet. Gynecol.*, 153, 885, 1985.
29. **Goldenberg, R. L. and Nelson, K. G.**, The premature breech, *Am. J. Obstet. Gynecol.*, 127, 240, 1977.

30. **Mann, L. J. and Gallant, J. M.,** Modern management of the breech delivery, *Am. J. Obstet. Gynecol.,* 134, 611, 1979.

31. **Bowes, W. A., Taylor, E. S., O'Brien, M., and Bowes, C.,** Breech delivery: evaluation of the method of delivery on perinatal results and maternal morbidity, *Am. J. Obstet. Gynecol.,* 135, 965, 1979.

32. **Woods, J. T.,** Effects of low-birthweight breech delivery on neonatal mortality, *Obstet. Gynecol.,* 53, 735, 1979.

33. **Effer, S. B., Saigal, S., Rand, C., Hunter, D. J. S., Stockopf, B., Harper, A. C., Nimrod, C., and Milner, R.,** Effects of delivery methods on outcome in the very low-birthweight breech infant: is the improved survival related to cesarean section or other perinatal care maneuvers?, *Am. J. Obstet. Gynecol.,* 145, 123, 1983.

34. **Main, D. M., Main, E. K., and Maurer, M. M.,** Cesarean section versus vaginal delivery for the breech fetus weighing less than 1500 grams, *Am. J. Obstet. Gynecol.,* 146, 580, 1983.

35. **Westgren, M., Sangster, J., and Paul, D.,** Preterm breech delivery: another retrospective study, *Obstet. Gynecol.,* 66, 481, 1985.

36. **Rosen, M. G. and Chik, L.,** The effect of delivery route on outcome in breech presentation, *Am. J. Obstet. Gynecol.,* 148, 909, 1984.

37. **Smith, M. L., Spencer, S. A., and Hull, D.,** Mode of delivery and survival in babies weighing less than 2000 g at birth, *Br. Med. J.,* 281, 1118, 1980.

38. **Duenholter, J. H., Wells, C. R., Reisch, J. S., Santos-Ramos, R., and Jimenez, J.,** A paired controlled study of vaginal and abdominal delivery of the low birth weight breech fetus, *Obstet. Gynecol.,* 54, 310, 1979.

39. **Sachs, B. P., McCarthy, B. J., Rubin, G., Burton, A., Terry, J., and Tyler, C. W., Jr.,** Cesarean section: risks and benefits for the mother and fetus, *JAMA,* 250, 2157, 1983.

40. **Yu, V. Y. H., Bajuh, B., and Cutting, D.,** Effect of mode of delivery on outcome of very-low-birthweight infants, *Br. J. Obstet. Gynaecol.,* 91, 633, 1984.

41. **Ingemarsson, I., Westgren, M., and Svenningsen, N. W.,** Long-term follow-up of preterm infants in breech presentation delivered by cesarean section: a prospective study, *Lancet,* 2, 172, 1978.

42. **Crowley, P. and Hawkins, D. F.,** Premature breech delivery — the cesarean section debate, *J. Obstet. Gynecol.,* 1, 2, 1980.

43. **Westgren, M. and Paul, R.,** Delivery of the low birth weight infant by cesarean section, *Clin. Obstet. Gynecol.,* 28, 752, 1985.

44. **Lagercrantz, H. and Bistoletti, P.,** Catecholamine release in newborn, *Pediatr. Res.,* 11, 889, 1981.

45. **Westgren, M., Lindahl, S., and Norden, N.,** Maternal and fetal endocrine stress response at vaginal delivery with and without epidural block, *J. Perinat. Med.,* 14, 235, 1986.

46. **Falconer, A. D. and Lake, D. M.,** Circumstances influencing umbilical cord plasma catecholamines at delivery, *Br. J. Obstet. Gynaecol.,* 9, 44, 1982.

47. **Faxelius, G., Lagercrantz, H., and Yao, A.,** Sympathoadrenal activity and peripheral blood flow after birth: comparison in infants delivered vaginally and by cesarean section, *J. Pediatr.,* 105, 144, 1984.

48. **Olver, R. E.,** Of labour and lungs, *Arch. Dis. Child.,* 56, 659, 1981.

49. **Scanlon, J. W.,** Anesthetic management of the high-risk pregnancy: consequences in the newborn, *Clin. Obstet. Gynecol.,* 24, 671, 1981.

50. **Nielsen, T. F. and Hökegård, K. H.,** Cesarean section and intraoperative surgical complications, *Acta Obstet. Gynecol. Scand.,* 63, 103, 1984.

51. **Daikoku, N. H., Kaltreider, F., Khouzami, V. A., Spence, M., and Johnson, J.,** Premature rupture of membranes and spontaneous preterm labor: maternal endometritis risks, *Obstet. Gynecol.,* 59, 13, 1982.

52. **Hurry, D. J., Larsen, B., and Charles, D.,** Effects of postcesarean section febrile morbidity on subsequent fertility, *Obstet. Gynecol.,* 64, 256, 1984.

53. **Kitchen, W. H., Yu, V. Y. H., Orgill, A. A., Ford, G., Richards, A., Astbury, J., Ryan, M. M., Russo, W., Lissenden, J. V., and Bajuk, B.,** Infants born before 29 weeks gestation: survival and morbidity at 2 years of age, *Br. J. Obstet. Gynaecol.,* 89, 887, 1982.

54. **Svenningsen, N.,** The pediatric approach to the premature breech, in *Perinatal Medicine,* Clinch, J. and Matthews, T., Eds., ETA Publications Ltd., Dublin, 1984, 209.

55. **Green, J. E., McLean, F., Smith, L. P., and Usher, R.,** Has an increased cesarean section rate for term breech delivery reduced incidence of birth asphyxia, trauma and death?, *Am. J. Obstet. Gynecol.,* 142, 643, 1982.

56. **Anon.,** Consensus in medicine: caesarean childbirth — summary of an NIH consensus statement, *Br. Med. J.,* 282, 1600, 1981.

57. **Yudkin, P. L. and Redman, C. W. G.,** Caesarean section dissected 1978—1983, *Br. J. Obstet. Gynaecol.,* 93, 134, 1986.

58. **Arulkumaran, S., Gibb, D. M. F., TambyRaja, R. L., Heng, S. H., and Ratnam, S. S.,** Rising caesarean section rate in Singapore, *Singapore J. Obstet. Gynaecol.,* 16, 6, 1985.

59. **Russel, J. K.,** Breech: vaginal delivery or caesarean section, *Br. Med. J.,* 285, 830, 1982.

60. **Hofmeyer, G. J.,** Effect of external cephalic version in late pregnancy on breech presentation and caesarean section rate: a controlled trial, *Br. J. Obstet. Gynaecol.,* 90, 392, 1983.

61. **Hay, D.,** Observations on breech presentation and delivery, *J. Obstet. Gynaecol. Br. Commonw.,* 66, 529, 1959.

62. **Bradley-Watson, P. J.,** The decreasing value of external cephalic version in modern obstetric practice, *Am. J. Obstet. Gynecol.,* 123, 237, 1975.

63. **Van Dorsten, J. P., Schifrin, B. S., and Wallace, R. L.,** Randomized controlled trial of external cephalic version with tocolysis in late pregnancy, *Am. J. Obstet. Gynecol.,* 141, 417, 1981.

64. **Fall, O. and Nilsson, B. A.,** External cephalic version in breech presentation under tocolysis, *Obstet. Gynecol.,* 53, 712, 1979.

65. **Stine, L. E., Phelan, P. J., Wallace, R., Eglinton, G. S., Van Dorsten, J. P., and Schifrin, B. S.,** Update on external cephalic version performed at term, *Obstet. Gynecol.,* 65, 642, 1985.

66. **Brocks, V., Philipsen, T., and Secher, N. J.,** A randomized trial of external cephalic version with tocolysis in late pregnancy, *Br. J. Obstet. Gynaecol.,* 91, 653, 1984.

67. **Ylikorkala, O. and Hartikainen-Sorri, A. L.,** Value of external version in fetal malpresentation in combination with use of ultrasound, *Acta Obstet. Gynecol. Scand.,* 56, 63, 1977.

68. **Muller-Holve, W.,** Ausserre Wendung unter Tocolysis, *Gynecol. Prat.,* 1, 425, 1977.

69. **Fianu, S. and Vaclavinkova, V.,** External cephalic version in the management of breech presentation with special reference to placental localization, *Acta Obstet. Gynecol. Scand.,* 58, 209, 1979.

70. **Duignan, N. M.,** The management of breech presentation, in *Progress in Obstetrics and Gynaecology,* Studd, J. W. W., Ed., Churchill Livingstone, London, 1983, 73.

71. **Ranney, B.,** The gentle art of external cephalic version, *Am. J. Obstet. Gynecol.,* 116, 239, 1973.

72. **Hibbard, L. T. and Schumann, W. L.,** Prophylactic external cephalic version in obstetric practice, *Am. J. Obstet. Gynecol.,* 116, 511, 1973.

73. **Kasule, J., Chimbira, T. H. K., and Brown, I. M.,** Controlled trial of external cephalic version, *Br. J. Obstet. Gynaecol.,* 92, 14, 1985.

74. **Benson, W. L., Voyce, D. C., and Vaughen, D. L.,** Breech delivery in the primigravida, *Obstet. Gynecol.,* 40, 417, 1972.

75. **Collea, J. V., Robin, S. C., Weghorst, G. R., and Quilligan, E. J.,** The randomized management of term frank breech presentation: vaginal delivery vs. cesarean section, *Am. J. Obstet. Gynecol.,* 131, 186, 1978.

76. **Ohlsen, H.,** Outcome of term breech delivery in primigravidae: a feto-pelvic breech index, *Acta Obstet. Gynecol. Scand.,* 54, 141, 1975.

77. **Friedman, E. A.,** *Labor — Clinical Evaluation and Management,* 2nd ed., Appleton-Century-Crofts, New York, 1967, 168.

78. **Joyce, D. N., Gime-Osagie, F., and Stevenson, G. W.,** Role of pelvimetry in active management of labour, *Br. Med. J.,* 4, 505, 1975.

79. **Ridley, J. W., Jackson, P., Stewart, J. H., and Boyle, P.,** The role of antenatal radiography in the management of breech deliveries, *Br. J. Obstet. Gynaecol.,* 89, 342, 1982.

80. **Bilodeau, R. and Marrier, R.,** Breech presentation at term, *Am. J. Obstet. Gynecol.,* 130, 555, 1978.

81. **Zatuchni, G. I. and Andros, G. J.,** Prognostic index for vaginal delivery in breech presentation at term, prospective study, *Am. J. Obstet. Gynecol.,* 98, 854, 1967.

82. **Borten, M.,** *Breech Presentation in Management of Labor,* Friedman, E., Ed., University Park Press, Baltimore, 1983, 241.

83. **Arulkumaran, S., Ingemarsson, I., Gibb, D. M. F., and Ratnam, S. S.,** Uterine activity in cases with breech presentation in spontaneous labour, *Aust. N.Z. J. Obstet. Gynaecol.,* in press.

84. **Gibb, D. M. F., Arulkumaran, S., Lun, K. C., and Ratnam, S. S.,** Characteristics of uterine activity in nulliparous labour, *Br. J. Obstet. Gynaecol.,* 91, 220, 1984.

85. **Arulkumaran, S., Gibb, D. M. F., Lun, K. C., Heng, S. H., and Ratnam, S. S.,** The effect of parity on uterine activity in labour, *Br. J. Obstet. Gynaecol.,* 91, 843, 1984.

86. **Eilen, B., Fleischer, A., Schilman, H., and Jagani, N.,** Fetal acidosis and the abnormal fetal heart rate tracing: the term breech fetus, *Obstet. Gynecol.,* 63, 233, 1984.

87. **Jenkins, D. N.,** Breech delivery, *Clin. Obstet. Gynecol.,* 7, 561, 1980.

88. **Taylor, J.,** Breech presentation with hyperextension of the neck and intrauterine dislocation of cervical vertebrae, *Am. J. Obstet. Gynecol.,* 56, 381, 1948.

89. **Caterini, H., Langer, A., Sama, J. C., Devaneson, M., and Pelosi, M.,** Fetal risk in hyperextension of the fetal head in breech presentation, *Am. J. Obstet. Gynecol.,* 123, 632, 1975.

90. **Wilcox, H. and Mo, B.,** The attitude of the fetus in breech presentation, *Am. J. Obstet. Gynecol.,* 58, 478, 1949.

91. **Ballas, S., Toaff, R., and Jaffa, A.,** Deflexion of the fetal head in breech presentation, *Obstet. Gynecol.,* 52, 653, 1978.

92. **Westgren, M., Grundsell, H., Ingemarsson, I., Muhlow, A., and Svenningsen, N.,** Hyperextension of the fetal head in breech presentation, a study with long-term follow-up, *Br. J. Obstet. Gynaecol.,* 88, 101, 1981.

92a. **Ingemarsson, I., Arulkumaran, S., and Westgren, M.,** unpublished observations.

93. **Crothers, B. and Putnam, M. C.,** Obstetrical injuries to the spinal cord, *Medicine,* 6, 41, 1927.

94. **Bresnan, M. J. and Abroms, I. F.,** Neonatal spinal cord transsection secondary to intrauterine hyperextension of the neck in breech presentation, *J. Pediatr.,* 84, 734, 1974.

95. **Daw, E.,** Management of the hyperextended fetal head, *Am. J. Obstet. Gynecol.,* 1224, 113, 1976.

96. **Bhagwanani, S., Price, H., Laurence, K., and Ginz, B.,** Risks and prevention of cervical cord injury in the management of breech presentation with hyperextension of the fetal head, *Am. J. Obstet. Gynecol.,* 115, 1159, 1973.

97. **Stem, W. and Rand, R.,** Birth injuries to the spinal cord: a report of two cases and review of the literature, *Am. J. Obstet. Gynecol.,* 78, 498, 1959.

98. **Behrman, S.,** Fetal cervical hyperextension, *Clin. Obstet. Gynecol.,* 5, 1018, 1962.

99. **Towbin, A.,** Latent spinal cord and brain stem injury at birth, *Dev. Med. Child Neurol.,* 11, 54, 1969.

100. **Towbin, A.,** Spinal cord and brain stem injury at birth, *Arch. Pathol.,* 77, 620, 1964.

101. **Gilles, F., Bina, M., and Satrel, A.,** Infantile atlantroccipital instability, the potential danger of extreme extension, *Am. J. Dis. Child.,* 133, 30, 1979.

102. **Hagberg, B. and Kyllerman, M.,** Epidemiology of mental retardation — a Swedish survey, *Brain Res.,* 5, 441, 1983.

103. **Hagberg, B., Hagberg, G., and Olow, I.,** The changing panorama of cerebral palsy in Sweden. IV. Epidemiological trends 1959—1978, *Acta Paediatr. Scand.,* 73, 433, 1984.

104. **Luterkort, M.,** The Natural History of Breech Pregnancy and its Consequences, Ph.D. thesis, University of Lund, Lund, Sweden, 1986.

105. **Schutte, M. F., Van Hemel, O. J., Van de Berg, C., and van de Pol, A.,** Perinatal mortality in breech presentations as compared to vertex presentations in singleton pregnancies: an analysis based upon 57,819 computer-registered pregnancies in the Netherlands, *Eur. J. Obstet. Gynecol. Reprod. Biol.,* 19, 391, 1985.

106. **Manzke, H.,** Morbidity among infants born in breech presentation, *J. Perinat. Med.,* 6, 127, 1978.

107. **Hambert, G. and Akesson, H. O.,** A sociopsychiatric follow-up study of 200 breech-born children, *Acta Psychiatr. Scand.,* 49, 264, 1973.

108. **Nilsson, S. T. and Bergsjo, P.,** Males born in breech presentation 18 years after birth, *Acta Obstet. Gynecol. Scand.,* 64, 323, 1985.

109. **Hohlweg-Majert, P. and Willard, M.,** Nach Untersuchungen der aus beckenendlage geborenen Kinder im Lebensalter von 3—7 Jahren auf ihre geistige und motorische Entwicklung, *Z. Geburtshilfe Perinatol.,* 179, 441, 1975.

110. **Neligan, G. A.,** The quality of the survivors of breech delivery in a geographically defined population, in *Perinatal Medicine,* Rooth, G. and Bratteby, L. E., Eds., Almqvist & Wiksell, Stockholm, 1976, 61.

111. **Bolte, A., Steinmann, H. W., Bensch, C. H., Putz, H. J., and Schraven, G. A.,** Kindliche Hirnschaden nach operativen Geburten, *Arch. Gynaekol.,* 205, 110, 1968.

112. **Fianu, S. T.,** Fetal mortality and morbidity following breech delivery, *Acta Obstet. Gynecol. Scand.,* 56, 1976.

113. **Muller, P. F., Campbell, H. E., Graham, W. E., Brittain, H., Fitzgerald, J. A., Hogan, M. A., Muller, B. H., and Rittenhouse, A. H.,** Perinatal factors and their relationship to mental retardation and other parameters of development, *Am. J. Obstet. Gynecol.,* 109, 1205, 1971.

114. **Sadowski, R. and Staemmler, H. J.,** Zum Einfluss der Beckenendlagengeburt auf die geistige und korperliche Entwicklung der Kinder, *Z. Geburtshilfe Perinatol.,* 178, 104, 1974.

115. **Hochuli, E., Dubler, O., Bornhauser, E., and Schoop, E.,** Die kindliche Entwicklung nach vaginaler und abdominaler Entbindung bei beckenendlagen, *Geburtshilfe Frauenheilk.,* 37, 4, 1977.

116. **Frenzel, J., Krause, W., Sander, I., and Michels, W.,** Early and late morbidity of underweight (LBW) newborn infants following breech presentation in relation to the mode of delivery, *Z. Geburtshilfe Perinatol.,* 188, 261, 1984.

117. **Cox, C., Kendall, A. C., and Hommers, M.,** Changed prognosis of breech-presenting low birthweight infants, *Br. J. Obstet. Gynaecol.,* 11, 881, 1982.

118. **Faber-Nijholt, R., Huisjes, H. J., Tonwen, B. C. L., and Fidler, V. J.,** Neurological follow-up of 281 children born in breech presentation: a controlled study, *Br. Med. J.,* 9, 286, 1983.

119. **Rosen, M. G., Debanne, S., Thompson, K., and Bilenker, R. N.,** Long-term neurological morbidity in breech and vertex births, *Am. J. Obstet. Gynecol.,* 151, 718, 1985.

Chapter 11

A CRITICAL ANALYSIS OF THE LONG-TERM SEQUELAE OF MIDCAVITY FORCEPS DELIVERY

Uma L. Verma

TABLE OF CONTENTS

I. INTRODUCTION

Current medical and medicolegal dogma maintain that birth trauma is largely responsible for long-term neurological handicap. The term "birth trauma" is loosely applied as a catchall diagnosis for asphyxial, metabolic, and mechanical factors, and long-term neurological handicaps include cerebral palsy, mental retardation, and seizures. The concept originated more than a century ago, when Little[1] described 47 children with a syndrome characterized by spastic rigidity, very similar to what we now term cerebral palsy. Little was convinced that the disorder was linked to difficulties surrounding the birth process.

Despite major changes in perinatal and neonatal practices which have resulted in significant reduction in perinatal mortality[2] and immediate neonatal morbidity,[3] the incidence of cerebral palsy and mental handicap has basically remained the same.[3-5] Forceps deliveries (in particular, midcavity forceps deliveries) have long been held accountable as a major factor in "birth trauma" and subsequent neurological sequelae.[6-9] The controversy surrounding this issue can only be settled by a well-controlled prospective study, which both the proponents[10,11] and opponents[6-9] of midcavity forceps deliveries agree is difficult, if not impossible, to execute because of moral, medical, and legal constraints. This chapter is not designed to take sides, but to critically evaluate the published reports so as to put the issue in its proper perspective.

Since the obstetric antecedents of long-term sequelae in the low birth weight neonates are a separate issue, they will be analyzed in a subsequent review.

II. MAGNITUDE OF THE PROBLEM

A summary of the report from the Task Force on Joint Assessment of Prenatal and Perinatal Factors Associated with Brain Disorders[12] gave the following estimates of the prevalence of neurological handicap. A total of 780,000 school-age children have mental retardation, another 750,000 Americans have cerebral palsy, and nearly 2,000,000 others have epilepsy. The estimates of the prevalence of the individual components of neurological sequelae in primary school children 7 to 10 years old are even more sobering:[13] (1) cerebral palsy in 2 per 1000, with 20 to 30% affected by severe mental retardation, 20 to 30% with mild mental retardation, and 30 to 40% with epilepsy; (2) severe mental retardation (IQ <50) in 4 per 1000, with <20% affected by cerebral palsy and 13% affected with epilepsy; (3) epilepsy in 5 in 1000, with 19% affected by cerebral palsy and 27% affected by mental retardation.

Paneth and Kiely,[5] commenting on the trends in frequency of cerebral palsy from a review of population studies in developed nations since 1950, concluded that cerebral palsy rates have not shown any evidence of decline in the last 30 years. There is some evidence[3] that there may be a slight increase in the incidence of cerebral palsy, mainly because of improved survival rates in the very low birth weight neonates. Important changes in obstetric practices occurring during these 30 years include an increase in the cesarean section delivery rate (from <5 to ≥25%) and a corresponding decrease in the forceps delivery rate (from >25% to <5%).[14] High forceps procedures are no longer done, and many centers have abandoned midcavity forceps deliveries altogether. If forceps deliveries played any significant role in the causation of neurological handicap, one would have anticipated a decline in the incidence of the sequelae, with the concurrent decrease in high and midcavity forceps deliveries, to <1% of all deliveries.[15] As previously discussed, the incidence of neurological sequelae has shown no change over this time.

III. NEUROPATHOLOGICAL CORRELATES

A. MECHANICAL TRAUMA

Traumatic lesions described in cases of difficult vaginal maneuvers, high and midcavity forceps deliveries, rotations, and extractions classically include neonatal skull fractures, subdural hematomas, and tentorial tears. These lesions have been documented during autopsies of neonates dying during or following difficult deliveries.[16] An excellent discussion of birth trauma associated with forceps deliveries is found in Munro Kerr's text on operative obstetrics, published in 1964.[17] More recently, O'Driscoll et al.[6] discussed the role of forceps in traumatic intracranial hemorrhage. Of a total of 36,420 primiparous births, 44 showed signs of intracranial hemorrhage at autopsy; 27 were cephalic presentations, and all were forceps deliveries. Analysis of these 27 cases showed that the occurrence of intracranial hemorrhage was independent of ease or difficulty of application, indications for the procedure, and the experience of the operator. These findings prompted the authors to recommend a radical reduction in the practice of forceps deliveries, to condemn the use of Kiellands forceps, and to liberalize the use of abdominal delivery. Of note is the fact that during the same period there were 9682 forceps births where the neonatal course was uneventful and where at least major injuries apparently did not occur.

Whether minor forms of these intracranial injuries are a cause of cerebral palsy and mental deficit in the survivors is open to conjecture, since no intracranial imaging techniques were available during the time period when complicated vaginal delivery was practiced more frequently. Certainly, if one substitutes clinical suspicion of neurological injury, then birth trauma associated with forceps deliveries may have been an important factor; however, the clinical basis for suspecting traumatic brain injury has included widely divergent neonatal conditions such as the need for resuscitation, neonatal oxygen therapy for reasons other than resuscitation, poor condition at birth, and abnormalities of respiration. Nevertheless, Eastman et al.[8] in 1962 examined the obstetric background of 753 cases of cerebral palsy and found that 50 of 474 mature neonates (10.5%) had been delivered by midcavity forceps, compared to 31 (4.9%) of the 634 historically normal controls.

B. NONTRAUMATIC BRAIN INJURY

Several important points must be stressed before describing the various lesions associated with neurological deficits.

1. The developing fetal and neonatal brain shows a complex sequence of events highlighted by cell proliferation, cell migration, differentiation, synapse formation, cell death, process alimentation, and myelination.[18] A variety of events, including hypoxia, infection, hemorrhage, and trauma, have the potential to alter the timely sequence of events and, therefore, produce functional deficits.
2. Irrespective of the precipitating event, the pathological lesions produced are the same. These may be loss of tissue due to necrosis, hemorrhage and infarction leading to atrophy and cyst formation, and varying combinations of disruption of either cell migration, dendritic formation, or myelinization.
3. The lesions seen at autopsy must be interpreted with care, keeping in mind the normal features of organogenesis and the nonspecific nature of the end results.

The pathological lesions found in autopsies of infants with cerebral palsy have consistently shown damage to the basal ganglia. Vogt and Vogt,[19] German neuropathologists, first described the relationship of basal ganglia lesions and cerebral palsy. Subsequently, Benda,[20] Towbin,[21] and Malamud et al.[22] all described similar findings, notably chronic scarring and cavitation in the basal ganglia and the surrounding white matter. Recent imaging techniques utilizing ultrasound[23-25] have also demonstrated the correlation of periventricular leucomalacia and the presence of cerebral palsy. However, neither the autopsy findings nor the radiological imaging techniques are specific as far as etiological factors are concerned. Identical lesions have been described with hypoxia, ischemia,[23,26] viral infection,[27] and endotoxemia.[28]

The brains of children with isolated mental retardation not due to genetic causes may be entirely normal, or they may be microcephalic but structurally normal. Recent studies by Purpura[29] have shown abnormalities of dendritic and synapse formation in the brains of children with mental retardation. However, similar findings[30] have also been described in the brains of animals who were environmentally deprived. There is no strong evidence that the abnormalities in the dendritic process seen in association with mental retardation are the cause of the handicap. It is quite conceivable that the environmental deprivation of the children with mental handicaps caused the dendritic abnormalities.

When mental retardation coexists with cerebral palsy, the brain lesions of scarring, fibrosis, and cavitation of the periventricular areas are more extensive and extend into the cerebral cortex and the sulci.[31]

IV. CLINICAL STUDIES

A. GENERAL CONSIDERATIONS

The potential for mechanical trauma with instrumental vaginal deliveries has been known and written about since the first description of forceps deliveries almost 300 years ago.[32] As a matter of fact, forceps were originally designed to affect delivery in the presence of pelvic obstruction. Since their first use, several reports have described serious maternal and fetal injuries resulting in maternal and fetal mortality and morbidity.[33-35] It has also been recognized that the more complicated the vaginal procedure, the greater the potential for trauma.[36] Additionally, the higher the station of the fetal head at which forceps are used, the higher the risk for malapplication and compression injuries of the fetal skull.[34,37,38] Therefore, there is good reason for abandoning high forceps deliveries and complicated rotational maneuvers. However, there is no evidence that all midforceps deliveries deserve the same condemnation, and the majority of authors maintain that there is still a place for a carefully executed midforceps vaginal birth.[11,15] The recent American College of Obstetricians and Gynecologists (ACOG) Committee on Obstetrics has very eloquently summarized the current thinking in their opening statement, which reads, "Controversy has surrounded the use of obstetric forceps since the 18th century and continues to the present. The apparently arbitrary nature of the various opinions and policies adopted by individuals and organizations through the years has contributed to the controversy and can be traced to a number of reasons, including inadequate definitions and studies with small sample size, improper matching and lack of proper controls."[39]

A major problem in evaluating the role of midforceps delivery in long-term neurological deficit has been to isolate the effects of the operative procedure from other confounding variables, the most important of which is the indication for the procedure. The importance of this point has been stressed by several authors and has yet to be resolved. An equally important issue is the commonality of the cerebral lesions seen with all varieties of prenatal, perinatal, and neonatal insults. In addition, similar brain lesions have been described following normal deliveries, forceps deliveries, and cesarean sections. Indeed, findings of peri- or intraventricular hemorrhage, other intracerebral hemorrhages, periventricular leucomalacia, and gliosis have been observed at autopsy in cases of antepartum stillbirth.[40] Since there is no unique lesion associated with forceps delivery per se, it has been impossible to define the role of forceps in the etiology of neurological deficit.

Several important points must be kept in mind during interpretation of the published data on long-term consequences of midforceps births.

Study design — The clinical reports describing the relationship between midforceps deliveries and long-term neurological deficit are either retrospective or prospective. With a few exceptions, the vast majority are retrospective, without controls, or with inadequate controls. The retrospective strategy, beginning at a defined outcome and tracing backward to earlier exposures, is useful in the study of rare diseases, and data can be collected rapidly and inexpensively. However, the temporal relationship of cause and effect is invariably obscured, especially if adequate controls are not selected. Prospective studies, also called cohort, follow-up, or longitudinal studies, begin with a single population divided into exposed and unexposed, both of which are longitudinally followed up for the development of adverse outcomes. The most important advantage of a cohort study is that it may provide a clearer temporal relationship between the exposure and outcome, reducing the problem of investigative bias. The main disadvantage is the potential for misinterpretation when a large segment of subjects is lost to follow-up. These considerations and the need for a large sample involve considerable financial and personal commitments. For the purposes of this discussion, all studies which start with abnormal neurological findings and work backward on obstetric and other antecedents will be defined as "retrospective", while all studies that start at delivery mode and then correlate this with sequelae will be termed "prospective". It should be emphasized that in many of these prospective studies the actual data collection was made retrospectively, often many years later from birth records.

Significant differences — The mere fact that the various groups are statistically significantly different does not necessarily imply clinical significance. For instance, when the sample size is sufficiently large, a very small difference may be statistically significant and yet be clinically meaningless. A good example is the three- to eight-point difference in intelligence quotients (IQs) seen between midcavity forceps delivery and spontaneous vaginal delivery in the National Collaborative Perinatal Project (NCPP) data.[41]

Significant correlations — The mere presence of a statistical correlation or association does not, cannot, and should not be interpreted as cause and effect. Cause and effect can only be defined by a prospective randomized, blinded, laboratory type of investigation, which is rarely possible when dealing with a complicated biological process such as birth.

Importance of confounding variables — Several reports have clearly shown that the level of mental performance as established by IQs of children is strongly correlated with socioeconomic status, maternal education, and race.[42-44] Therefore, it is mandatory that these variables be controlled for by stratification in any study which evaluates the role of midforceps and subsequent mental ability.

Selection of proper controls — A multitude of complications during pregnancy, labor, delivery, and the postnatal period have been shown to be associated with an increased risk of developmental and neurological handicap. Therefore, the control population must be appropriately selected if one must isolate the role of the forceps delivery from the complications which led to the performance of a forceps delivery. In view, however, of the multiplicity of known and unknown variables in the causation of sequelae, selection of a controlled population may be impossible.

Problems of follow-up losses, errors in data, and missing values — Investigators in this field are well aware of these frustrating sources of error and bias. The extensively used and quoted NCPP illustrates that these problems persist in spite of extensive organization and financial investment. The project consisted of 45,192 first-time enrollers.[41] During the index pregnancy, 4% of the subjects were lost; 15%[41] were lost by the first year of follow-up, 25% were lost by the fourth year of follow-up,[41] and almost 50% were lost by the seventh year of evaluation.[45] The data were entered into a computer immediately after collection, yet a computer search for possible erroneous labor data entry was identified in 33% of the NCPP population.[45] In spite of cases lost to follow-up and the problems associated with errors in data entry, there were 1745 and 2328 midforceps deliveries in primiparae and

TABLE 1
Frequency of Delivery Method in Various IQ Subgroups[47]

IQ subgroup	No.	SVD (%)	Forceps (%)	CS (%)	Other (%)
<50	117	92.3	4.3	2.6	0.9
>50, <64	189	93.1	2.1	3.2	1.6
≥65, <74	277	96	1.1	1.8	1.1
Control	69,693	93.7	3.8	2.2	0.2

Note: SVD — spontaneous vaginal delivery; CS — cesarean section; other — breech deliveries.

multiparae, respectively, in the definitive study group.[45] However, a statistical analysis of delivery variables and outcome could not be done for midcavity forceps deliveries because of insufficient numbers,[41,45] probably due to missing data.

B. RISK ASSESSMENT OF SPECIFIC STUDIES

One of the main goals of research is to assign risk of adverse outcome. A useful relationship is relative risk (RR), i.e., risk of disease in the exposed population relative to the risk in the control (unexposed, referent) population. An RR of less than one implies a protective effect, whereas an RR greater than one implies a deleterious effect. Besides the level of RR, its statistical significance must also be evaluated. Here, too, the sample size can produce clinically meaningless figures. It is possible to have a large RR which is not significant because of small sample size, the opposite effect being a small RR, which may be significantly different, where the sample size is too large.

C. SINGLE-CENTERED STUDIES

Fairweather[46] reported on the obstetric and social origins of mentally handicapped children. A total of 66 infants who had intelligence quotients of <75 and attended a special school were identified. Eight of them were either dead or lost to follow-up. The final group of 58 was compared to all births occurring in Aberdeen in 1948 for obstetric and social factors. The authors concluded that there were marked excesses of low birth weight births and adverse social factors in the backgrounds of infants with mental handicaps. The families were characterized by a high frequency of instability, poor socioeconomic status, and previous connections with special schools. The direct contribution of recognized obstetric complications to the total volume of mental handicap was small. Only one case of difficult forceps delivery was identified. However, the patient also exhibited preeclampsia, meconium-stained amniotic fluid, fetal distress, and deep transverse arrest.

Barker[47] investigated the association between low intelligence and obstetric complications by analyzing all children born in Birmingham, England between 1950 and 1954 and who lived in that city until the age of 5 years. Obstetric data had been recorded for all births, and visiting nurse records provided the subsequent histories. Exclusions were stillbirths, infant deaths prior to age 5, children lost to follow-up, and multiple births. The remaining study group comprised 73,687 infants, of whom 753 were noted to be mentally retarded. Of these children, 146 had identifiable causes for the deficit and were therefore also excluded, leaving 607 children in whom there was seemingly no cause for the low intelligence. The abnormal population was ascertained from public health agencies and schools for special children, and individuals were said to be subnormal based on an IQ of <75. The subnormal group was divided into three subgroups based on IQ, and these three groups were compared to the rest of the population for factors relating to pregnancy, labor, and delivery. Table 1 shows the relationship between IQ subgroup and mode of delivery. There was no excess of

TABLE 2
Frequency of Obstetrical Risk Factors in Various Groups[48]

Group	No.	Uncomplicated labor/delivery (%)	LBW %	IUGR (%)	Forceps %
Postnatal	24	75	12.5	8.3	8.3
MR — mild	112	68.5	2.8	10.2	10.2
MR — severe	35	74.3	17.1	8.6	2.9
Mongolism	71	85.7	17.1	11.4	1.4
MR and major anomalies	125	56.4	26.8	22.5	7
Controls	NA	NA	5.8	NA	4.7

Note: MR — mental retardation; LBW — low birth weight; IUGR — intrauterine growth retardation; NA — not available.

forceps deliveries in any of the IQ subgroups. The distribution of mode of delivery within each of these IQ subgroups was remarkably similar to the control population.

Barker also commented on 28 infants with low IQs who had "birth injury and/or asphyxia".[47] Both birth trauma and fetal distress were coded together, and it is impossible to separate the two. In 5 of these 28 cases there may have been trauma. All were either cases of breech presentation or precipitate labor. He concluded that recognized abnormalities of pregnancy and delivery seemed to play only a minor part in determining mental subnormality.

In 1968 Drillien[48] compared a group of 406 children who had IQs of <70 with historical controls obtained from the British Perinatal Mortality Survey for births occurring in 1958. The study group was divided into categories based on probable etiology as follows: (1) postnatal, (2) mild retardation of unknown origin, (3) severe retardation of unknown origin, (4) mongolism, and (5) mental retardation with other major anomalies. These subgroups were compared to the control population for factors pertaining to reproductive history, labor and delivery complications, low birth weight, intrauterine growth retardation, and forceps birth. The results are summarized in Table 2.

Important points which must be stressed are that 31% of the infants had major anomalies and that this group had markedly elevated incidences of labor complications, low birth weight, and intrauterine growth retardation. In addition, 29% of the infants with pure mental retardation also had minor developmental anomalies. The author commented, "In any attempt to assess the significance of obstetric factors in the etiology of mental handicap, an immediate difficulty arises from the fact that the same clinical picture may result from developmental malformation originating in early pregnancy; from adverse factors operating on a potentially normal central nervous system during later pregnancy and perinatal period; from environmental factors after birth; or from a combination of adverse factors operating at different times on infants who for other reasons may be predisposed to suffer damage. The presence of major developmental anomalies which must have arisen at an early stage of fetal life in almost 50% of cases with mental handicap suggests that the total picture is more likely to be due to an adverse event early in pregnancy."

The author concluded that obstetric factors are not implicated to any noticeable extent. The study shares the problems of retrospective design and inappropriate controls. However, it highlights the multifactorial nature of mental handicap.

Corston[49] compared the immediate and long-term consequences of high and midforceps deliveries to spontaneous vaginal deliveries occurring over a period from 1922 to 1936. Cases were identified from birth records. A total of 430 forceps births were compared to 500 spontaneously delivered controls who were selected randomly. The study and controls

TABLE 3
Frequency of Adverse Outcome According to Mode of
Delivery[49]

Group	Total no.	No. evaluated	SB (%)	Neonatal death (%)	Mean IQ
SVD	3711	76	5.7	2.8	115
Midforceps	323	73	8.3	5.8	124
High forceps	107	17	27	10	118

Note: SVD — spontaneous vaginal delivery; SB — stillbirth; IQ — intelligence quotient.

were 17 to 31 years old at the time of the follow-up evaluation. Only 90 of the forceps delivery cases and 76 of the control cases completed the study. Both groups underwent physical, neurological, and psychological testing. The results are shown in Table 3.

He concluded that if a baby survives the operative delivery then no physical or mental impairment is to be expected.

As previously defined this would qualify as a prospective study; however, the large numbers of cases lost to follow-up present a major problem. Additionally, data collected after the event from "birth records" are known to be inadequate even today.

Fuldner,[50] in a paper entitled "Labor Complications and Cerebral Palsy", presented information on 204 children with cerebral palsy institutionalized in a home for crippled children. The children were selected from a total number of 667 on the basis of unknown etiology and adequate birth records. The obstetric background was compared to a "control population" obtained from New York City data for births for the year 1948. His findings suggested that cerebral palsy was more frequent in males, premature infants, victims of antepartum hemorrhage or arrest of labor, breech deliveries, and cesarean section and forceps births. He concluded that prematurity and complications of labor are significant factors for the incidence of cerebral palsy. However, the retrospective nature of the study, with inappropriate controls and no statistical testing, makes this report questionable.

Steer and Bonney[51] described a series of 317 cases of cerebral palsy attending special clinics. Of these cases, 41 had other causes of cerebral palsy and the remaining 276 were labeled as "possible obstetrical etiology". The obstetric backgrounds of these cases were compared to "usual" incidences of sex, multiple births, prematurity, method of delivery, birth injury, asphyxia, maternal complications, and cesarean section. Their findings included a higher incidence of prematurity, twinning, and breech deliveries in the study group. They commented that "birth injury" was a catchall term which included both mechanical and hypoxic injury and that it was difficult to separate these two.

A retrospective study design and inadequate controls are evident in this study; their conclusions are intuitively, if not statistically, well founded.

Chefetz[52] commented on the role of reproductive insufficiency and the multiplicity of factors while investigating the etiology of cerebral palsy. The study patients were identified by enrollment in centers for crippled children and were compared to controls selected from births occurring directly before or after the index cases. Of 275 cases of cerebral palsy, 190 formed the study group after exclusions due to known causes of cerebral palsy and inadequate records. The control group was comprised of 260 "normal" infants (as determined by their personal physicians). The two groups were compared for presence of (1) "reproductive insufficiency", which was defined as infertility, prior fetal loss, and antepartum hemorrhage; (2) factors operating during labor; (3) type of delivery; and (4) condition at birth. The frequency of midforceps deliveries was not statistically different in the two groups.

Interestingly, the incidence of reproductive insufficiency was significantly higher in the obstetric background of the cerebral palsy group. Almost 80% of the study patients had at least one prenatal abnormality, compared to 30% of the controls. He concluded that the etiology of cerebral palsy is probably multifactorial and that it is unusual to find just one cause in any given case.

Forceps deliveries were not implicated. However, this retrospective case controlled study had 14 cases in the study and 7 in the control group. Therefore, conclusions regarding safety of forceps are somewhat questionable.

Amiel-Tison[53] reported a series of 41 neonates who were born in the years 1962 to 1964 and had neonatal seizures suggestive of cerebral damage. Of the 41, 25 were followed up for 2 to 5 years; 15 of the 25 were normal, 4 had mild disabilities, and 6 had moderate to severe deficits. In addition, four neonates died; one who had been delivered by elective cesarean section died within 48 h and exhibited subdural hematoma and multiple areas of leucomalacia at autopsy. The prenatal and intrapartum events were obtained by chart review. The author found that in 11 of 25 cases there was evidence of "obstetric trauma", as evidenced by dystocia, breech extraction, difficult forceps birth, difficult cesarean section, precipitate labor, cord accidents, and postmaturity. She concluded that "long-standing fetal distress, whatever its cause, leads to severe permanent damage. On the other hand, obstetric trauma, causing an acute but brief distress, may lead to brain damage from which complete recovery is possible, provided the baby does not have status epilepticus."

Extremely small numbers, a catchall definition of obstetric trauma, and the uncontrolled nature of the study are major problems. Additionally, this represents a selective group since cases were entered only if seizures occurred, thus not addressing the majority of cases of neurological sequelae which occur in the absence of neonatal seizures.

Dierker et al.[15] compared a group of 110 midcavity forceps births to a matched control group of cesarean births. Matching was done for indications for procedure, birth weight ± 200 g, gestational age ± 2 weeks, sex, and race. Obstetric information was obtained by chart review. By study design all infants had been followed up for at least 2 years. The infant information was obtained from charts and maternal interviews and was confirmed by managing pediatricians. There was no difference in the incidence of clinically apparent abnormal outcomes at this age. This study was performed prospectively, and it adequately controlled for major confounding variables. However, an interesting new problem is presented in this relatively recent report. The number of cases of midcavity forceps delivery performed has been reduced substantially; the cases seen today represent the "easy" midcavity forceps delivery. The authors recognized this fact and commented, "One cannot conclude from this study that midcavity forceps are safe. The operative procedure was infrequently used (0.8%) and generally from +2 station or lower. One might interpret this as selection of only the relatively "easy" midcavity forceps candidates."

D. MULTICENTRIC STUDIES

The NCPP[54] was undertaken from 1957 to 1965. The broad objectives of the study were "by means of prospective and retrospective approaches, with suitable controls, to:

1. Determine the relationship between factors in the perinatal environment and the continuum of human reproductive failure, with particular reference to the central nervous system for:
    a. Early manifestations of deficits (infancy and early childhood)
    b. Later manifestations of deficits (5 to 15 years).
2. Study the effect of the extra-uterine environment on infant development (e.g., family situation, socioeconomic factors).
3. Determine the relationship of prematurity to factors in the perinatal environment and

to the continuum of human reproductive failure, with particular reference to the central nervous system.

4. Determine the relationship between factors in the postnatal environment up to 15 years, and the development of neurological and sensory disorders.

5. Determine the relationship between genetic factors and continuum of human reproductive failure, with particular reference to the central nervous system.

6. Study clinico-pathological correlations in the continuum of human reproductive failure, with particular reference to the central nervous system.

7. Improve the classification, treatment, and prevention of cerebral palsy.''

A total of 55,908 pregnancies from 12 hospitals around the country were entered in the study. The sample was 45% white, 45% black, and 10% other ethnic groups. The mean socioeconomic status of the population was slightly lower than the general population of the U.S. For each patient-infant pair a set of 53 data sheets was completed and a massive data base generated. During the initial visit medical, obstetric, family, and socioeconomic histories were obtained. During subsequent visits the results of medical, obstetric, and laboratory examinations were noted. The course of labor and delivery was documented. Neonatal information was obtained from the labor and nursery records. After delivery a trained physician scrutinized the charts for documentation of all events.

The infants were examined at 1 year for the presence of malformations and neurological status. Follow-up examinations were conducted at 4 and 7 years and provided the basis for the diagnosis of neurological handicap.

The data base was computerized and was the source for a series of reports dealing with a variety of topics. Before analyzing the reports which describe the long-term consequences of midcavity forceps deliveries, it is important to discuss the data base and its usefulness in providing the information we are seeking. There is no doubt that the NCPP was a tremendous task and that its sample size is large enough that even rare conditions may be reliably studied. The information was prospectively generated before the outcomes were known so that adequate controls were available and no dependence was placed on patient or physician recall.

It must be remembered, however, that the project was initiated 30 years ago, and obstetric and neonatal practices have changed substantially during this time. The conclusions drawn from this considerable undertaking may well have lost their applicability today. Furthermore, even with this degree of effort there is the problem of patients lost to follow-up, amounting to 15, 25, and 50% at the end of the first, fourth, and seventh years, respectively. The possibility can be raised that the patients who had the follow-up examinations may have been self-selected because of the presence of disease or other factors. Equally important is the factor of missing data; for example, fetal presentation was not known in almost 2000 cases, birth weight was not available in 850 cases, and the mode of delivery was unknown in 1270 cases.[54] The problems with missing data may be fully appreciated given that Broman et al.[41] and Friedman and Neff[45] could not apply discriminate analysis for the relationship of midcavity forceps delivery to IQ because of inadequate numbers, when in fact there were more than 3000 mother-infant pairs at the end of the fourth and seventh years, respectively.

As in any observational study, the NCPP data generated associations between events during prenatal life and outcome, but cause and effect could not be established. In addition, similar outcomes can be produced by a variety of "events", making it absolutely important to control for these confounding variables.

Niswander[54] and Gordon reported on the total collaborative data at the end of the first year. The study population was divided into two groups based on the presence of definite neurological abnormalities at 1 year of age. The results are presented as rates per 1000 live

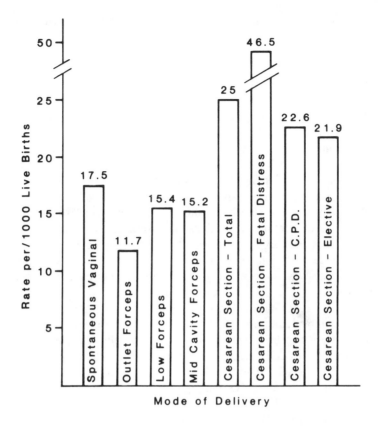

FIGURE 1. Effect of mode of delivery on prevalence of neurological abnormality at 1 year of age.[54]

births. The prevalence of neurological abnormalities under different labor circumstances is shown in Figure 1.

This figure shows that all types of forceps deliveries have a lower rate of resultant abnormality than spontaneous vaginal deliveries and cesarean sections. No statistical analysis was applied, and no effort was made to control for race, birth weight, socioeconomic status, and indications for the procedure and for all variables known to influence outcome. The authors appreciate the importance of confounding factors, and in their statement on type of delivery and outcome they state:

Examination of the data relating the use of forceps to fetal outcome produces results which require considerable care in their interpretation. The perinatal mortality rates for white and negro babies delivered by forceps are substantially less than for those delivered spontaneously. This diminution in the rates of forceps-delivered infants is consistent for stillbirths and for neonatal deaths. The low birthweight rate is higher for the babies delivered spontaneously than for any of the forceps groups, for both races. The mean birthweights show the same trend. There is a slight tendency for the neurologic abnormality rate to be highest for the spontaneously delivered babies.

The effects on the fetus of the use of forceps is a matter of debate in the medical profession. The wide variation in the use of this procedure suggests that the issue is, as yet, unresolved.

The fact of the matter is that the characteristics of the gravidas delivered by forceps differ considerably from those delivering spontaneously. The birthweight data indicate that the smaller babies, for example, are more frequently found in the no-forceps groups, which is logical. Gestational age, age of gravida, and parity differ between the forceps and no-forceps groups. Since all of these factors are known to have an effect on the outcomes of pregnancy, they must be considered in any assessment of the effects of the use of forceps. A detailed study including these and possibly other factors is required to determine the value to the fetus of delivery by outlet and elective low forceps delivery.[54]

The report is a factual presentation of the NCPP data, and no effort is made to reach conclusions.

Bishop et al.,[55] while discussing obstetric influences on the premature infant's first year of development, also based on NCPP data, described the results of the neurological and psychological examinations which showed that all classes of forceps deliveries were protective against the subsequent development of neurological and psychological abnormalities. This protective effect was seen in all birth weight subgroups. Their conclusion on the protective value of forceps delivery, particularly in the low birth weight neonates, influenced obstetrical practice extensively, and it has only been recently that some studies[56-58] have challenged this view. We feel the conclusions were invalid because the factor of race was not controlled. Forceps were used more frequently in the white population, which is known to have a lower incidence of long-term neurological abnormality. Additionally, the factor of socioeconomic status was not controlled. The influence of environment on outcome is a well-documented factor.

Friedman et al.,[59] reporting on long-term effects on infants of dysfunctional labor, selected 656 mother-infant pairs from the total NCPP population and presented information on the 3- to 4-year IQ and speech, hearing, and language results. The patients were stratified into labor patterns, mode of delivery, and labor plus mode of delivery groups and controlled for race and parity. The results showed that the infant delivered by midforceps after arrest of labor had a significantly lower IQ and significantly abnormal speech, language, and hearing results. The abnormalities with midforceps were independent of the labor pattern. There are several major problems with these conclusions.

The total NCPP midforceps group that came for the 4-year follow-up evaluation included over 3000 infants, but the author selected only 74. It is not possible based on these data to determine if these 74 cases were representative of the total group. In addition, a comparison has been made between midcavity forceps delivery cases and normal deliveries. A more appropriate control would have been cesarean section controlling for the indication for the procedure, particularly in the case of fetal distress. Another problem with this presentation is illustrated in Table 4. A comparison of the mean IQs of the various delivery groups in the total NCPP 4-year data and in this report shows basic differences in the control groups.

The table shows that the controls in Friedman et al.'s study had higher IQs than the controls in the total data base and that the cases of midcavity forceps delivery had lower IQs in this group compared to the total NCPP group. This degree of change in IQ is not explained by eliminating the low birth weight neonates, and it suggests that some other selection basis may have been introduced inadvertently. Most importantly, the authors did not control for the confounding variables shown in Table 5. These variables are seen to have a much greater effect on IQ differences than the decrease in IQ with midcavity forceps deliveries.

In a subsequent report, Friedman et al.[60] describe 680 patient-infant groups taken from the NCPP data base and evaluate the mean IQ at 4 years of age. This study is controlled for parity, birth weight, race, site of delivery, type of delivery, and labor pattern, and it is a matched pair analysis. However, the mean IQ in the midcavity forceps births is compared to that of spontaneous vaginal deliveries. The previous criticisms apply to this report as well; i.e., controls should have been other than spontaneous vaginal delivery cases so that indications such as fetal distress could be controlled. Additionally, socioeconomic status must be controlled. The importance of socioeconomic status and IQ in the context of mode of delivery is highlighted in Figure 2.

TABLE 4

**Mean 4-Year IQ According to Race, Mode of Delivery in
the NCPP Data Base,[41] and Data of Friedman et al.[59]**

	White			Black		
Group	No.	LBW	IQ	No.	LBW	IQ
NCPP						
SVD	4561		102.3	8696		91.1
		} 721			} 1718	
MCF	1420		106.1	662		92.1
Friedman						
Primiparous						
SVD	36		106.2	56		93.2
		} 0			} 0	
MCF	74		99.8	52		83.3
Multiparous						
SVD	44		102.8	99		94.8
		} 0			} 0	
MCF	20		99.7	13		85.8

Note: NCPP — National Collaborative Perinatal Project; SVD — spontaneous
vaginal delivery; MCF — midcavity forceps; LBW — low birth weight;
IQ — intelligence quotient.

TABLE 5

Difference in Mean IQs by Race for Different Confounding Variables[41]

	White		Black	
Variable	Mean	Difference	Mean	Difference
SES (I vs. III)	95.6—110.9	15.3	88.0—98.1	10.1
Education of mother (years) (<8 vs. college)	96.1—116.1	20.0	87.1—98.4	11.3
Maternal MR (yes vs. no)	92.4—104.8	12.4	85.2—91.4	6.2
No. prenatal visits (<5 vs. >14)	98.2—108.8	10.6	88.5—93.8	5.3
GA at registration (weeks) (<13 vs. >26)	108.9—100.5	8.4	93.1—89.7	3.4
GA at delivery (weeks) (<28 vs. >37)	95.3—105.0	9.7	81.5—91.8	10.3
SVD vs. MCF	102.3—106.1	3.8	91.1—92.1	1

Note: SES — socioeconomic status; MR — mental retardation; GA — gestational age; SVD — spontaneous
vaginal delivery; MCF — midcavity forceps.

In a book titled "Labor and Delivery: Impact on Offspring", Friedman and Neff[45]
updated the total NCPP data and utilized extensive statistical evaluation and manipulation
to assign a role for labor and delivery variables including midcavity forceps and long-term
deleterious effects. This time the controls (or the referent group) were outlet forceps cases,
which (as seen from previous figures) have shown the highest IQ at 4 years of any group.
They go further and classify low forceps deliveries as midcavity forceps deliveries, and in
comparing them to outlet forceps they conclude that they too are hazardous. The confounding
effect of socioeconomic status is not examined, and evaluation of these findings is therefore
difficult. Valid conclusions from this study are that (1) difficult midcavity forceps cases
have the potential for serious consequences, (2) the more difficult the forceps delivery the
greater the hazard to the newborn, and (3) rotations are also hazardous. Additionally, for
the first time this report provides information relating to the indications for the forceps
delivery. This report clearly shows that forceps deliveries done for fetal distress, arrest, or
cephalopelvic disproportion have worse outcomes than spontaneous vaginal or elective for-

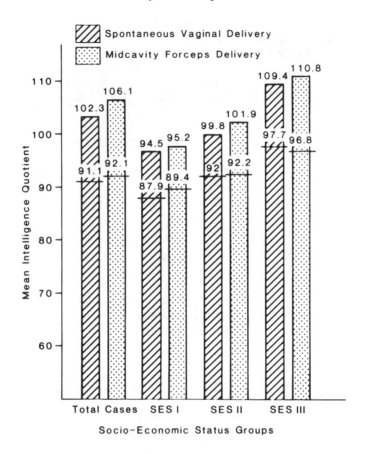

FIGURE 2.   Effects of mode of delivery, socioeconomic status, and race on IQ at 4 years of age.[41] Transverse bars indicate IQ in blacks.

ceps deliveries, thus emphasizing that indications for the procedure must be controlled for before valid conclusions may be made.

Broman et al.[41] describe the 4-year IQs of offspring of NCPP patients. The cohort from which the 4-year sample was drawn consisted of 37,945 live-born single births to white or black mothers registering for the first time. The sample consisted of 26,760 children who came for the 4-year evaluation. Of the 11,185 children excluded, 9.6% were dead and 88.1% missed the exam, and in the remainder the IQs could not be determined. The sample, cohort, and total population did not differ in any of the demographic or neonatal characteristics.

Each child was administered the Stanford-Binet Intelligence Scale as close to his/her fourth birthday as possible. The IQ scores were first correlated with 169 selected demographic, genetic, obstetric, pediatric, neurological, and psychological variables. Three of these variables — race, sex, and socioeconomic status — were strongly associated with IQ and were therefore used for stratification so as to reduce the "error" variance in the relationship of other factors to IQ. Second, a forward stepwise multiple regressive technique was used to assess the effect of all variables which were significantly associated with IQ in the first step of the analysis. Finally, the ability of predictors to discriminate between children with low and normal IQs was examined by discriminant function analysis.

Results from this extensive analysis failed to reveal deleterious effects of midcavity forceps deliveries when examined via univariate analysis. Stepwise multiple regression initially showed that forceps delivery was associated with higher IQ in the white population. However, this effect was not seen when controlled for socioeconomic status and parity.

Finally, the only factors which discriminated between low and normal IQ were maternal education, socioeconomic status, birth weight, and neonatal brain abnormality. Mode of delivery had little power to discriminate between low and normal IQ.

This report has examined at length the determinants of mental performance; it has shown that labor and delivery have very little to do with mental development and that apart from major central nervous system (CNS) malformations the social environment in which the child grows probably plays a most important role.

In 1977, Nelson and Broman[61] examined the relationship between severe motor and mental handicap and perinatal factors in a sample of 38,260 patients enrolled in the NCPP. At 7 years of age, 64 infants had IQs below 50 and moderate or severe motor deficits. Additionally, 26 children with handicaps noted at 1 year who had died prior to their seventh birthday were also studied; i.e., 1 in 575 liveborns who lived at least 1 year were studied and compared to the rest of the NCPP children. Of the 90 children with severe handicaps, 40 had other causes of disability, including meningitis, trauma, CNS malformations, and metabolic chromosomal and other syndromes, leaving 50 cases without discernible causes. A total of 133 antecedent variables were examined, initially by univariate analysis and later by linear discriminant analysis, to identify independent discriminators. The variables tested included 27 prenatal, 33 antenatal, 26 labor and delivery, and 47 neonatal characteristics. None of the prenatal or antenatal variables, four of the labor variables, and seven neonatal variables were significantly different on univariate analysis. The handicapped group had significantly higher incidences of fetal distress, forceps deliveries, arrest of labor, and small placenta. Additionally, the handicapped group had significantly different Apgar scores, gestational age, birth weight, and evidence of respiratory insufficiency.

When the data was subjected to discriminate analysis, eight antecedents emerged as significant factors. All except one (namely, midforceps delivery) were neonatal. The most significant discriminators were intracranial hemorrhage and neonatal seizures. The eight-variable linear discriminant function correctly classified only 30% of the handicapped group; i.e., 70% of the cases could not be identified by the presence of these antecedents. The authors concluded, "It is impressive that in the present study so few maternal risk factors could be identified for so grave an outcome."[61]

The study is a retrospective analysis of the NCPP data and suggests that midforceps births are associated with neurological deficits. The strength of the association, however, is somewhat limited, with neonatal factors showing stronger associations. In addition, the handicapped group also had evidence of fetal distress and arrest of labor, both factors known to be deleterious in themselves.

Nelson and Ellenberg[62-64] have three major reports generated from the NCPP data base that are designed to assess obstetric complications as risk factors for the development of cerebral palsy. Of the 51,285 singleton live births in the data base, outcome at 7 years was known for 45,559. A total of 189 children had cerebral palsy, and 323 had seizures. The first report[62] describes the role of pregnancy, labor, and delivery variables as risk factors for the subsequent development of cerebral palsy and nonfebrile seizure disorders. The concept of relative risk as a measure of forward risk assessment was used to predict the development of adverse outcome in the exposed vs. the nonexposed populations. They further evaluated the obstetric variables and various subsets of Apgar scores to see if the predictive value for adverse outcome was enhanced. They found that one or more obstetric complications was present in more than 60% of the pregnancies and was not associated with increased risk of cerebral palsy unless Apgar score was also depressed. In addition, low birth weight was a dominant factor for both mortality and long-term deficits, especially in breech delivery, which was the only complication in which the rate of cerebral palsy significantly exceeded the cerebral palsy rate in uncomplicated pregnancies. For infants with birth weights >2500 g, none of the pregnancy and labor variables, including midforceps deliveries, were associated with a cerebral palsy risk in excess of the rate in uncomplicated pregnancies. Finally, none of the obstetric complications evaluated separately or jointly were associated with increased risk of nonfebrile seizure disorder. They concluded that in infants weighing >2500 g, the group of children with one or more risk factors and a depressed 5-min Apgar score (1.5% of the population) accounted for 17% of deaths and 13% of cerebral palsy cases — 11 times as many infant deaths and 8 times as much cerebral palsy incidence as in the control population. In contrast, the group of infants weighing >2500 g with one or more risk factors and Apgar scores of >6 at 5 min did not show an increased rate of cerebral palsy.

The second report, entitled "Antecedents of Cerebral Palsy",[63] describes a univariate analysis of risk for 400 maternal characteristics of the prenatal, antenatal, and perinatal periods. The findings revealed a relatively large increase in cerebral palsy rates in association with maternal mental retardation, seizure disorders, and hyperthyroidism, as well as with the use of thyroid hormones and estrogens during pregnancy. Midforceps delivery was one of several factors not associated with an increased risk of cerebral palsy.

The final report of Nelson and Ellenberg[64] utilized a multivariate analysis of risk of cerebral palsy. Prenatal and perinatal factors related to cerebral palsy on univariate analysis, described in the second report, were examined by multivariate techniques. All potential risk factors were entered into a stepwise multiple regressive analysis so as to define the most suitable variables for entry into the logistic regression analysis, which was the final step in the analytical procedure. The results may be summarized as follows. Maternal mental retardation, low birth weight, and fetal malformations were the leading predictors of cerebral palsy; breech presentation (but not breech delivery) was also a predictor. A third of the children with cerebral palsy who presented as breech had major non-CNS malformations. Of the 189 infants with cerebral palsy, 40 had clinical evidence suggestive of asphyxia; only 17 of the 40 were free of major congenital defects that might have contributed to the deficits. Of the cases of cerebral palsy, 34% could have been predicted correctly prior to the onset of labor. The addition of risk factors present during labor, delivery, and the neonatal periods increased the prediction minimally, to 37%. Two important conclusions were made by the authors: "First, if we do not know the cause or causes of most cerebral palsy, or if the causes are numerous or onset very early in development and no one cause contributes too much of the outcome, then no foreseeable single intervention is likely to prevent a large proportion of cerebral palsy. Second, information about events during labor, delivery and the newborn period did not identify a substantially larger number of cases than information limited to major characteristics determined before labor began. These results suggest a relatively small role for factors of labor and delivery in accounting for cerebral palsy in this population. The data further suggest that an association of birth events with poor neurologic outcome may sometimes be misleading, since in a substantial proportion of cases the outcome may have been related partly or wholly to defects intrinsic to the fetus."[64]

The conclusions reached by the authors succinctly describe the state of current thinking concerning the relationship between obstetric factors and long-term neurological deficits. These remarks are also an excellent summary of the contributions which the NCPP data base has provided concerning the determinants of long-term childhood disability.

Besides the studies generated by the NCPP, the only other report of a multicentric study comes from Australia. McBride et al.[65] examined the impact of delivery method on developmental outcome of the infant at 5 years of age. The births occurred in the 4-year period from 1970 to 1974. Obstetric information was recorded prospectively, as was maternal IQ and socioeconomic status. Patients were selected so as to control for complications of pregnancy and for low birth weight. Socioeconomic status was controlled for by selecting only English-speaking patients. The infants were tested between 4 and 5 years of age for physical skills, motor skills, and IQ. The modes of delivery investigated were low forceps delivery (188 infants), midcavity forceps delivery (51 infants), forceps rotation with forceps delivery (57 infants), manual rotation with forceps delivery (67 infants), elective cesarean section (101 infants), and spontaneous vaginal delivery (control, 207 infants). Breech presentation (100 infants) was compared separately to the vertex presentation groups.

The six vertex groups were subjected to analysis of variance, covariance, stepwise regression analysis, and chi-square tests. A p value of <0.01 was accepted as significant. There were no statistically significant differences in physical and motor skills in the various vertex delivery groups. Analysis of IQ scores revealed significant differences, children with complicated deliveries having higher IQs than those with spontaneous vaginal deliveries. However, when family background variables were taken into account, this difference no longer existed. Results of a stepwise multiple linear regression indicated that family background variables were the most important predictors of intellectual ability in the offspring. Perinatal factors and delivery method did not contribute significantly to intellectual ability.

This was a well-controlled prospective study, and the conclusions reached were similar to those described by Nelson and co-workers[61-64] from the NCPP data base.

V. SUMMARY AND CONCLUSIONS

Pertinent studies of the past 30 years concerning the long-term consequences of midcavity forceps deliveries have been reviewed and their strengths and weakness stressed. The concensus of the majority of the studies is that the probable etiology of long-term neurological handicap is multifactorial, that events prior to and during early pregnancy have more to do with the deficits than labor and delivery, that the association between midforceps deliveries and long-term deficit cannot be separated from the confounding effects of indications for the forceps, and that environmental factors are extremely important. An in-depth analysis of the major reports does not support the statements that midforceps are an anachronism and that all midforceps are hazardous. It is the general concensus that difficult midcavity rotations and extractions are better forgotten; however, there is still a place for selected midcavity forceps delivery in modern obstetric practice.

An equally important message from this analysis is the importance of study design, of appropriate controls, and the need to adequately evaluate the role of confounding variables. Clinical and, particularly, observational studies may often lack these aspects, in which case interpretation should be guarded. There are, unfortunately, many examples of obstetric practices being influenced by over-interpreted data. The premature death of midcavity forceps delivery threatens to go this route.

REFERENCES

1. **Little, W. J.,** On the influence of abnormal parturition, difficult labors, premature birth, and asphyxia neonatorum on the mental and physical condition of the child, especially in relation to deformities, *Trans. Obstet. Soc. London,* 2, 293, 1862.
2. HEW, From Facts of Life and Death, Publ. No. 79-1222, U.S. Department of Health, Education, and Welfare, Washington, D.C., 1979, 8.
3. **Stanley, F. J. and Watson, L.,** The cerebral palsies in Western Australia: trends, 1968 to 1981, *Am. J. Obstet. Gynecol.,* 138, 89, 1988.
4. **Jarvis, N., Holloway, J. S., and Hey, E. N.,** Increase in cerebral palsy in normal birthweight babies, *Arch. Dis. Child.,* 60, 1113, 1985.
5. **Paneth, N. and Kiely, J.,** The frequency of cerebral palsy: a review of population studies in industrialised nations since 1950, in *The Epidemiology of the Cerebral Palsies,* Clin. Dev. Med., No. 87, Stanley, F. and Alberman, E., Eds., Lippincott, New York, 1984, chap. 6.
6. **O'Driscoll, K., Meagher, D., MacDonald, D., and Geoghegan, F.,** Traumatic intracranial haemorrhage in firstborn infants and delivery with obstetric forceps, *Br. J. Obstet. Gynaecol.,* 88, 577, 1981.

7. **Friedman, E. A.,** Midforceps delivery: no?, *Clin. Obstet. Gynecol.,* 30, 93, 1987.
8. **Eastman, N. J., Kohl, S. G., Maisel, J. E., and Kavaler, F.,** The obstetrical background of 753 cases of cerebral palsy, *Obstet. Gynecol. Surv.,* 17, 459, 1962.
9. Midforceps delivery: is it an anachronism?, *Contemp. Obstet. Gynecol.,* 15, 82, 1980.
10. **Hayashi, R. H.,** Midforceps delivery: yes?, *Clin. Obstet. Gynecol.,* 30, 90, 1987.
11. **Richardson, D. A., Evans, M. I., and Cibils, L. A.,** Midforceps delivery: a critical review, *Am. J. Obstet. Gynecol.,* 145, 621, 1983.
12. Summary of the Report from the Task Force on Joint Assessment of Prenatal and Perinatal Factors Associated with Brain Disorders, What causes mental retardation and cerebral palsy?, *Pediatr. Neurosci.,* 12, 175, 1986.
13. **Susser, M., Hauser, W. A., Kiely, J. L., Paneth, N., and Stein, Z.,** Quantitative estimates of prenatal and perinatal risk factors for perinatal mortality, cerebral palsy, mental retardation and epilepsy, in Prenatal and Perinatal Factors Associated with Brain Disorders, NIH Publ. No. 85-1149, U.S. Department of Health and Human Services, Washington, D.C., 1985, 53.
14. The national experience: complication-specific changes in cesarean delivery rates — an analysis of data from the Commission on Professional and Hospital Activities, in Cesarean Childbirth, NIH Publ. No., 82-2067, U.S. Department of Health and Human Services, Washington, D.C., 1981, 119.
15. **Dierker, L. J., Rosen, M. G., Thompson, K., and Lynn, P.,** Midforceps deliveries: long-term outcome of infants, *Am. J. Obstet. Gynecol.,* 154, 764, 1986.
16. **Towbin, A.,** Central nervous system damage in the human fetus and newborn infant, *Am. J. Dis. Child.,* 119, 529, 1970.
17. **Kerr, M.,** Injuries to the brain, spinal cord and peripheral nerves, in *Operative Obstetrics,* 8th ed., Moir, J. C. and Myerscough, P. R., Eds., Balliere Tindall, London, 1971, 934.
18. **Giles, F. H. and Green, B. E.,** Neuropathologic indicators of abnormal development, in Prenatal and Perinatal Factors Associated with Brain Disorders, NIH Publ. No. 85-1149, U.S. Department of Health and Human Services, Washington, D.C., 1985, 53.
19. **Vogt, C. and Vogt, A.,** Zur Lehre der Erkrankungen des striaren Systems, *J. Psychiatr. Neurol.,* 25, 627, 1920.
20. **Benda, C. E.,** *Development Disorders of Mentation and Cerebral Palsies,* Grune & Stratton, New York, 1952.
21. **Towbin, A.,** Cerebral intraventricular hemorrhage and subependymal matrix infarction in the fetus and premature newborn, *Am. J. Pathol.,* 52, 121, 1968.
22. **Malamud, N., Itabsi, H. H., Castor, J., et al.,** An etiologic and diagnostic study of cerebral palsy, *J. Pediatr.,* 65, 270, 1964.
23. **Slovis, T. L., Shandaran, S., Bedard, M. P., and Poland, R. L.,** Intracranial hemorrhage in the hypoxic-ischemic infant: ultrasound demonstration of unusual complications, *Radiology,* 151, 163, 1984.
24. **Trounce, J. Q., Fagan, D., and Levene, M. I.,** Intraventricular haemorrhage and periventricular leucomalacia: ultrasound and autopsy correlation, *Arch. Dis. Child.,* 61, 1203, 1986.
25. **Weindling, A. M., Rochefort, M. J., Calvert, S. A., Fok, T.-F., and Wilkinson, A.,** Development of cerebral palsy after ultrasonographic detection of periventricular cysts in the newborn, *Dev. Med. Child Neurol.,* 27, 800, 1985.
26. **Pape, K. E. and Wigglesworth, J. S.,** *Haemorrhage, Ischaemia and the Perinatal Brain,* Lippincott, New York, 1979.
27. **Seay, A. R. and Griffin, D. E.,** Effects of viral infections on the developing nervous system, in *Progress in Perinatal Neurology,* Vol. 1, Korobkin, R. and Guillerminault, C., Eds., Williams & Wilkins, Baltimore, 1981, chap. 5.
28. **Faix, R. G. and Donn, S. M.,** Association of septic shock caused by early-onset Group B streptococcal sepsis and periventricular leukomalacia in the preterm infant, *Pediatrics,* 76, 415, 1985.
29. **Purpura, D. P.,** Dendritic spine dysgenesis and mental retardation, *Science,* 186, 1126, 1974.
30. **Colemen, P. D. and Riesen, A. H.,** Environmental effects on cortical dendritic fields. I. Rearing in the dark, *J. Anat.,* 102, 363, 1968.
31. **Towbin, A.,** Obstetric malpractice litigation: the pathologist's view, *Am. J. Obstet. Gynecol.,* 155, 927, 1986.
32. **Laufe, L. E.,** The ancients, the evolution of obstetric forceps, in *Obstetric Forceps,* Harper & Row, New York, 1968, chap. 1.
33. **Finechel, G. M., Webster, D. L., and Wong, W. K. T.,** Intracranial hemorrhage in the term newborn, *Arch. Neurol.,* 41, 30, 1984.
34. **Chiswick, M. L. and James, D. K.,** Kielland's forceps: association with neonatal morbidity and mortality, *Br. Med. J.,* 1, 7, 1979.
35. **Cyr, R. M., Usher, R. H., and McLean, F. H.,** Changing patterns of birth asphyxia and trauma over 20 years, *Am. J. Obstet. Gynecol.,* 148, 490, 1984.
36. **Cook, W. A. R.,** Evaluation of the midforceps operation, *Am. J. Obstet. Gynecol.,* 99, 327, 1967.

37. **Bowes, W. A. and Bowes, C.,** Current role of the midforceps operation, *Clin. Obstet. Gynecol.,* 23, 549, 1980.
38. **Taylor, E. S.,** Can mid-forceps operations be eliminated?, *Obstet. Gynecol.,* 2, 302, 1953.
39. Obstetric Forceps, ACOG Comm. Opinion No. 59, American College of Obstetrics and Gynecology, Washington, D.C., 1981.
40. **Sims, M. E., Turkel, S. B., Halterman, G., and Paul, R. H.,** Brain injury and intrauterine death, *Am. J. Obstet. Gynecol.,* 151, 721, 1985.
41. **Broman, S. H., Nichols, P. L., and Kennedy, W. A.,** *Preschool IQ: Prenatal and Early Development Correlates,* L. Eelbaum, Hillsdale, NJ, 1975.
42. **Lesser, G. S., Fifer, G., and Clark, D. H.,** Mental abilities of children from different social-class and cultural groups, *Monogr. Soc. Res. Child Dev.,* 4(102), 30, 1965.
43. **Honzik, M. P.,** Development studies of parent-child resemblance in intelligence, *Child Dev.,* 28, 215, 1957.
44. **Kennedy, W. A., VanDeRiet, V., and White, J. C.,** A normative sample of intelligence achievement of Negro elementary school children in the southeastern United States, *Monogr. Soc. Res. Child Dev.,* 6(90), 28, 1963.
45. **Friedman, E. A. and Neff, R. K.,** *Labor and Delivery: Impact on Offspring,* PSG Publishing, Littleton, MA, 1987.
46. **Fairweather, D. V. I.,** Obstetric and social origins of mentally handicapped children, *Br. J. Prev. Soc. Med.,* 14, 149, 1960.
47. **Barker, D. J. P.,** Low intelligence and obstetric complications, *Br. J. Prev. Soc. Med.,* 20, 15, 1966.
48. **Drillien, C. M.,** Studies in mental handicap, *Arch. Dis. Child.,* 43, 283, 1968.
49. **Corston, J. M.,** The end results in children delivered by mid or high forceps, *Am. J. Obstet. Gynecol.,* 67, 263, 1954.
50. **Fuldner, R. V.,** Labor complications and cerebral palsy, *Am. J. Obstet. Gynecol.,* 74, 159, 1957.
51. **Steer, C. M. and Bonney, W.,** Obstetric factors in cerebral palsy, *Am. J. Obstet. Gynecol.,* 83, 526, 1962.
52. **Chefetz, M. D.,** Etiology of cerebral palsy, *Obstet. Gynecol.,* 25, 635, 1965.
53. **Amiel-Tison, C.,** Cerebral damage in full-term newborn aetiological factors, neonatal status and long-term follow-up, *Biol. Neonate,* 14, 234, 1969.
54. **Niswander, K.R. and Gordon, M.,** The women and their pregnancies, in The Collaborative Perinatal Study of the National Institute of Neurological Diseases and Stroke, DHEW Publ. No. 73-379, U.S. Department of Health, Education, and Welfare, Washington, D.C., 1972.
55. **Bishop, E. H., Israel, S. L., and Briscoe, C. C.,** Obstetric influences on the premature infant's first year of development, *Obstet. Gynecol.,* 26, 628, 1965.
56. **Schwartz, D. B., Miodovnik, M., and Lavin, J. P.,** Neonatal outcome among low birth weight infants delivered spontaneously or by low forceps, *Obstet. Gynecol.,* 62, 283, 1983.
57. **Barrett, J. M., Boehm, F. H., and Vaughn, W. K.,** The effect of type of delivery on neonatal outcome in singleton infants of birth weight of 1,000 g or less, *JAMA,* 250, 625, 1983.
58. **Tejani, N., Verma, U. L., Hameed, C., and Chayen, B.,** Method and route of delivery in the low birth weight vertex presentation correlated with early periventricular/intraventricular hemorrhage, *Obstet. Gynecol.,* 69, 1, 1987.
59. **Friedman, E. A., Sachtleben, M. R., and Bresky, P. A.,** Dysfunctional labor. XII. Long-term effects on infant, *Am. J. Obstet. Gynecol.,* 127, 779, 1977.
60. **Friedman, E. A., Sachtleben-Murray, M. R., Dahrouge, B. A., and Neff, R. K.,** Long-term effects of labor and delivery on offspring: a matched-pair analysis, *Am. J. Obstet. Gynecol.,* 150, 941, 1984.
61. **Nelson, K. B. and Broman, S. H.,** Perinatal risk factors in children with serious motor and mental handicaps, *Ann. Neurol.,* 2, 371, 1977.
62. **Nelson, K. B. and Ellenberg, J. H.,** Obstetric complications as risk factors for cerebral palsy or seizure disorders, *JAMA,* 251, 1843, 1984.
63. **Nelson, K. B. and Ellenberg, J. H.,** Antecedents of cerebral palsy. I. Univariate analysis of risks, *Am. J. Dis. Child.,* 139, 1031, 1985.
64. **Nelson, K. B. and Ellenberg, J. H.,** Antecedents of cerebral palsy, *N. Engl. J. Med.,* 315, 81, 1986.
65. **McBride, W. G., Black, B. P., Brown, C. J., Dolby, R. M., Murray, A. D., and Thomas, D. B.,** Method of delivery and developmental outcome at five years of age, *Med. J. Aust.,* 1, 301, 1979.

Chapter 12

OBSTETRICAL ANTECEDENTS OF PERIVENTRICULAR/ INTRAVENTRICULAR HEMORRHAGE AND PERIVENTRICULAR LEUCOMALACIA: LONG-TERM SEQUELAE

Eric Garfinkel and Uma L. Verma

TABLE OF CONTENTS

I. INTRODUCTION

The magnitude of the contribution of low birth weight (LBW) to neonatal mortality[1-5] and long-term neurological handicap[6-8] has been documented repeatedly. Compared to the normal birth weight neonate, LBW neonates are 40 times more likely to die[4] and 3 times more likely to survive with neurodevelopmental handicaps.[8] The risk for mortality and handicap increases in the lower birth weight subsets. Over the last 20 years there has been a rapid decline in neonatal mortality, mainly due to increased survival in all weight subsets of LBW neonates including those with birth weights <1000 g.[9,10] The increased survival rate of the very small neonate has generated concern regarding the possibility of an increase in the incidence and severity of neurological handicap.[11-14] Some recent reviews have concluded that the prevalence of neurological handicap among graduates of neonatal intensive care nurseries appears to be decreasing,[9] while others have shown an increase in the incidence and severity of handicap, especially in the lowest birth weight survivors.[15-19] The logical solution to this problem would be prevention of preterm birth. However, recent efforts to decrease the overall incidence of preterm birth by emphasis on early diagnosis and the use of tocolytic agents have been shown to be unsuccessful.[20] Extraordinary emphasis is being placed on the intrapartum management of labor and delivery of these tiny neonates in the somewhat simplistic belief that this may improve outcome.

With the introduction of routine bedside transfontanelle cranial ultrasonography, the definition of periventricular/intraventricular hemorrhage (PV/IVH) became clear. It was evident that this type of bleeding was common, affecting up to 50% by some reports, and it was assumed that this finding would be predictive of long-term neurological sequelae. However, with time this correlation proved tenuous, especially for Grades I and II and even with more severe grades of hemorrhage.[21,22] The definition of periventricular leucomalacia (PVL), seen on ultrasound imaging, has been described more recently. Its incidence in the LBW neonates has not yet been fully assessed; however, recent reports suggest a better correlation with long-term outcome.[22,23]

The failure to detect anatomical lesions by the currently available imaging techniques does not rule out functional impairment. Newer imaging techniques for greater anatomical detail and better assessment of functional integrity may reveal a different correlation and predictive power. Prediction of the neonate at risk for neurological sequelae by recognition of anatomical or functional abnormalities on imaging would eliminate uncertainty for patients and their physicians. Additionally, it would allow a more definite end point in researching the antecedents of neurodevelopmental impairment.

II. PATHOGENESIS

PV/IVH and PVL are the two most common findings at autopsies in premature neonates. Although it has been customary to describe them as separate entities, it is likely that they are both manifestations of hemodynamic instability in the immature developing brain. Pape and Wigglesworth[24] and Ment et al.[25] suggest that PV/IVH and PVL are the result of interaction of (1) the vascular anatomy of the immature brain, (2) the susceptibility of the blood brain barrier, and (3) failure in autoregulation of cerebral blood flow. However, both groups have based their hypotheses on the assumption that factors which control cerebral blood flow and maintain the integrity of the blood brain barrier in the perinatal period are similar to those found in adults. There is little information on whether this is a valid premise. Despite this assumption, the hypothesis provides a starting point for future studies and a possible basis for clinical applications.

PV/IVH occurs in the germinal matrix, a specialized, highly vascular area present only in the premature brain, almost disappearing by the 34th week of gestation. The germinal matrix occurs in a layered fashion around the ventricular system just external to the delicate ependyma. However, its thickest and most vascular cap lies between the head and body of the caudate nucleus and the lateral ventricles. It consists of layers of immature precursors of neurons and glial cells which migrate centrifugally to their definitive locations in the brain. Migration is virtually complete in the human fetus by the 26th week of gestation, leaving the fragile capillary bed of the germinal matrix poorly supported and, therefore, vulnerable to rupture. Hyperperfusion, irrespective of etiology, would increase the risk of hemorrhage, and hypoperfusion would increase the risk of ischemic neurosis. In addition, the area is rich in fibrinolytic substances which would tend to increase the size and spread of the hemorrhage.

Metabolic factors known to increase cerebral blood flow, such as hypoxia, hypercarbia, and acidosis, frequently occur in the perinatal period of LBW neonates. Additionally, autoregulation in these neonates may be impaired, resulting in a pressure-passive situation contributing to both hyperperfusion and hemorrhage or to both hypoperfusion and ischemia.[26] These problems have been well substantiated clinically in neonates with idiopathic respiratory distress syndrome.[26] Although the same metabolic imbalance may occur in the intrapartum period, a correlation with outcome is unclear. Even less clear is whether these situations play a role in the antepartum period.

Recent reports state that PVL may occur in as many as 20% of all preterm babies.[27] The location of these lesions in the periventricular white matter is anatomically determined by the boundary zone between the centripedal and centrifugal arteries of the developing brain.[24] The proximity of the zone to the ventricles places it in jeopardy for hypoperfusion and ischemia in the neonates who develop PV/IVH. Additionally, in the premature brain these boundary zones are vulnerable to ischemic damage from hypotension in the presence of defective autoregulation. PVL may appear on sonography as a shining hyperechoic area described as a flare which may regress, persist, or later show cystic change. The latter two situations represent permanent tissue damage and would be expected to correlate with long-term sequelae.

Several other factors have been shown to correlate with PV/IVH and PVL. Hyperosmolar states and cerebral edema may compromise the integrity of the blood brain barrier. A significant and possibly important correlate that may be operative in all phases of the perinatal period is infection. Intrauterine infection, even in the presence of intact membranes, is probably a frequent cause of preterm labor.[28-30] Its association with PVL has recently been observed,[31] suggesting that at least some of these lesions are initiated in the antepartum period.

III. OBSTETRICAL CORRELATES OF PERIVENTRICULAR/ INTRAVENTRICULAR HEMORRHAGE AND PERIVENTRICULAR LEUCOMALACIA

The majority of reports describing risk factors for PV/IVH and PVL have dealt with neonatal factors, with very little analysis of antepartum or intrapartum events. With few exceptions, all are retrospective, have small numbers, and differ in study populations. Premature (and perhaps unwarranted) speculations and conclusions based on these reports need to be critically examined. From these studies, certain clinically relevant obstetric factors have been shown to correlate with PV/IVH; these will be discussed. To our knowledge, only one study[31] dealing with obstetric correlates of PVL has been published, and it will be discussed.

A. FETAL OR NEONATAL TRANSPORT

There is convincing evidence that *in utero* transport has a significantly better immediate and long-term neonatal outcome than neonatal transport.[32-34] Older reports did not specifically address the issue of PV/IVH as the outcome. Recent reports have documented a decreased incidence of PV/IVH in inborn compared to outborn neonates.[32,33] In addition, there are data showing that the earlier in labor the patient is transferred, the better the neonatal outcome.[34] It is therefore critical for the obstetrician to identify the pregnant patients at risk for premature delivery and make arrangements for care to be delivered at a facility with a Level III neonatal intensive care unit. Several screening protocols for patients at risk for preterm birth have been explored and shown to be effective in identifying the parturiant at risk.[35] However, it must also be stressed that the etiology of preterm labor is multifactorial, with different risk factors acting in different populations, so that no one single protocol can be universally effective. However, certain factors such as prior preterm delivery, multiple gestations, and maternal medical disorders are universally applicable.

Education of the patient on the symptoms of preterm labor and home monitoring of uterine activity in patients at risk for premature labor are increasingly being utilized with some success, but the data are still preliminary. In addition, this approach is probably impractical and logistically impossible in inner-city populations, which have the highest incidence of preterm births.

B. ROLE OF LABOR

The impression that premature neonates who were delivered prior to the onset of labor because of severe maternal disease have a lower incidence of PV/IVH was first suggested by Bejar et al.[36] in 1981. None of the neonates delivered without labor developed major PV/IVH, compared to 20% of the neonates delivered after the onset of labor. They hypothesized that labor seems to be important in the pathogenesis of large hemorrhages. Similar findings have been reported by Barrett et al.[37] and most recently by Tejani et al.[38] Although the three studies have similar conclusions, they are retrospective, have small numbers, and the birth weight and gestational age ranges are too wide, resulting in a questionable control population.

The pathophysiological basis for labor predisposing a fetus to PV/IVH is unknown. Novy[39] monitored fetal blood pressure in the pregnant primate model and showed that each uterine contraction resulted in increased mean blood pressure, which presumably in the presence of impaired autoregulation would result in waves of increased cerebral blood flow.

Although the concensus of opinion holds that PV/IVH and PVL are the end results of the vulnerability of the preterm brain to fluctuations of cerebral blood flow initiated by neonatal hemodynamic instability, an alternative hypothesis suggested by Tejani et al.[38] merits further testing. The authors, commenting on their findings of the absence of PV/IVH in neonates delivered prior to labor and on the findings of antepartum initiation of PV/IVH described by Bejar,[36] hypothesized that an "event" in the antepartum period may be responsible for both the onset of preterm labor and for the PV/IVH. The findings of PV/IVH and PVL in stillbirths[40] and in the antenatal period indirectly support this hypothesis.

The concept that brain injury may have been initiated in the antepartum (rather than the intrapartum) period is further suggested by Bardeguez et al.'s[41] recent study on cord blood creatinine phosphokinase brain band isoenzymes. The authors found that neonates destined to develop PV/IVH had markedly elevated levels of this enzyme, indicating neuronal and neuroglial injury prior to the development of PV/IVH and in the absence of intrapartum markers of hypoxia.

C. ROLE OF CHORIOAMNIONITIS

Another interesting aspect of premature labor is its association with silent and overt intra-amniotic infection[28-30] and failed tocolysis.[42] A recent report by Bejar et al.[31] has documented the development of PVL immediately after birth in neonates with possible chorioamnionitis. The authors feel that the origins of the PVL are in the antepartum period and suggest the possible role of intrauterine sepsis.

This concept is further supported by the findings of the National Collaborative Perinatal Project (NCPP),[7] which showed that one of few factors significantly associated with a higher risk for development of cerebral palsy was chorioamnionitis. The findings are, however, preliminary and need to be further documented.

D. ROLE OF INTRAPARTUM HYPOXIA

Hypoxia, hypercarbia, and acidosis are known to increase cerebral blood flow. These factors are known to be operative during labor; however, in the retrospective studies that were published, there was no observed correlation between fetal heart rate changes suggestive of hypoxia and PV/IVH.[38,43] Additionally, there was no correlation between umbilical arterial pH, pCO_2, or base excess and PV/IVH.[38,44] While fetal hypoxia/acidosis should be avoided, there appear to be no ill effects associated with the fluctuations in acid-base status within the normal range, as seen in labor. One may conclude from this and the preceding discussions that once spontaneous labor has occurred there is no advantage to delivery by cesarean section, except for accepted obstetric indications.

E. ROUTE AND MODE OF DELIVERY

No other aspect of preterm birth has received as much attention as the route and mode of delivery. However, as yet the best method of delivery remains to be determined. Arbitrary opinions, often based on poorly documented retrospective studies, have recommended abdominal delivery for all LBW neonates, especially those in the subset <1500 g birth weight, as least traumatic for the neonate.[45,46] Others, however, have questioned the wisdom of this aggressive approach and are recommending cesarean section only for accepted obstetric indications.[47-50] The subsequent discussion will be limited to cephalic presentations, since malpresentations (breech in particular) are a different issue and have been adequately dealt with elsewhere in this book.

Prior to diagnostic imaging of the perinatal brain, the clinical diagnosis of PV/IVH was understandably limited to severe cases with classical signs of intracranial bleeding. The majority of earlier studies used autopsy material for elucidating the diagnosis of both PV/IVH and PVL. Therefore, the earlier studies are not suitable for any reliable evaluation of antecedent risk factors and will not be discussed.

The suggestion that the mode of delivery may influence long-term outcome of the LBW neonate was first made by Bishop et al.[51] while commenting on the 1-year outcome of infants enrolled in the NCPP. The report suggested that the preterm neonates delivered by forceps had higher intelligence quotients (IQs) compared to spontaneous vaginal delivery cases. The authors recommended prophylactic forceps in preterm births to protect the soft, pliable skull and its contents. The recommendations were adopted quickly without adequate analysis of the findings. A critical review of the NCPP data showed that forceps deliveries were more common in whites and in socioeconomically advantaged populations and that these two factors have a marked influence on IQ and therefore must be controlled.[52] The authors' conclusions were, therefore, premature and probably invalid. Recent reports, although retrospective, have shown that forceps deliveries offer no advantage for survival,[37,53] PV/IVH,[47] or long-term outcome.[53]

Clark et al.[33] analyzed risk factors for PV/IVH in 63 neonates with birth weights of <1250 g. PV/IVH (as diagnosed by computerized axial tomography [CT] scan) was present in 19 neonates. There was no correlation between route of delivery and the development of PV/IVH. The only factor associated with an increased risk of PV/IVH was birth outside the perinatal center. Levene et al.[32] studied 146 neonates at <34 weeks gestation by real-time ultrasound and evaluated 32 risk factors, including route of delivery; they concluded that, except for site of birth, obstetric factors did not appear to influence the risk of PV/IVH.

Kitchen et al.,[54] reporting on the Australian Collaborative Project, evaluated survival and long-term outcome in 166 neonates with gestational age <29 weeks born in the years 1977 to 1978 where brain imaging techniques had not been used. The route of delivery did not significantly influence the incidence of handicap in the survivors. Not unexpectedly, long-term survival increased and the incidence of major handicap decreased with advancing gestational age. The authors updated their data in 1985 with a report on 326 neonates, the later part of the study including diagnostic imaging.[50] Obstetric factors independently associated with improved outcome were gestational age, absence of hypertension, singleton pregnancy, and the use of maternal steroids. The slight advantage with cesarean section delivery disappeared when confounding obstetric variables were controlled. There was no association between route of delivery and frequency of handicap in the survivors. The authors concluded that there was little evidence from mortality or morbidity data to support routine delivery of infants of borderline viability by cesarean section.

Barrett et al.[37] retrospectively analyzed the relationship between mode of delivery and neonatal outcome in 109 singleton neonates weighing <1000 g at birth. The study failed to reveal any association between route of delivery and mortality/morbidity. The only significant factor was the association of spontaneous labor with PV/IVH. The frequency of PV/IVH was not influenced by route of delivery.

Worthington et al.[55] analyzed factors influencing survival and morbidity of 214 consecutive neonates weighing <1500 g at birth. Neither survival nor PV/IVH was influenced by the route of delivery. The authors questioned the current trend of liberalized cesarean section for the very low birth weight neonate.

Tejani et al.[38] analyzed obstetric factors associated with early PV/IVH diagnosed by sonography within 24 h of birth. They found that fetal heart rate (FHR) patterns, umbilical acid base, and route of delivery did not influence early PV/IVH. However, infants delivered prior to the onset of labor were significantly less likely to develop PV/IVH. In 1987 the authors[47] updated their material, this time reporting on the association between route and mode of delivery in the LBW vertex presentation and PV/IVH. No correlation was evident between route or mode of delivery and the development of early PV/IVH.

Bada et al.[56] evaluated the relative risk of obstetric factors for early and late PV/IVH in 155 inborn neonates weighing <1500 g. Early PV/IVH identified within 24 h of life was seen in 55% of cases, and late hemorrhages occurred in another 24%. None of the obstetric factors analyzed, including the presence of labor, presentation, and route of delivery, appeared to increase the risk of early or late PV/IVH.

Morales and Koerten[48] determined the effects of obstetric management on PV/IVH in 488 very low birth weight neonates. The authors' conclusions reflect the current consensus of opinion and a summary statement for the role of route of delivery and PV/IVH. ''While the pathogenesis of intraventricular hemorrhage in the very-low-birth-weight infant is likely to be multifactorial, its occurrence is inversely related to gestational age and birth weight. Hence, all efforts to prolong intrauterine life through aggressive tocolysis and expectant management of premature rupture of membranes should be used.'' In addition, the authors recommend the antenatal use of corticosteroids in gestations between 28 and 33 weeks to enhance lung maturation and decrease the incidence of one of the contributing factors in the etiology of intraventricular hemorrhage.

When faced with the unavoidable delivery of a low birth weight infant, we conclude that for cephalic presentations a carefully monitored vaginal delivery may be allowed. The monitoring systems should include FHR as well as acid-base monitoring. Cesarean section is indicated for obstetric reasons and not for prematurity alone. Where spontaneous labor has not occurred and delivery is indicated, as in some cases of preterm premature rupture of membranes and maternal disorders, policy is yet unclear. It is not known if induced labor holds the same association with PV/IVH as spontaneous labor. For these cases at this time, the choice between elective cesarean section and induction of labor is governed by the obstetric situation.

F. PHARMACOLOGICAL APPROACHES

Steroids — About one third of preterm births occur in patients without any risk factors. In addition, preterm births will occur in spite of the availability of tocolytic drugs. Since one of the major correlates of PV/IVH and PVL appears to be the presence and the severity of RDS and its complications, the use of steroids must be considered. There is sufficient evidence in the literature showing the efficacy of steroids in enhancing lung maturity and some evidence suggesting a decreased incidence of PV/IVH. Clark et al.[33] prospectively analyzed 25 risk factors for PV/IVH in 63 newborns weighing <1250 g. The only factor which correlated with PV/IVH was birth outside the center. The groups of inborn and outborn infants were comparable from obstetric, neonatal, and asphyxial points of view. There was, however, a significant difference in the frequency of therapeutic intervention between the two groups. Prenatal administration of glucocorticoids was used more frequently in the inborn group. Additionally, if PV/IVH did occur, it was usually limited to Grade I hemorrhages. Similar findings of decreased incidence and severity of PV/IVH with antenatal steroids have been independently reported by Kitchen et al.[50] and Morales and Koerten.[48]

Barbiturates — Shankaran et al.[57] recently reported a prospective randomized study of maternal phenobarbital administration for the prevention of neonatal PVH/IVH. A total of 46 women were randomly assigned to control or study groups. The study group received 500 mg of phenobarbital intravenously 5 to 8 h prior to delivery. Although the total incidence of PV/IVH was not significantly different in the two groups, the incidence of moderate and severe hemorrhages was higher in the control group. The major problems with the study were the very small numbers and the fact that the control group received alkali therapy more frequently. Additionally, the control group had a higher incidence of PV/IVH than was reported by other groups. The possible protective action of barbiturates in the prevention of PV/IVH is not understood well, even though its benefits in the treatment of birth asphyxia, seizures, and meningitis are well established. The possible mechanism for the neuroprotective effects may be decreased cerebral metabolic needs or elimination of the hypertensive peaks produced by neonatal activity and therapeutic procedures.

G. SUMMARY AND CONCLUSIONS

In summary, the low birth weight infant is best delivered in a center with a state-of-the-art neonatal intensive care unit. Spontaneous labor is associated with PV/IVH, although not causative of it, and this suggests that antepartum injury may cause both preterm labor and PV/IVH. This is further substantiated by finding PVL and some other old standing brain injury immediately after birth both on imaging and autopsy. Once labor ensues, cesarean section (except for obstetric reasons) provides no advantage over monitored vaginal delivery. The role of chorioamnionitis in the causation of PVL needs further documentation. Pharmacological agents, such as maternal administration of steroids and barbiturates, require larger and better-controlled prospective studies before any conclusions may be made.

IV. BRAIN IMAGING IN THE NEONATE

Prediction of developmental disability based on imaging of the neonatal brain is a new and promising technology. There are limitations to our ability to accurately predict developmental outcome, mainly due to the inability of earlier equipment to accurately image the full spectrum of perinatal brain injury. PV/IVH was easily recognized very early, whereas the diagnosis of PVL has only recently been made possible.

Several excellent review articles and monograms have documented the value of the CT scan[58-60] and ultrasound[58,61] in providing accurate, reliable, and reproducible anatomical details of the normal and injured perinatal brain. Both provide excellent anatomical details of ventricular and periventricular hemorrhages. Ultrasound appears to be superior to the CT scan for the early manifestations of periventricular ischemia, especially in the premature brain, where hypodense areas normally may be seen in the absence of ischemic necrosis.[58] The later manifestations of ischemia with cystic PVL can be identified easily by both modalities. It must be emphasized that the timing of the brain imaging for PVL is critical since these lesions evolve later than PV/IVH. Of the two modalities, ultrasound is better suited to the neonatal intensive care situation, as it is portable, relatively inexpensive, noninvasive, and does not involve radiation exposure. Most importantly, it provides imaging without disturbing the sick neonate. The main shortcoming of both ultrasound and the CT scan is their capability of providing an anatomical diagnosis which does not always conform to functional deficits.

The technology for noninvasive, cribside diagnosis of PV/IVH and ventricular dilatation (VD) was developed in the mid-1970s. These conditions were generally classified according to the system devised by Papile et al.[60] Grade I hemorrhage is defined as bleeding into the subependymal germinal matrix. Grade II refers to extravasation of blood into the lateral ventricles, which remain normal in size. Grade III denotes a hemorrhage with accompanying dilatation of the ventricles, and grade IV is described as intraventricular hemorrhage with extension of the hemorrhage into the cerebral parenchyma.

It later became evident that VD frequently occurs in the low birth weight, preterm neonate in the absence of observable hemorrhage.[63-65] These cases could then be followed and their outcomes compared with those of VD occurring with periventricular or intraventricular hemorrhage.

The refinements of ultrasound apparatus and techniques necessary for imaging of PVL were developed in the mid-1980s. With this technological advance it became clear that a small but clinically significant proportion of cases previously described as having hemorrhage and/or dilatation manifest leucomalacia as well.[66,67]

There are two main stages of PVL. The first stage is seen as a flare of increased echodensity representing infarction, typically extending from the subependymal region into the substance of the white matter. This finding may regress or persist as an echodensity. If it persists for more than 2 weeks it may be termed the persistent flare type of PVL.[27] In other cases the central area of density liquifies, leaving one or more cavity visible on ultrasound. These are referred to as cavitary or cystic leucomalacia. These cysts may persist or be reabsorbed. Reabsorption is often associated with mild compensatory VD.[68,69]

V. NEWER IMAGING TECHNIQUES

Recent improvements have facilitated the use of nuclear magnetic resonance (NMR) for diagnostic imaging in medicine. NMR currently provides two modalities for evaluating structure and function, namely, NMR imaging and *in vivo* nuclear magnetic resonance spectroscopy (NMRS) for monitoring of high-energy phosphorus metabolism. The initial results of NMR imaging of the central nervous system promise both greater anatomical detail and physiological data, particularly on myelination. Recently, McArdle et al. have used NMR in neonates and have described developmental features of the neonatal brain with normal patterns of gray-white matter differentiation and myelination,[70] ventricular size, and anatomy of the extra cerebral space.[71] Additionally, the authors have provided data on the of NMR for the diagnosis of PV/IVH[72] and PVL.[73] Several other reports have also the feasibility of using NMR in the neonatal situation.[74-76]

The second application of NMR is spectroscopic (NMRS) investigation of cerebral energy metabolism.[77] Preliminary studies using NMRS in normal neonates and in neonates with asphyxia, PV/IVH, or PVL have provided valuable biochemical information.[77] However, the results are preliminary, and much more data on the normal and abnormal neonatal brain is needed in order to establish normal ranges for gestational age and to determine cerebral energy metabolism changes under pathological situations.

VI. NEONATAL CEREBRAL BLOOD FLOW MEASUREMENTS

The central role of cerebral blood flow (CBF) in the pathogenesis of PV/IVH and PVL emphasizes the need for accurate, reliable, and noninvasive methods of evaluating CBF during the neonatal period. Jugular venous plethyesmography,[78,133] xenon clearance,[79] and positron emission tomography[80] have all been investigated for this purpose, but have not been found to be universally applicable in the neonatal situation. The usefulness and applicability of Doppler blood flow velocimetry in neonates was initially described by Bada et al.[81] and, more recently, by Perlman et al.[82] The findings of Perlman and associates on the relationship of fluctuating flow through the anterior cerebral arteries and the development and prevention of PV/IVH with the use of pancurare are exciting, but they need to be substantiated further.

VII. LONG-TERM OUTCOME OF PERIVENTRICULAR/ INTRAVENTRICULAR HEMORRHAGE AND PERIVENTRICULAR LEUCOMALACIA

Having considered obstetric antecedents of PV/IVH and PVL and having briefly surveyed imaging techniques, we will now summarize the long-term outcome in neonates with PV/ IVH and PVL. Most of the outcome studies of PV/IVH and VD published to date do not account for the effects of PVL; this confounds interpretation of their findings. However, by examining the data across studies, we are able to make some preliminary prognostic formulations concerning the effects of each of these disorders as they occur in isolation and in combination with each other.

Two other complications in the interpretation of data across different outcome studies of hemorrhage, dilation, and leucomalacia are the lack of comparability of different outcome measures used by different researchers and the failure of some researchers to include adequate control groups. Operational definitions of developmental disabilities vary widely across studies, making generalizations regarding the true incidence of sequelae difficult.[83] When adequately matched control groups are not employed, it becomes impossible to differentiate the effects of a specific brain injury from those otherwise associated with prematurity and its complications.

Despite these complications, we are able to extrapolate some preliminary prognostic information from the relevant follow-up literature. We begin with a discussion of the sequelae of isolated PV/IVH. This is followed by consideration of the sequelae to cerebroventricular dilatation in the preterm neonate, with and without concurrent hemorrhage. Finally, we will summarize the most recent research on PVL and make some tentative inferences concerning the interface of the sequelae described for leucomalacia with those described for hemorrhage and dilatation.

Grades I and II PV/IVH seem to be relatively benign. While mild developmental disabilities do occur with relative frequency in this population, they do not seem to be attributable to or specifically predicted by isolated subependymal or intraventricular hemorrhage.

Studies which have failed to include control groups have sometimes falsely attributed sequelae to isolated hemorrhages. Where adequate control groups have been used, the relatively benign nature of isolated PV/IVH has generally been apparent. An example may be illustrative.

Papile et al.[84] followed 51 subjects with grades I and II PV/IVH and 115 comparable preterm control subjects. Major developmental disabilities were seen in 10% of both the clinical (grades I and II PV/IVH) and control groups. Minor disabilities were found in 41% of the clinical group and in 41% of the control group. Multiple handicaps were present in 4% of the clinical group and in 6% of the control group. Therefore, the difficulties observed in these children could not be attributed to the isolated hemorrhage per se and were most likely due to other factors associated with prematurity and its complications. Other studies using adequate control groups have supported this finding.[85-88] At this point, it is not clear to what extent PVL may play a role in these problems. However, it is established that an isolated finding of periventricular hemorrhage does not suggest increased developmental risk for preterm newborns.

There is evidence of a specific pattern of developmental risk associated with VD whether or not hemorrhage is present. The finding of VD indicates a markedly increased risk of focal neuromuscular dysfunction and a slightly increased risk of mental developmental delay and developmental language disorder.[85-88]

Garfinkel et al.[88] diagnosed focal neuromuscular disorders in 67% of low birth weight, preterm infants surviving grade III or IV PV/IVH (vs. 14% of matched control subjects) and in 63% of infants with isolated VD (vs. 13% of control subjects). Upon repeat evaluation at 30 to 48 months of age, 30% of subjects with a history of grade III and IV PV/IVH and 83% of those having shown dilatation in the absence of hemorrhage continued to display disorders of motor function and of muscle tone. There were no longer any serious and persisting motor disabilities present in the matched control groups.

The typical site of neuromuscular affectation following VD is in the lower extremities. Pape and Wigglesworth[24] explain that the major corticospinal tracts innervating the lower extremities are closer to the ventricles than those innervating the upper extremities. In most cases the dysfunction is relatively mild (i.e., hypertonicity or mild spastic diparesis). By early childhood most of these children are walking, although many will have an awkward gait and will require physical therapy and/or orthopedic support.

Mental development seems to be mildly affected in some cases of VD; however, severe mental retardation is not the characteristic outcome of this neuropathology. In our own research we found mental developmental delays (Bayley Mental Developmental Index <70) in 27% of infants with grade III or IV hemorrhage (vs. 7% of control subjects) and 12% of infants exhibiting VD without hemorrhage (vs. zero control subjects). By early childhood, mental delays (McCarthy General Cognitive Index <70) were evident in 15% of children who had grade III or IV hemorrhage (vs. zero controls) and in 33% of those exhibiting VD without hemorrhage (vs. zero controls). VD is indicative of an increased risk of mental developmental delay. However, this is to a much lesser extent than is the predisposition to focal neuromuscular disturbance. Mental retardation in the absence of neuromuscular impairment is rarely found in cases of VD. In most cases the developmental delays observed are of a borderline to mild degree of mental retardation. Severe retardation is the exception in this group. Therefore, while VD increases the probability of mild intellectual deficit to some extent, the characteristic outcome of the lesion remains motor disability.[88]

A third common sequelae to VD is a mild specific language delay during early childhood. This was found in 44% of our clinical sample and in 10% of controls.[88] Clinical experience suggests that most of these specific language difficulties will resolve within a few years, particularly as the children enter school. However, continued longitudinal research is needed to ascertain whether these early language difficulties persist or resolve and whether other specific learning disabilities emerge as the children are faced with more complex academic tasks.

Overall, the typical 3-year-old child with a history of neonatal VD, with or without hemorrhage, is walking (although a disturbance of gait is common), talking (possibly with some immaturity of speech or language), and functioning within grossly normal limits of intelligence.

Although the statistics reported above have been taken from our own research, similar findings concerning the sequelae of grades III and IV PV/IVH have been reported by others.[60,84-87,89,91] Most studies have neither identified nor followed neonatal VD separately from hemorrhage. However, our data are consistent with that of Vaucher et al.[65] in suggesting that the pattern of disabilities found in this group is very similar to that found with hemorrhage plus dilatation.

In most groups of survivors of PV/IVH and/or VD there are a few severely disabled children who do not fit the pattern described above. It is hypothesized that these severe disabilities result from neuropathologies other than simple hemorrhage or dilatation. In some cases, these more severe sequelae may be the result of cystic PVL. In addition, persistent noncystic PVL may account for some of the milder disabilities seen in preterm infants with or without PV/IVH as well.

McMenamin et al.[92] screened 460 preterm neonates with birth weights of <2250 g. PV/IVH was found in 39%, and 34% of those with hemorrhage also displayed intraparenchymal echodensity.

Of the latter infants, 52% had large echodensities extending into major portions of the frontal and parietal lobes, and 48% had small echodensities extending only a few millimeters into the parenchymal white matter. Mortality rates for infants with large and small intraparenchymal echodensities varied dramatically. Of the infants born at <1000 g, 94% with large echodensities and 38% with small echodensities expired. Of the infants born at 1000 to 1250 g, 53% of those with large echodensities and 26% of those with small echodensities expired.

All survivors of large intraparenchymal echodensities developed cystic lesions. Only 13% of those who survived small echodensities developed cysts. Large echodensities typically occurred in the presence of VD, and small echodensities were more often found with hemorrhage in the absence of dilatation.

All infants surviving large intraparenchymal echodensities developed significant neurological deficits; 63% of these were severe and 37% were moderately severe. Of those surviving small echodensities, there were no severe deficits; 9% had moderate deficits and 27% had mild ones. In cases of moderate to severe disability, both mental retardation and cerebral palsy were usually present. The most common form of cerebral palsy was spastic quadraparesis, as opposed to diparesis, which is typical of VD in general.[92]

Bozynski et al.[93] report essentially similar data. Of 100 infants born at <1200 g and surviving the neonatal period, 5 developed cystic PVL. Of these, three had both hemorrhage and dilatation and two had isolated dilatation with leucomalacia. One infant expired 1 month following discharge. The other four were all developmentally disabled; three (75%) had severe multiple disabilities and one (25%) had moderate spastic diparesis.

Weindling et al.[69] diagnosed PV/IVH in 46% of 102 neonates weighing <2000 g at birth. Status with regard to VD was not specified. Of those with hemorrhage, 15% developed cystic PVL, and there was one case of cystic leucomalacia in the absence of hemorrhage. All children with cavitary PVL developed cerebral palsy (five spastic quadraparesis and three spastic diparesis), six of eight had visual problems (all had squinting and four had hypermetria), and all had developmental delays (four borderline to mild and four moderate to severe).

The data from the above studies suggest that a small but clinically significant subgroup of infants surviving PV/IVH and VD may also have some form of PVL. Cystic leucomalacia tends to occur with VD (with or without hemorrhage), while noncystic echodensities tend to occur with hemorrhage in the absence of dilatation. Cavitary leucomalacia seems to be almost invariably associated with moderate to severe disabilities, and the modal outcome is multiple disability affecting motoric, mental, and visual function, in that order of severity. Noncavitary leucomalacia seems to result in milder problems, along the lines of those seen with VD.

Graham et al.[23] present data challenging the notion that all periventricular cysts lead to cerebral palsy. They have found that the number and location of cysts may be important factors in the prediction of outcome. Their data suggest that single cysts in front of the anterior horn of the lateral ventricle or in the area of the corona radiata adjacent to the body of the lateral ventricle may only be associated with mild cerebral palsy, and this occurs only in about 20% of cases. Multiple cysts and/or cysts in the region of the occipital horn of the lateral ventricle were associated with moderate to severe disability in 87% of cases. While these data are based on a rather small sample, they do highlight the importance of considering the size and location of cystic lesions in studying the outcome of PVL.

Overall, an isolated finding of PV/IVH in the absence of dilatation or leucomalacia is generally benign. VD is associated with an increased risk of mild to moderate motor developmental problems, particularly those affecting the lower extremities, and with a slight increase in the probability of borderline to mild mental retardation and developmental language delay. More severe problems are occasionally seen with PVH and/or VD, and further study is needed to determine to what extent PVL plays a role in these cases.

Cystic PVL is a more ominous finding associated with high mortality and morbidity. Moderate to severe neurodevelopmental sequelae would be expected in survivors. Most will have multiple handicaps with cerebral palsy and mental retardation. Concerning cerebral palsy, spastic quadraparesis is more common in this group than spastic diparesis. Borderline to profound mental developmental delays may be found. In addition, cavitary leucomalacia may be associated with problems of the visual system, particularly when the lesions occur in the region of the occipital horn of the lateral ventricle. Noncystic leucomalacia is associated with a better prognosis; the majority of these infants may be spared functional disability. When sequelae are seen with noncystic leucomalacia, they are relatively mild, primarily affecting motoric function.

In future clinical and research applications, it will be important to continue ultrasound screening of the preterm neonate for at least 3 to 6 weeks to take into account cavitary leucomalacia when studying or predicting outcome.[93]

REFERENCES

1. **Susser, M., Marolla, F. A., and Fleiss, J.,** Birth weight, fetal age and perinatal mortality, *Am. J. Epidemiol.,* 96, 197, 1972.
2. **Abramowicz, M. and Kass, E. H.,** Pathogenesis and prognosis of prematurity, *N. Engl. J. Med.,* 275, 878, 1966.
3. **Lee, K., Paneth, N., Gartner, L. M., and Pearlman, M.,** The very low-birth-weight rate: principal predictor of neonatal mortality in industrialized populations, *J. Pediatr.,* 97, 759, 1980.
4. **Shapiro, S., McCormick, M. C., Starfield, B. H., Krischer, J. P., and Bross, D.,** Relevance of correlates of infant deaths for significant morbidity at 1 year of age, *Am. J. Obstet. Gynecol.,* 136, 363, 1980.
5. **Koops, B. L., Morgan, L. J., and Battaglia, F. C.,** Neonatal mortality risk in relation to birth weight and gestational age: update, *J. Pediatr.,* 101, 969, 1982.
6. **Lilienfeld, A. M. and Parkhurst, E.,** A study of the association of factors of pregnancy and parturition with the development of cerebral palsy: a preliminary report, *Am. J. Hyg.,* 53, 262, 1951.
7. **Niswander, K. R. and Gordon, M.,** The women and their pregnancies, in *The Collaborative Perinatal Study of the National Institute of Neurologic Diseases and Stroke,* W.B. Saunders, Philadelphia, 1972.

8. **Hardy, J. M. B., Drage, J. S., and Jackson, E. C.,** The first year of life, in *The Collaborative Perinatal Study of the National Institute of Neurological and Communicative Disorders and Stroke,* The Johns Hopkins Press, Baltimore, 1979.

9. **Stewart, A. L., Reynolds, E. O. R., and Lipscomb, A. P.,** Outcome for infants of very low birth weight: survey of the world literature, *Lancet,* 1, 1038, 1971.

10. **Kitchen, W. H., Ryan, M. M., Rickards, A., Astbury, J., Ford, G., Lissenden, J. V., Keith, C. G., and Keir, E. H.,** Changing outcome over 13 years of very low birthweight infants, *Semin. Perinatol.,* 6, 373, 1982.

11. **Britton, S. B., Fitzhardinge, P. M., and Ashby, S.,** Is intensive care justified for infants weighing less than 801 gm at birth?, *J. Pediatr.,* 6, 937, 1981.

12. Editorial, Quality not quantity of babies, *Br. Med. J.,* 280, 347, 1980.

13. Editorial, The fate of the baby under 1500 g at birth, *Lancet,* 1, 461, 1980.

14. **Kirley, W. H.,** Fetal survival — what price. Presidential address, *Am. J. Obstet. Gynecol.,* 137, 873, 1980.

15. **Drillien, C. M.,** *The Growth and Development of the Prematurely Born Infant,* Churchill Livingstone, Edinburgh, 1964.

16. **Stanley, F. J. and Atkinson, S.,** Impact of neonatal intensive care on cerebral palsy in infants of low birthweight, *Lancet,* 2, 1162, 1981.

17. **Stanley, F. J. and Watson, L.,** The cerebral palsies in Western Australia: trends, 1968 to 1981, *Am. J. Obstet. Gynecol.,* 158, 89, 1988.

18. **Kitchen, W. H., Orgill, A., Rickards, A., Ryan, M. M., Lissenden, J. V., Keith, C. G., Yu, V. Y., Ford, G. W., Astbury, J., Russo, W., Bajuk, B., and Nave, J. R. M.,** Collaborative study of very-low-birthweight infants: outcome of two-year-old survivors, *Lancet,* p. 1457, 1982.

19. **Hagberg, B., Hagberg, G., and Olow, I.,** The changing panarama of cerebral palsy in Sweden 1954—1970, *Acta Paediatr. Scand.,* 64, 187, 1975.

20. **Tejani, N. and Verma, U. L.,** Effect of tocolysis on incidence of low birth weight, *Obstet. Gynecol.,* 61, 556, 1983.

21. **Stewart, A. L., Thorburn, R. J., Hope, P. L., Goldsmith, M., Lipscomb, A. P., and Reynolds, E. O. R.,** Ultrasound appearance of the brain in very preterm infants and neurodevelopmental outcome at 18 months of age, *Arch. Dis. Child.,* 58, 598, 1983.

22. **DeVries, L. S., Dubowitz, V., Lary, S., Whitelaw, A., Dubowitz, L. M. S., Kaiser, A., Silverman, M., and Wigglesworth, J. S.,** Predictive value of cranial ultrasound in the newborn baby: a reappraisal, *Lancet,* p. 137, 1985.

23. **Graham, M., Levene, M. I., Trounce, J. Q., and Rutter, N.,** Prediction of cerebral palsy in very low birthweight infants: prospective ultrasound study, *Lancet,* 2, 593, 1987.

24. **Pape, K. E. and Wigglesworth, J. S.,** Physiological and pathological interactions of cerebral blood flow in the preterm newborn infant, in *Haemorrhage, Ischaemia and the Perinatal Brain,* Lippincott, New York, 1979.

25. **Ment, L. R., Duncan, C. C., and Stewart, W. B.,** Perinatal cerebral insults: hemorrhage and ischemia, *Pediatr. Neurosci.,* 12, 168, 1985—86.

26. **Lou, H. C., Lassen, N. A., and Friis-Hansen, B.,** Impaired autoregulation of cerebral flow in the distressed newborn infant, *J. Pediatr.,* 94, 118, 1979.

27. **Trounce, J. Q., Rutter, N., and Levene, M. I.,** Periventricular leucomalacia and intraventricular haemorrhage in the preterm neonate, *Arch. Dis. Child.,* 61, 1196, 1986.

28. **Bobitt, J. R., Hayslip, C. C., and Damato, J. D.,** Amniotic fluid infection as determined by transabdominal amniocentesis in patients with intact membranes in premature labor, *Obstet. Gynecol.,* 136, 796, 1980.

29. **Miller, J. M., Jr., Pupkin, M. J., and Hill, G. B.,** Bacterial colonization of amniotic fluid from intact fetal membranes, *Am. J. Obstet. Gynecol.,* 136, 796, 1980.

30. **Minkoff, H.,** Prematurity: infection as an etiologic factor, *Obstet. Gynecol.,* 62, 2, 1983.

31. **Bejar, R., Wozniak, P., Allard, M., Benirschke, K., Vaucher, Y., Coen, R., Berry, C., Schragg, P., Villegas, I., and Resnik, R.,** Antenatal origin of neurologic damage in newborn infants. I. Preterm infants, *Am. J. Obstet. Gynecol.,* 159, 357, 1988.

32. **Levene, M. I., Fawer, C.-L., and Lamont, R. F.,** Risk factors in the development of intraventricular haemorrhage in the preterm neonate, *Arch. Dis. Child.,* 57, 410, 1982.

33. **Clark, C. E., Clyman, R. I., Roth, R. S., Sniderman, S. H., Lane, B., and Ballard, R. A.,** Risk factor analysis of intraventricular hemorrhage in low-birth-weight infants, *J. Pediatr.,* 99, 625, 1981.

34. **Yu, V. Y. H., Wong, P. Y., Bajuk, B., Orgill, A. A., and Astbury, J.,** Outcome of extremely-low-birthweight infants, *Br. J. Obstet. Gynaecol.,* 93, 162, 1986.

35. **Hobel, C. J., Youkeles, L., and Forsythe, A.,** Prenatal and intrapartum high-risk screening. II. Risk factors reassessed, *Am. J. Obstet. Gynecol.,* 135, 1051, 1978.

36. **Bejar, R., Curbelo, V., Coen, R., et al.,** Large intraventricular hemorrhage (IVH) and labor in infants ≥1000 g, *Pediatr. Res.,* 15, 649, 1981.

37. **Barrett, J. M., Boehm, F. H., and Vaughn, W. K.,** The effect of type of delivery on neonatal outcome in singleton infants of birth weight of 1,000 g or less, *JAMA,* 250, 625, 1983.

38. **Tejani, N., Rebold, B., Tuck, S., DiTroia, D., Sutro, W., and Verma, U.,** Obstetrical factors in the causation of early periventricular-intraventricular hemorrhage, *Obstet. Gynecol.,* 64, 510, 1984.

39. **Novy, M. J.,** The effect of sustained uterine contractions on myometrial and placental blood flow in the rhesus monkey. Respiratory gas exchange and blood flow in the placenta, in Proc. 25th Int. Congr. Physiological Sciences, Publ. No. (NIH) 73-361, Hannover, Federal Republic of Germany, 1971.

40. **Sims, M. E., Turkel, S. B., Halterman, G., and Paul, R. H.,** Brain injury and intrauterine death, *Am. J. Obstet. Gynecol.,* 151, 721, 1985.

41. **Bardeguez, A., Tejani, N., Verma, U. L., and Kim, S. J.,** Umbilical artery creatinine phosphokinase brain band isoenzyme as a predictor of neonatal periventricular/intraventricular hemorrhage, *Am. J. Obstet. Gynecol.,* in press.

42. **Hameed, C., Tejani, N., Verma, U. L., and Archbald, F.,** Silent chorioamnionitis as a cause of preterm labor refractory to tocolytic therapy, *Am. J. Obstet. Gynecol.,* 149, 726, 1984.

43. **Rayburn, W. F., Johnson, M. Z., Hoffman, K. L., Donn, S. M., and Nelson, R. J., Jr.,** Intrapartum fetal heart rate patterns and neonatal intraventricular hemorrhage, *Am. J. Perinatol.,* 4, 98, 1987.

44. **Hameed, C., Tejani, N., Tuck, S., Novotny, P., Verma, U., and Chayen, B.,** Correlation of fetal heart rate monitoring and acid-base status with periventricular/intraventricular hemorrhage in the low birth weight neonate, *Am. J. Perinatol.,* 3(1), 24, 1986.

45. **Haesslein, H. C. and Goodlin, R. C.,** Delivery of the tiny newborn, *Am. J. Obstet. Gynecol.,* 134, 192, 1979.

46. **Fairweather, D. V. I.,** Obstetric management and follow-up of the very-low-birth-weight infant, *J. Reprod. Med.,* 26, 387, 1981.

47. **Tejani, N., Verma, U., Hameed, C., and Chayen, B.,** Method and route of delivery in the low birth weight vertex presentation correlated with early periventricular/intraventricular hemorrhage, *Obstet. Gynecol.,* 69, 1, 1987.

48. **Morales, W. J. and Koerten, J.,** Obstetric management and intraventricular hemorrhage in very-low-birth-weight infants, *Obstet. Gynecol.,* 68, 35, 1986.

49. **Olshan, A. F., Shy, K. K., Luthy, D. A., Kickok, D., Weiss, N. S., and Daling, J. R.,** Cesarean birth and neonatal mortality in very low birth weight infants, *Obstet. Gynecol.,* 64, 267, 1984.

50. **Kitchen, W., Ford, G. W., Doyle, L. W., Rickards, A. L., Lissenden, J. V., Pepperell, R. J., and Duke, J. E.,** Cesarean section or vaginal delivery at 24 to 28 weeks' gestation: comparison of survival and neonatal and two-year morbidity, *Obstet. Gynecol.,* 66, 149, 1985.

51. **Bishop, E. H., Israel, S. L., and Briscoe, C. C.,** Obstetric influences on the premature infant's first year of development, *Obstet. Gynecol.,* 26, 628, 1965.

52. **Broman, S. H., Nichols, P. L., and Kennedy, W. A.,** *Preschool IQ: Prenatal and Early Development Correlates,* L. Eelbaum, Hillsdale, NJ, 1975.

53. **Nelson, K. B. and Ellenberg, J. H.,** Obstetric complications as risk factors for cerebral palsy or seizure disorders, *JAMA,* 251, 1843, 1984.

54. **Kitchen, W. H., Yu, V. Y. H., Orgill, A. A., Ford, G., Rickards, A., Astbury, J., Ryan, M. M., Russo, W., Lissenden, J. V., and Bajuk, B.,** Infants born before 29 weeks gestation: survival and morbidity at 2 years of age, *Br. J. Obstet. Gynaecol.,* 89, 887, 1982.

55. **Worthington, D., Davis, L. E., Grausz, J. P., and Sobocinski, K.,** Factors influencing survival and morbidity with very low birth weight delivery, *Obstet. Gynecol.,* 62, 550, 1983.

56. **Bada, H. S., Korones, S. B., Anderson, G. D., Magil, H. L., and Wong, S. P.,** Obstetric factors and relative risk of neonatal germinal layer/intraventricular hemorrhage, *Am. J. Obstet. Gynecol.,* 148, 798, 1984.

57. **Shankaran, S., Cepeda, E. E., Ilagan, N., Mariona, F., Hassan, M., Bhatia, R., Ostrea, E., Bedard, M. P., and Poland, R. L.,** Antenatal phenobarbital for the prevention of neonatal intracerebral hemorrhage, *Am. J. Obstet. Gynecol.,* 154, 53, 1986.

58. **Rumack, C. M. and Johnson, M. L.,** *Perinatal and Infant Brain Imaging,* Year Book Medical Publishers, Chicago, 1984.

59. **Flodmark, O., Becker, L. E., Harwood-Nash, D. C., Fitzhardinge, P. M., Fitz, C. R., and Chuang, S. H.,** Correlation between computed tomography and autopsy in premature and full-term neonates that have suffered perinatal asphyxia, *Radiology,* 137, 93, 1980.

60. **Papile, L., Burstein, J., Burstein, R., and Koffler, H.,** Incidence and evolution of subependymal and intraventricular hemorrhage: a study of infants with birthweights less than 1,500 gm, *J. Pediatr.,* 92, 529, 1978.

61. **Allan, W. C. and Philip, A. G. S.,** Neonatal cerebral pathology diagnosed by ultrasound, in *Clinics in Perinatology,* Vol. 12, Philip, A. G. S., Ed., W.B. Saunders, Philadelphia, 1985, 195.

62. **Bejar, R., Curbelo, V., Coen, R. W., Leopold, G., James, H., and Gluck, L.,** Diagnosis and follow-up of intraventricular and intracerebral hemorrhages by ultrasound studies of infant's brain through the fontanelles and sutures, *Pediatrics,* 66, 661, 1980.

63. **Garfinkel, E.,** Intraventricular Hemorrhage and Variants in the Premature Newborn: Neurologic and Developmental Consequences during Infancy, Ph.D. thesis, Hofstra University, Hempstead, NY, 1984.

64. **Sinha, S. K., Sims, D. G., Davies, J. M., and Cheswick, M. L.,** Relation between periventricular haemorrhage and ischemic brain lesions diagnosed by ultrasound in very pre-term infants, *Lancet,* 2, 1154, 1985.

65. **Vaucher, Y. E., Bejar, R. F., Jones, B. L., and Merritt, T. A.,** Neurologic outcome: effects of ventricular dilatation (VENT DIL), intraventricular hemorrhage (IVH) and white matter necrosis (WMN) in preterm infants, *Pediatr. Res.,* 21(4), 405A, 1987.

66. **Rushton, D. I., Preston, P. R., and Durbin, G. M.,** Structure and evolution of echo dense lesions in the neonatal brain: a combined ultrasound and necropsy study, *Arch. Dis. Child.,* 60, 798, 1985.

67. **Weindling, A. M., Wilkinson, A. R., Cook, J., Calvert, S. A., Fok, T.-F., and Rochefort, M. J.,** Perinatal events which precede periventricular haemorrhage and leucomalacia in the newborn, *Br. J. Obstet. Gynaecol.,* 92, 1218, 1985.

68. **Dubowitz, L. M. S., Bydder, G. M., and Mushin, A.,** Developmental sequence of periventricular leucomalacia, *Arch. Dis. Child.,* 60, 349, 1985.

69. **Weindling, A. M., Richefort, M. J., Calvert, S. A., Fok, T.-F., and Wilkinson, A.,** Development of cerebral palsy after ultrasonographic detection of periventricular cysts in the newborn, *Dev. Med. Child Neurol.,* 27, 800, 1985.

70. **McArdle, C. B., Richardson, C. J., Nicholas, D. A., Mirfakhraee, M., Hayden, C. K., and Amparo, E. G.,** Developmental features of the neonatal brain: MR imaging. I. Gray-white matter differentiation and myelination, *Radiology,* 162, 223, 1987.

71. **McArdle, C. B., Richardson, C. J., Nicholas, D. A., Mirfakhraee, M., Hayden, C. K., and Amparo, E. G.,** Developmental features of the neonatal brain: MR imaging. II. Ventricular size and extracerebral space, *Radiology,* 162, 230, 1987.

72. **McArdle, C. B., Richardson, C. J., Hayden, C. K., Nicholas, D. A., Crofford, M. J., and Amparo, E. G.,** Abnormalities of the neonatal brain: MR imaging. I. Intracranial hemorrhage, *Radiology,* 163, 387, 1987.

73. **McArdle, C. B., Richardson, C. J., Hayden, C. K., Nicholas, D. A., and Amparo, E. G.,** Abnormalities of the neonatal brain: MR imaging. II. Hypoxic-ischemic brain injury, *Radiology,* 163, 395, 1987.

74. **Dubowitz, L. M. S. and Bydder, G. M.,** Nuclear magnetic resonance imaging in the diagnosis and follow-up of neonatal cerebral injury, in *Clinics in Perinatology,* Vol. 12, Philip, A. G. S., Ed., W.B. Saunders, Philadelphia, 1985, 243.

75. **Wilson, D. A. and Steiner, R. E.,** Periventricular leukomalacia: evaluation with MR imaging, *Radiology,* 160, 507, 1986.

76. **DeVries, L. S., Regev, R., Connell, J. A., Bydder, G. M., and Dubowitz, L. M. S.,** Localized cerebral infarction in the premature infant: an ultrasound diagnosis correlated with computed tomography and magnetic resonance imaging, *Pediatrics,* 81, 36, 1988.

77. **Hope, P. L. and Reynolds, E. O. R.,** Investigation of cerebral energy metabolism in newborn infants by phosphorus nuclear magnetic resonance spectroscopy, in *Clinics in Perinatology,* Vol. 12, Philip, A. G. S., Ed., W.B. Saunders, Philadelphia, 1985, 261.

78. **Sankaran, K., Peters, K., and Finer, N.,** Estimated cerebral blood flow in term infants with hypoxic ischemic encephalopathy, *Pediatr. Res.,* 15, 1415, 1981.

79. **Ment, L. R., Duncan, C. C., Ehrenkranz, R. A., Lange, R. C., Taylor, K. J., Kleinman, C. S., Scott, D. T., Sivo, J., and Gettner, P.,** Intraventricular hemorrhage in the preterm neonate: timing and cerebral blood flow changes, *J. Pediatr.,* 104, 419, 1984.

80. **Volpe, J. J., Herscovity, P., Perlman, J. M., and Raichle, M. E.,** Positron emission tomography in the newborn: extensive impairment of regional cerebral blood flow with intraventricular hemorrhage and hemorrhagic intracerebral involvement, *Pediatrics,* 72, 589, 1983.

81. **Bada, H. S., Hajiiar, M. S., Chan, C., et al.,** Noninvasive diagnosis of neonatal asphyxia and intraventricular hemorrhage by Doppler ultrasound, *J. Pediatr.,* 95, 775, 1979.

82. **Perlman, J. M., Goodman, S., Kreusser, K. L., et al.,** Reduction in intraventricular hemorrhage by elimination of fluctuating cerebral blood-flow velocity in preterm infants with respiratory distress syndrome, *N. Engl. J. Med.,* 312, 1353, 1985.

83. **Brann, A.,** Factors during neonatal life that influence brain disorders, in Perinatal and Prenatal Factors Associated with Brain Disorders, Freeman, J., Ed., National Institutes of Health, Bethesda, MD, 1985.

84. **Papile, L., Munsick-Bruno, G., and Schaefer, A.,** Relationship of cerebral intraventricular hemorrhage and early childhood neurologic handicaps, *J. Pediatr.,* 103, 273, 1983.

85. **Schub, H. S., Ahman, P., Bain, R., et al.,** Long-term developmental follow-up of premature infants with subependymal intraventricular hemorrhage: reason for optimisim, *Clin. Res.,* 28, 874A, 1980.

86. **Smith, Y., Sostek, A., Katz, K., and Subramanian, S.,** Intraventricular hemorrhage. A limited predictor of outcome in premature infants, *Pediatr. Res.,* 18, 383A, 1984.

87. **Papile, L., Munsick, G., Weaver, N., and Pecha, S.,** Cerebral intraventricular hemorrhage (CVH) in infants ≤1500 gms: developmental follow-up at one year, *Pediatr. Res.,* 13, 528, 1979.

88. **Garfinkel, E., Tejani, N., Boxer, H. S., Levinthal, C., Atluru, V., Tuck, S., and Vidyasaga, S.,** Infancy and early childhood follow-up of neonates with periventricular or intraventricular hemorrhage or isolated ventricular dilatation: a case controlled study, *Am. J. Perinatol.,* 5(3), 214, 1988.

89. **Hoffman-Williamson, M., Bernbaum, J., Daft, A., and Rosenberg, H.,** Early developmental sequelae of intraventricular hemorrhage (IVH) in preterm infants, *Pediatr. Res.,* 18, 105, 1988.

90. **Gaiter, J.,** The effects of intraventricular hemorrhage on Bayley developmental performance in preterm infants, *Semin. Perinatol.,* 6, 305, 1982.

91. **Williams, M., Lewandowski, L., and D'Eugenio, D.,** Evaluation at 4—5 years of survivors of neonatal intraventricular hemorrhage, *Pediatr. Res.,* 18, 116A, 1984.

92. **McMenamin, J. B., Shackelford, G. D., and Volpe, J. J.,** Outcome of neonatal intraventricular hemorrhage with periventricular echodense lesions, *Ann. Neurol.,* 15, 285, 1984.

93. **Bozynski, M. E. A., Nelson, M. N., Matalon, T. A. S., Genaze, D. R., Rosati-Skertich, C., Naughton, P. M., and Meier, W. A.,** Cavitary periventricular leucomalacia: incidence and short term outcome in infants weighing ≤1200 grams at birth, *Dev. Med. Child Neurol.,* 27, 572, 1985.

INDEX